HANDBOOK OF PSYCHIATRIC EMERGENCIES

Second Edition

Andrew E. Slaby, M.D., Ph.D., M.P.H.
Professor of Psychiatry and Human Behavior
Brown University;
Psychiatrist-in-Chief
Rhode Island Hospital, Providence

Julian Lieb, M.D.
Associate Clinical Professor of Psychiatry
Yale University School of Medicine
Woodbridge, Connecticut

Laurence R. Tancredi, J.D., M.D.
Associate Professor of Law and Psychiatry
New York University, New York

 Medical Examination Publishing Co., Inc.
an Excerpta Medica company

Slaby, Andrew Edmund.
  Handbook of psychiatric emergencies.

  Bibliography
  Includes index.
    1. Crisis intervention (Psychiatry) — Handbooks,
manuals, etc. I. Lieb, Julian, joint author.
II. Tancredi, Laurence R., joint author. III. Title.
RC480.6.S53 1981 616.89'025 80-26575
ISBN 0-87488-655-4 hardcover
ISBN 0-87488-645-7 paperback

SIMULTANEOUSLY PUBLISHED IN:

Europe   : HANS HUBER PUBLISHERS
                          Bern, Switzerland

South and East Asia : TOPPAN COMPANY (S) Pte. Ltd.
                          Singapore

United Kingdom   : HENRY KIMPTON PUBLISHERS
                          London, England

Preface

A psychiatric emergency is defined by an individual, or by his family or community, as an event requiring immediate attention for a psychiatric or psychosocial problem. A belligerent intoxicated person is brought to the emergency room by the police; a depressed man undergoing a divorce rings up his therapist at three o'clock in the morning thinking he wants to kill himself; a young law student is brought to a university health service by her roommate, psychotic after smoking marijuana that is contaminated with phencyclidine — all these events are instances where prompt and decisive intervention is called for. They are times of crises where the attending clinicians must summon all of their professional skills to obviate the possibility of a catastrophic or even fatal outcome for the patients or someone close to them. Emergency clinicians must have a knowledge of psychodynamics, diagnostic psychiatry, psychopharmacotherapy, brief psychotherapy and interviewing skills, as well as general medical and administrative know-how in order to provide effective management at the time of human crisis. In emergency situations they must use common sense, reasoning skills, empathy and intuitive resources in such a way as to resonate best with each unique clinical situation. An ability to tolerate anxiety and ambiguity and to blend flexibility and firmness, as well as a readiness to tactfully contend with fear and anger, are needed to stand the clinician in good stead.

Emergency psychiatry requires careful listening and observation, as well as a certain element of risk taking and pragmatism. A diplomatic cautiousness tempered with courage is required to handle the threats to personal safety and self-esteem that sometime occur. Emergency clinicians must constantly guard against being too provocative or too permissive. Much can be gained by consistently maintaining a professional demeanor and a necessary degree of authoritarianism. Clinicians who divest themselves of their dignity or invite a patient to do this to them court trouble both for themselves and their patients.

It is ironic that while emergency psychiatry is the one area wherein the possibility to do good or harm is most immediate and greatest, less emphasis is placed on training and supervision in this area than on the more traditional, longer psychotherapies. Clinicians who choose or are assigned to work in emergency facilities often feel demoralized and emotionally and physically drained. Burnout is a recurrent problem and staff turnover is frequently high. Emergency psychiatry is extremely taxing and time consuming. The drain on psychological resources that occurs in the practice of emergency psychiatry explains to some degree why it is so difficult "to shift gears" to this approach when necessary. It is more convenient and less emotionally taxing for a therapist practicing in the community to tell a patient in distress to go to the emergency room of a nearby hospital or CMHC than to attend to the emergency himself. In order to be fully effective at a time of crisis, it is sometimes necessary to move from a more highly stylized mode of therapy to more active intervention.

The second edition of this book has been expanded from the earlier edition to enhance its value for the spectrum of mental health clinicians dealing with psychiatric emergencies encountered both in community and general medical hospital settings. Emphasis is placed on essential historical and clinical data that leads to appropriate diagnosis and management. An outline format has been employed in order to provide clinicians with direct and concise information that is practical in the emergency setting, with updated references at the end of the book. Doses and routes of administration of standard medications have been included, and, wherever possible, alternate approaches to particular emergencies suggested.

This book is divided into six general sections. The first two deal with basic principles of emergency psychiatry practice and psychopharmacology. Requirements in terms of the physical plant are discussed, as well as pragmatics of record keeping, development of management plans, interviewing and emergency psychopharmacotherapy. The third section provides a guide to the management of the most frequently encountered psychiatric emergencies in the delivery of mental health services. The fourth and fifth sections deal respectively with the occupational hazard of crisis interventionists, burnout, and planning for disasters. The sixth and final section has been expanded from the first edition to include not only legal aspects of emergency psychiatric care, but also a discussion of some of the ethical principles guiding the providers of such care. Although the majority of emergency psychiatric care is rendered in the emergency room of general medical hospitals, or on crisis units of CMHC's, the material presented here is equally applicable to clinicians working in health maintenance organizations, university health centers, outpatient clinics, inpatient treatment facilities, private offices and as part of home visit teams. The emphasis is consistently pragmatic with theory introduced only to the degree that it will help clinicians function in the environment they must and should provide the care in. It is our hope that by reading this volume clinicians will not only be able to enrich their skills in handling psychiatric emergencies, but will also acquire a renewed awe of the complexity of human response to internal and external stresses.

A.E.S.

*For those who have
shared with us their moments of crisis
and taught us what we know*

Acknowledgments

Crisis intervention is learned on the front lines, by intervening in human crises. Every good crisis therapist has learned foremost from those with whom he or she shared the sacred moments of a crisis, and secondly, from the recounting of such moments by fellow interventionists. We thank both those who have come to us at the time of personal crises, as well as those workers on the front lines who have shared with us their feelings on how they have best served others; what we have learned from both is reflected in the content of this book. The Task Force on Emergency Care Issues of the American Psychiatric Association (Drs. Gail Barton, Clothilde Bowen, John Petrich and Andrew E. Slaby), working together with Drs. Betsy Comstock, Beverly J. Fauman, Michael Fauman and J. Michael Foxworth, have struggled over the past two years to develop standards for provision of emergency psychiatric care. Some of the outgrowths of their work are reflected in this book. Finally, we would also like to thank Ms. Alicia Jordan, Ms. Joan Freiberger, Ms. Erica Fritz and Ms. Carol Maxfield who struggled with the crises of scrutinizing the rough copy of this book and typing it to reach the deadline for publication.

Contents

notice

The editor(s) and/or author(s) and the publisher of this book have made every effort to ensure that all therapeutic modalities that are recommended are in accordance with accepted standards at the time of publication.

The drugs specified within this book may not have specific approval by the Food and Drug Administration in regard to the indications and dosages that are recommended by the editor(s) and/or author(s). The manufacturer's package insert is the best source of current prescribing information.

I

BASIC PRINCIPLES OF EMERGENCY PSYCHIATRIC CARE

GENERAL PRINCIPLES OF
EMERGENCY ROOM PSYCHIATRY

Major Sources of Anxiety for Emergency Psychiatric Clinicians

When psychiatric clinicians first begin to work in emergency rooms of a hospital, they often find themselves anxious and with pervasive senses of uncertainty as to what the future may bring. It is at this time that a psychiatric clinician may first entertain thoughts of dropping out of a training program. Alternatively, they may develop distressing somatic or psychological symptoms. In one instance, a second-year psychiatric resident had recurrent diarrhea throughout the course of his three-month rotation on an emergency service. Another, worried over her decision not to hospitalize a patient who had suicidal ideation, found herself reading the obituary column of a local newspaper.

In the following section, major sources of anxiety for psychiatric clinicians will be discussed and we will outline some of the measures which can be implemented to combat them.

Violence

It cannot be denied that some patients, particularly acutely intoxicated alcoholic males and actively psychotic paranoid schizophrenics present a great potential for violence. The actual risk of physical harm coming to the clinician, however, is usually exaggerated. In many instances, potentially violent patients who have already perpetrated a violent act are brought to the emergency room by police officers or friends who serve to reduce patient's immediate potential for violence. In other instances, there are certain precautions that psychiatric clinicians may take to protect themselves against potential harm. These techniques include:

1) meeting patients outside the office to determine whether it is prudent to see them alone in the confines of an office
2) interviewing patients with a member of the hospital security force present
3) leaving the door open during the interview
4) allowing patients access to the door so that they do not feel

1

"trapped" (obviously, in such instances, if there is a real concern for violence, a security officer should be made aware of the fact that the patient may attempt to escape and should station him- or herself outside the door waiting inconspicuously for such a possibility)
5) medicating the patient appropriately
6) taking care to avoid touching the patient who might react to physical contact as a threatened physical assault or, in the case of some paranoid patients, as a sexual advance

Suicide

Psychiatric clinicians often fear that they may fail to recognize a truly suicidal patient, who if not hospitalized, might successfully complete the self-destructive act. Fortunately, there are many guiding clinical, epidemiologic and sociologic correlates of suicidal behavior which help to distinguish people who represent major suicidal risks from those who manipulatively threaten suicide. Other guideposts serve to distinguish that subgroup whose self-destructive behavior may be classified as a "gesture" from those who more accurately could be defined as attempters. It is usually those in the latter group who require immediate hospitalization. No criteria are infallible, and as surgeons are taught early in their careers, "Man proposes, but God disposes." Suicide is particularly difficult to predict in some groups, especially schizophrenics and in that subpopulation variously referred to as "borderline personality", "latent schizophrenia" or "pseudoneurotic schizphrenia." It is usually easy to recognize the antecedents of an act after it has been executed. It is less easy to identify with precision those same features in individuals before they attempt to take their life. A thorough assessment using the format outlined in this book will generally serve to identify those individuals who constitute "high suicide risk" and who generally should be hospitalized.

Difficult Dispositions

Dispositions are often a problem in the emergency room setting. As in many other localities, it is frequently difficult or impossible to find a setting which offers a treatment program that is consistent with what we feel best suits the patient's needs. Additionally, lack of funds or inadequate insurance may necessitate that patients be hospitalized far from their home setting. Knowledge of available facilities in the immediate area and of possible sources of payment for the services they will render will facilitate the best disposition, given the realistic limitations that exist in any community setting.

Commitment Against a Patient's Will

Psychiatric clinicians may be concerned by the occasional necessity of committing patients against their will. Such concern is usually strongest at the beginning of work on a crisis unit, but no one ever becomes entirely immune to a patient's protestations. The realization, however, that failure to hospitalize suicidal patients may result in their untimely death leaves the evaluating clinician with no other ethical choice but to commit. Patients' motivation to take their own or another's life often results in part from factors that are a part of their illness, factors that we hope will be positively influenced by treatment, e.g. antipsychotic agents in the treatment of paranoid patients. Obviously not all destructive behavior is a consequence of psychosis; and if a person brought to an emergency service, following a violent act, is not found to be psychotic, he or she may need to be handed over to the appropriate legal authorities. This action protects both the innocent patients and the psychiatric staff in hospitals from the violence of such people. It also serves to reduce the inaccurate belief held by some that in its therapeutic armanentarium, psychiatry harbors answers for all forms of violence. We do not, and cannot afford to, pretend to have such answers.

Too Many Patients to Evaluate

The number of patients who present to an emergency room varies from setting to setting and, in any given setting, from day to day. There is nothing that can guarantee that a psychiatric clinician will not be inundated. If a number of patients arrive in rapid succession, it may be necessary for clinicians to personally triage the patients. Generally speaking, they should see the most disturbed patients first. It is also feasible to be involved with the management of more than one patient concurrently. One should also be pragmatic, e.g. enlist the aid of other emergency room personnel in tasks such as arranging transportation, hospitalization, or administering medication. Ideally, an emergency room psychiatric team consisting of a psychiatrist, psychiatric social worker, a psychiatric nurse, and mental health workers can serve to reduce the pressure brought to bear on any one clinician, when an unexpected number of patients arrive.

It frequently happens that patients are inappropriately triaged into psychiatry. For instance, a patient who presents with shortness of breath and anxiety may be triaged to psychiatry by an emergency room nurse. These symptoms, however, should alert the psychiatric clinician to seek alternate explanations for the behavior. One such patient, with a history of four myocardial infarctions, was sent to psychiatry only to be found to have a pulmonary embolus as the basis of her anxiety.

Uncertainty

To the novice, the element of uncertainty as to what the next patient will be like is a constant source of anxiety. Only experience can provide one with a sufficient repertoire of psychotherapeutic, socio-therapeutic and chemotherapeutic techniques that can be generalized to most of the patients that one sees. As will become clear in this book, the usual lot of the emergency psychiatric clinician is a group of patients who are predominantly schizophrenic, alcoholic or depressed, and a smaller group of patients with neuroses, character disorders, or in transient situational stress.

On the whole, patients with mental organic syndromes infrequently present to psychiatry. Therefore, the psychiatric clinician should always keep a high level of suspicion for fear of missing the occasional patient with an amphetamine or bromide psychosis, a subdural hematoma, or hypoglycemia.

Demand for Rapid Decision Making

Emergency room psychiatry is unique in the demand it places upon psychiatric clinicians to arrive at quick decisions regarding the diagnosis of the cause of a patient's altered behavior, thought, or mood, its immediate management, and the patient's disposition. There is no easy way to learn this other than by working in an emergency room setting for a period of time under adequate supervision and supplementing the experience by directedly reading in the area of pharmacotherapy, crisis intervention, brief psychotherapy and diagnostic psychiatry.

Responsibility

Other than in those situations where it is absolutely clear that no further treatment will be required or where a patient has been hospitalized, the psychiatric clinician should assume the responsibility of maintaining a supportive and guiding contact with the patient, and at times, with the patient's family members, until the crisis has approached or achieved resolution, or until the patient has become involved in outpatient treatment. Studies have shown that when a psychiatric clinician helps the patient follow through with treatment recommendations, there is a greater incidence of successful linkage to treatment than when a patient is just given the name of a treatment center or another psychiatric clinician.

Sleep Deprivation

Some of the psychiatric clinicians' anxiety, while working on an emergency room service, result from the real loss of sleep they experience during hours on duty. Emergency room psychiatry is extremely taxing; and if psychiatric clinicians are working twenty-four hour shifts, they may find themselves exhausted, tense, and irritable by the time they see their twentieth patient. It is unreasonable to assume that any individual can perform at peak efficiency throughout a twenty-four hour shift, especially a psychiatric clinician who is very dependent upon subtle cues in work with patients. Therefore, wherever possible, arrangements should be made, either by the psychiatric clinician or by the administration, to limit emergency room work to 8- to 12-hour shifts.

Financing for Outpatient Treatment

Often, as lamentable as it is, a key factor in determining disposition is patient's ability to pay for treatment. Anxiety is often greatly reduced if one is fortunate enough to have available for referral a city, state, or federally funded community mental health center. In such circumstances, psychiatric clinicians who are concerned that the patients be treated within their communities rather than sent to a remote state hospital are usually able to provide patients with what they believe is the most viable treatment program. Nonetheless, the number of beds available in such hospitals and in psychiatric units of general hospitals is often limited. It may become necessary, therefore, to hospitalize patients elsewhere. If there is medical coverage available through medicare, welfare, insurance, or personal funds, then private psychiatric hospitalization should be considered. Failing such resources and depending upon the availability of beds, it may be necessary to send a patient to a remote, and often poorly staffed state hospital. In such circumstances, one is often placed in the unfortunate situation of having to rationalize this state of affairs to oneself or to the patient and his family. An intonation of guilty explanations at 4 A.M. does not improve self-esteem or disposition. Conversely, momentary exhilaration experienced after obtaining a bed on a favored unit is frequently followed by the helpless realization that a clinician has just filled that unit and that the next patient requiring hospitalization will, in all probability, have to be sent to an inferior unit or to a state hospital. Such experiences certainly do not mitigate anxiety early in the morning.

The Receiving Staff's Reactions to the Psychiatric Clinician's Presumptive Diagnosis and Decision to Hospitalize

Obviously, the psychiatric clinician must do what is best for each patient and use the full store of his diagnostic and treatment acumen in arriving at each clinical decision. Often, however, the need to hospitalize is equivocal, for the diagnosis is based on inadequate or poorly assimilated information. Also, and not infrequently, patients with a variety of presenting symptoms recover dramatically within a day or two following hospitalization. Clinicians must be prepared to tolerate a certain amount of criticism from receiving clinicians concerning admission, but should not allow this to interfere with the resolve to hospitalize patients when it is felt that there are clear indications for doing so.

Medical Problems Superimposed on Psychiatric Problems

Psychiatric patients may be hypochondriacal, having somatic delusions, or present with conversion symptoms. In addition, real somatic illnesses such as migraine headaches, bronchial asthma and ulcerative colitis may exacerbate at times of stress. Of great significance in an emergency room setting, are the myriads of medical complications consequent to long-term ingestion of alcohol or drugs. Patients with localized or systemic organic disease will also present at times to psychiatry with symptoms of concurrent psychiatric disorders or with psychiatric symptoms, resulting from the underlying organic disease. Careful history taking including a medical, surgical and obstetrical history, clinical observation of the patient, and a physical examination will often serve as guideposts toward a correct diagnosis. One should never hesitate to make liberal use of available specialty consultations, e.g. neurology, internal medicine.

Resistance to Treatment Recommendations

Consequent to the primary task of arriving at an accurate diagnosis and deciding on an appropriate disposition comes the major challenge, at times, of dealing with patients' or their families' resistance in accepting a treatment plan. As in psychotherapy, such resistance needs to be diagnosed in its psychohistorical and current social contexts. Strong resistance might mean a treatment plan is indeed inappropriate. The clinician should be willing to reconsider with the patient how a decision was arrived at based on the information the patient or others provided about the various personality traits; psychopathology; social, cultural and economic factors; personal values; myths and taboos; and the ways in which the patient views his problem might militate against acceptance of a treatment recommendation (Lieb and Slaby, 1975). Concerns about being labelled "mentally ill" are often preeminent in importance in diverting a patient from considering either outpatient treatment or hospitalization. Additionally, uninformed notions about psychiatric hospitals frequently instill in patients or family a strong rejection of psychiatric hospitalization. Great patience, endurance, and a tolerance for anger are often required before it is possible to reach a point at which the patient and the family can accept recommendation. At times a firm, somewhat authoritarian approach will succeed where others have failed. A clinician may not, however, be able to reason with a schizophrenic in the midst of a psychotic break or with a patient with an organic psychosis; in such instances commitment may become necessary.

Difficult Families

At times of stress, all individuals tend to be curt, defensive, anxious, and short of temper. Family members of patients often have a greater amount of diagnosed and undiagnosed psychopathology which may make it difficult to work rationally with them to form a therapeutic alliance. Even if a family seems relatively healthy, guilt may militate against a smooth working relationship when time and resources are limited. Clinicians should present the results of their evaluation and their management recommendations to the family in as non-threatening and clear a manner as possible, with the awareness that the development of mental illness in a family member represents a crisis to a family, as does a sudden loss or other misfortune.

Concern that Patients Get the Care they Need

In some cases, it is painfully obvious that a single emergency room visit will have little or no effect on the trajectory of a patient's illness. A person who has been an alcoholic for several years, with recurrent emergency room visits when intoxicated, is unlikely to follow through on treatment recommendations. This situation obviously can tremendously frustrate psychiatric clinicians and engender anger in them at the realization that they are so helpless in the face of such obvious need for treatment. In other instances, despite the knowledge that hospitalization and the proper medication may guarantee some symptom reduction, it is impossible to guarantee that patients will continue on medication and in treatment once they are released from the hospital. A graphic example is that of the recurrently hospitalized paranoid schizophrenic patient who refuses to take medication once released from the hospital and will not consent to intramuscular injections of a long-acting phenothiazine. It is helpful if psychiatric clinicians recognize their own limitations in effecting a perfect disposition and treatment plan in all cases.

Use of Multiple Sources of Data in Evaluating Patients

Psychiatric patients in the emergency room are not always as able to provide as complete and coherent a history as are candidates for psychoanalysis. They may in fact be unable to provide a history at all because of an acute schizophrenic psychosis, a drug-induced state, or dementia. In such instances, the clinicians should not hesitate to contact other possible sources for historical information. These include:
1) patients' families
2) friends of the patients
3) their employer or fellow employees
4) their clergy
5) police officers who may have brought them in
6) their primary physician
7) their therapist

Charts may show that patients have long standing medical or psychiatric conditions which explain part or all of their present clinical picture. In addition, a former therapist or an old chart may provide baseline data to which the current clinical status can be compared.

Knowledge of Available Dispositions

Entry into treatment programs depends on good working relationships with individuals who are responsible for admissions to treatment systems. Clinicians should, in addition to acquiring a knowledge of public and private hospitals in the area, social agencies, church and school related treatment programs, community based crisis centers and private therapists, strive to develop personal working relationships with individuals from these resources at the first possible opportunity. Clinicians who have had long experience in the emergency room learn how an interested and appreciative attitude towards ambulance drivers can make a quantifiable temporal difference in how rapidly patients are picked up and brought to an inpatient ward. Clergy and community workers may know of several resources for alcoholism, or half-way houses for psychiatric patients in general.

Medication

In addition to the usual stock of routine psychiatric medications (e.g. hypnotics, major and minor tranquilizers, lithium carbonate, antidepressants and antiparkinson agents) that should be available to the patient whose prescription has run out at a time when all pharmacies are closed. a variety of liquid and parenteral medications should be readily available. These include thioridazine concentrate and liquid forms of chlorpromazine, haloperidol, perphenazine, and thiothixine. Intramuscular chlorpromazine, haloperidol, perphenazine and thiothixine should be kept in stock as well as parenteral Cogentin and Benadryl. Dalmane, Benadryl and Chloral Hydrate are helpful for patients presenting with sleeping difficulties. A smaller supply of the various antidepressants and lithium carbonate should be kept in stock to tide over patients whose supplies run out. It is not a recommended policy to commence antidepressant or lithium therapy in the emergency room setting. These drugs require time before their effect is felt and one day will make little difference as far as immediate effect is concerned. Baseline laboratory studies should be performed before therapy with these agents is begun.

Legal Backup

Legal consultation should be available for both patients and clinicians. When questions arise as to whether a patient can be committed when either her or his family opposes such a decision, a forensic psychiatrist can provide quick information that might facilitate the best care consistent with the civil rights of the patient. Other questions that frequently come up are in connection with appropriate disposition and treatment for individuals who are under arrest for homicidal or other criminal acts.

Appropriate Examining Equipment

A well-stocked examining room complete with a blood pressure cuff, ophthalmoscope and other instruments used for a complete medical and neurological examination should be available. A nurse or female attendant should be present during the physical examination of a woman patient.

Clinical Laboratory

Twenty-four hour availability of a laboratory which can perform basic blood and urine screening tests, as well as tests for toxic substances, is part of an ideal emergency psychiatric evaluation service. In addition, there should be access to the radiological department for x-rays and CAT scans if needed.

Distribution of Methadone

Attitudes toward the liberal distribution of methadone to addicts may vary from clinician to clinician but federal regulations governing methadone distribution are strict and are monitored regularly. Individuals who are in registered treatment programs may receive methadone, and these programs can have working relationships with the emergency room services to provide partial doses to those who have been recorded as having missed their doses that day. Methadone programs should make available a list of the medical backup for ready consultation if needed. In general, giving half the usual dose, or less, will be sufficient to prevent withdrawal symptoms when patients miss one of their daily doses.

Introduction to Patients

When patients present at the emergency room, they are usually quite upset and see their problem as requiring immediate attention. Although this will frequently prove not to be the case when the patient is interviewed, it is still good practice for clinicians to introduce themselves to a new arrival shortly after they have registered, even if this means that clinicians have to excuse themselves for a few minutes from a patient they are already interviewing. This tactic serves several functions:

1) Patients need to be evaluated as to their relative need for *immediate attention.* A patient with an acute brain syndrome secondary to a medical condition (e.g. transient cardiac arrhythmia) or a patient with an uncontrolled schizophrenic psychosis may require immediate attention.

2) A prompt introduction reduces the anxiety of more integrated patients who then know a clinician is aware of their presence, despite the fact that they cannot be seen immediately. (This is but common courtesy).

3) Nurses and other emergency room staff respect a clinician who is aware of the fact that "psych" cases are not a homogenous group and that some patients may need more immediate care than others. Prompt treatment of disruptive psychotic behavior reduces staff tensions in the emergency room.

4) The presence of a psychotic patient in the waiting room may frighten other patients who are waiting to be seen for medical or surgical problems. A grief stricken woman awaiting news as to whether her husband is still alive after being rushed to the hospital with chest pain is not comforted by a paranoid patient's delusions. A schizophrenic patient may respond in an exaggerated and bizarre manner to the sight of blood or mutilation.

Ready Accessibility of the Emergency Psychiatric Clinician

There are periods when the immediate presence of psychiatric clinicians is needed in the emergency room. If they are unavailable, patients may suffer unduly and staff morale may become reduced with the awareness that a compromised standard of medical care is being provided. The use of a paging system or portable "beepers" facilitates easy location, but should this fail, it is a recommended practice to give the charge nurse the telephone numbers where the psychiatric clinician may be contacted.

Index Cards on Frequent Visitors to the Emergency Room

Some patients appear in the emergency room so frequently that an index card file with data and diagnosis, current medication, available friends and relatives to call, and the therapist's phone number, becomes the only way to guarantee continuity of care. Such a filing system allows information to be fed into the emergency room by community workers, clergy, physicians and psychotherapists.

Pediatric Social Services

In instances when a single parent has to be hospitalized, the emergency room pediatric social workers should be contacted for help in temporary placement of the children. Additionally, should it become apparent that there is a history of child abuse, the pediatric social workers can help arrange intervention to protect the children.

Security

Hospital security officers may be needed to watch a suicidal patient who is being reluctantly hospitalized or to minimize the abusive and assaultive behavior of alcoholic and psychotic patients receiving immediate treatment or awaiting disposition. The more that security officers are made to feel that they are part of a medical treatment team, that their interventions are valued and that the clinicians are willing to explain the rationale of their interventions to them, the more they become willing to act in a prompt and humane way for the protection of patients and clinicians.

Neurological, Medical and Surgical Consultation

Ideally, there should be available in an emergency room opportunities for prompt consultation with other specialists would be particularly advised when there is:

1) a history of previous neurological disease which could explain the patient's present symptoms and signs
2) a physical examination suggestive of neurological dysfunction
3) a history of or the recent onset of seizures
4) a history suggestive of amnesia, head injury, unconsciousness or progressive deterioration of motor, sensory, or cognitive functioning

5) a mental status examination which suggests an organic mental syndrome

Medical consultation should be obtained for all patients with a history of recent alcohol abuse. These individuals represent a high risk for occult medical disease such as pneumonia, subdural hematomas, and gastrointestinal bleeding. Also, liver disease or alterations of central nervous system functioning may be responsible for the presentation to the psychiatrist. Additionally, referrals to medicine would include patients suspected of endocrine disturbances, cardiovascular disease, pulmonary problems, etc. Any suspicion of a problem which may require medical or surgical evaluation requires emergency room consultation before the patient is sent on to a hospital, *unless* the referring psychiatric clinician feels totally confident that the hospital to which they are sending the patient has adequate medical services.

Physical Examination

A complete physical examination is usually not part of the routine psychiatric emergency consultation. This relates in part to the fact that a psychiatrist's expertise lies in the performance and evaluation of parts of the physical examination that relate to alterations of mood, thought and behavior, much as a cardiologist's expertise lies in the examination of the heart. However, if either history or presentation suggests that there is some underlying disease requiring more careful medical, surgical, or neurological attention, then a physical examination should be performed. In all instances, vital signs should be taken (i.e. blood pressure, pulse, temperature and respiratory rate) and if organicity is suggested, a neurological exam should be performed by the psychiatrist before referral. Level of consciousness should be assessed as part of a determination of whether or not an organic etiology may be responsible for the changes in behavior. Any suggestion of a chronic or acute mental syndrome requires that the psychiatrist further evaluate the patient. One should be particularly alert to stigmata of endocrine disorders such as moonshaped face, buffalo hump, prognathism, large hands, etc. Changes in mental status may accompany a variety of alterations of cardiac rate or rhythm (e.g. bradycardia, tachycardia, or heart block), as well as radical changes in blood pressure.

Use of narcotics may be suggested by pupillary changes and needle marks on the arm. Withdrawal may be indicated by goose flesh, rhinorrhea, and lacrimation. Inspection of the skin and conjunctiva may reveal evidence of liver disease through the presence of jaundice. Scars on the head, especially fresh ones, should make one think of a subdural hematoma. The pupillary size, symmetry of pupils, and their reaction to light and accommodation are important. Pupillary inequality suggests the possibility of a subdural hematoma, which occurs not infrequently with a history of seizures or alcoholism. Cyanosis, dyspnea and pyrexia are also indicators of an organic process. A cachectic individual presenting with dementia may have an occult neoplasm, as yet undiagnosed, which has metastasized to the brain or have mental changes as the result of "distal effects" of a tumor without direct invasion of the brain. Examination of the breasts or a chest x-ray may reveal a mammary carcinoma or pulmonary tumor that may have metastasized and caused the changes. Smelling an obtunded individual's breath may suggest alcoholism, diabetes (acetone breath), or hepatic or renal disease (foul breath).

Laboratory Tests

Every alcoholic who presents with an altered mental status should have a serum alcohol level drawn to document that the changes *may* be explained by alcohol intoxication. A toxicology screen will help to identify what a patient might have overdosed on. Urine analysis and blood sugar help to identify patients presenting with mood or behavioral disturbances secondary to hyperglycemia or hypoglycemia. Blood can also be drawn for serology or thyroid function tests and the results used when a patient returns for a follow-up visit. A CBC should be drawn if an infection or anemia is suspected. An electrocardiogram should be performed in the emergency room if cardiac dysfunction is suggested by history or alteration of pulse.

Diagnostic Formulation

Following the evaluation, clinicians should integrate their data and write down a presumptive diagnosis and a reasonable differential diagnosis. The DSM III (Diagnostic and Statistical Manual III) of the American Psychiatric Association can serve as a guide to this task.

Diagnosis using the DSM III is made on five axes. Axis I is concerned with the clinical psychiatric syndromes. Axis II and III respectively are concerned with personality and specific developmental disorders (II) and physical disorders (III). The severity of psychosocial stress and the highest level of adaptive functioning during the past year are rated on Axes IV and V. For instance, if an obsessive compulsive lawyer who was a senior partner in a large international law firm without any medical or surgical illness presented acutely intoxicated after he was told that his wife and three children had just burned to death in the family home, his diagnosis using the five axes of the DSM III would be:

Axis I	303.00 Alcohol Intoxication
Axis II	301.40 Compulsive Personality Disorder
Axis III	None
Axis IV	Loss of wife and three children unexpectedly in a fire. Loss of house and all personal property
	Severity: 7 Catastrophic
Axis V	Highest level of adaptive functioning in the last year
	2 Very Good

We have attempted in this volume to comply with the guidelines of the nosological schema outlined in the DSM III.

Disposition

After diagnosis, there arises the question of what immediate psychotherapeutic or psychopharmacologic interventions should be employed or whether the patient should be hospitalized. Not hospitalizing a patient, as many clinicians well know, may require considerably more effort than that which is involved in expeditous hospitalization. Many chronically psychotic and some acutely psychotic patients can be managed as outpatients if clinicians themselves have the time or other agencies have resources to provide careful monitoring of pharmacotherapy and the individual and/or family therapy that may be needed. Many patients in the emergency room can be managed either by crisis intervention with one or two followup visits or by referral to an outpatient therapist or agency. The remainder may require hospitalization for alcohol or narcotic detoxification or because their behavior is so self- or other-destructive that they cannot be managed outside of a hospital. There is a group of patients who are hospitalized primarily because they lack the social supports of family and friends.

Hospitalization

It is a good policy for each clinician to maintain a list of hospitals, the types of services they provide, the specialty inpatient services available in the area and the types of financial or insurance coverage that are required. This allows the clinician to present to the patient and his family a number of treatment alternatives when hospitalization is necessary.

Inpatient psychiatric treatment may be required if there is an absence of adequate or responsible social support. In some cases, regardless of the nature of patients' social matrices and the degree of responsibility of their relatives and friends, hospitalization may be required. Such cases would include:
1) markedly suicidal patients
2) markedly homicidal patients
3) patients with psychosis without rapid remission
4) demented patients who can no longer be cared for at home
5) manic patients
6) stuporously depressed patients
7) patients in catatonic stupor or excitement
8) schizophrenic patients with command hallucinations

Disposition is always governed by the adequacy of social support. A moderately suicidal patient with supportive family and friends may not require inpatient care, whereas a mild suicidal patient who is middle-aged, divorced, male, friendless, homeless, and alcoholic, may well require hospitalization.

Outpatient Care

This varies according to the patient's needs and desires. A patient may only wish immediate reduction of anxiety. Another patient may seek long-term treatment, with the hope that future exacerbations of anxiety or depression may be avoided. Patients such as schizophrenics, manic-depressive patients and patients addicted to alcohol or drugs may require long-term programs because of the nature of the treatment of these problems. In many instances, exacerbations of illness in this last group occur without apparent cause.

Other

Dispositions other than outpatient or inpatient care are available, and in some cases are more effective than more traditional psychiatric care. These include:
1) Alcoholics Anonymous
2) Methadone maintenance programs
3) Drug treatment programs
4) Church groups

5) Women's and men's centers
6) Half-way houses
7) Family services
8) Ethnic and community health clinics

Compliance

Patient compliance with the recommendation to enter outpatient therapy varies. In one study (Wilder, et al., 1977), older Puerto Rican and white women usually carrying the diagnosis of depression, were most likely to follow through on emergency psychiatric clinicians recommendations to enter outpatient therapy. Blacks and patients diagnosed as schizophrenic were least likely to do.

Outcome Studies of Hospitalization

Outcome studies of the hospitalization of severely ill psychiatric patients provide conflicting results but on the whole, tend to favor briefer hospitalizations with emphasis on family therapy and community placement. Endicott, et al. (1979) found in general, standard treatment was inferior to brief hospitalization with or without day care. Herz et al. (1979) found little differential effect between brief and standard hospitalization on families but when a difference occurred it tended to favor brief hospitalization. Sylph and Kedward (1977) found that the hospital had a major role yet to play in the lives of all long-term patients regardless of the extra hospital facilities available. Lamb (1979) found that use of community social rehabilitation programs was directly related to provision and use of transportation. Board and care homes appeared in Lamb's study to offer asylum for life's pressures, a degree of structure and some treatment (usually in terms of medication supervision). Clearly success in the community following major psychiatric illness is the reuslt of a complex interplay of patients, illness, treatment and environmental variables.

CRISIS INTERVENTION

Many individuals present to emergency services with medical, psychiatric, or social crises. Every clinician should have at his or her command the necessary expertise to recognize a crisis situation and deal with it appropriately. Specific crises call for specific remedies; and thorough familiarity with both medical and social resources within and without the emergency setting is a must for clinicians working in emergency settings. Furthermore, it is essential to attempt to assess the exact nature of these crises. This will often require both a cross-sectional and longitudinal assessment of the patient, which will frequently provide the opportunity to effect more permanent changes than those possible by crisis intervention alone. For instance, individuals with manic depressive illness or relapsing schizophrenia will often decompensate under environmental circumstances, which for them, have untoward real or symbolic connotations. A patient's presenting symptoms might include flights of ideas, elation, and an infectious gaiety; the most likely diagnosis would, of course, be a manic psychosis. On interviewing a family member, one might then learn that the patient has had similar episodes in the past but has responded well to phenothiazines and has never required hospitalization. One might also learn that no one has ever taken the trouble to discuss maintenance lithium carbonate with the patient and his or her family. Let us say also, that another family member explains that the patient has always responded poorly to anniversaries, and his fortieth birthday is upcoming. All this data would provide a clinician with the groundwork for an immediate plan. A phenothiazine or butyrophenone to obliterate or reduce acute symptoms; referral to an outpatient clinic for lithium carbonate therapy; and some supportive psychotherapy now and perhaps later with the patient, around his upcoming birthday, would probably be all that was immediately needed.

The basic techniques used in crisis intervention work and the theoretical formulations that underlie them are described in detail by us in *The Crisis Team: A Handbook for Mental Health Professionals* (Lieb, et al., 1973) and will therefore be discussed only synoptically here.

Pragmatism and Innovation are the Keynotes of Successful Crisis Intervention

Successful resolution of crises requires pragmatism with a knowledge of and willingness to employ a variety of therapeutic techniques. This may involve supportive psychotherapy, with or without the use of antianxiety or antipsychotic agents, in the emergency service, coupled with a few follow-up visits. At other times, it may be necessary to bring in other family members, friends, or a lover, either heterosexual or homosexual. A brief hospitalization for one to a few days may be required for chronically ill psychiatric patients for diagnostic reassessment, or a reinstitution or readjustment of medication. In other instances, an intensive inpatient or outpatient workup may be needed to differentiate medical or neurological problems from the more purely psychiatric causes of behavioral disturbances.

Confidentiality

Effective crisis intervention sometimes requires a broadening of the definition of confidence to include, with the patient's permission, their families, spouses, friends or lovers so that a clearer picture of what is troubling them may be obtained. A quick resolution of a crisis may at times then be facilitated by sociotherapeutic manipulations when such are indicated. Obviously, if a patient is obtunded, psychotic, comatose, suicidal, or homicidal, the psychiatric clinician must decide who should be contacted to best effect speedy and accurate diagnostic assessment so that definitive therapeutic interventions may be initiated without undue delay. When possible, however, written consent should be obtained before others are contacted.

Ready Availability of the Clinician Involved in the Crisis Intervention

What appear to be insurmountable crises or therapeutic impasses are often resolvable to a considerable degree if the patients and their families feel that the clinician seeing them in the emergency room setting is available for consultation and an extra visit, if indicated. One often finds that when a patient or family feels that a clinician is available, seemingly urgent matters seem less pressing.

Awareness of What was Previously Effective when a Patient was in Crisis

It has been said that one who fails to know the past is doomed to repeat it. An awareness of what has contributed in the past to successful resolution of the patient's crises often reduces a need to attempt therapeutic manipulations that are doomed to failure. One might, for instance, call a patient's therapist or a family member in order to learn what may have been used effectively in the past to resolve a crisis. Calling the patient's therapist, in addition to being an obvious courtesy, is part of all ideal emergency care systems. In the first place, it allows the therapist to be aware of his patient's crisis. Then, it provides for continuity of care and allows the emergency room clinician more information (e.g. the doses of medication a patient is on). Lastly, patients often feel that with the involvement of their own therapist and the setting up of a follow-up appointment, there is less need for hospitalization or other more dis-rupting therapeutic interventions.

Responsibility

For effective crisis intervention, clinicians must have a strong sense of personal responsibility to patients so that they can provide the best care possible, given obvious social or environmental limita-tions at the time of crisis. This responsibility must be sensed by pa-tients, their families, and other members of patient care teams in the community.

Decision to Enter Therapy

In some instances, intervention in a crisis results in the identifi-cation by individuals or their families of chronic problems that have been overlooked but have contributed to bringing about the crisis. During the crisis, the clinicians may serve the role of one who clarifies and articulates the problem felt by all and guides the pa-tient or patients into a long-term therapy arrangement. This may prevent further crises and reduce the progression to a state where hospitalization can be avoided. If a patient is showing evidence of an endogenous depression, referral to a therapist for antidepressant medication may prevent the development of a full-blown psychotic depressive state, especially if a patient has a history of previous psy-chotic depressive episodes or has a family history of affective illness. Likewise, involvement in couples therapy or family therapy after a patient presents with a drinking problem and depression of a few weeks or months may serve to turn the tide of a potential alcoholic career. Both of these are examples of secondary prevention (i.e. stop-ping the progression of an illness early in its course).

Differential Diagnosis

Part of crisis intervention involves the establishment of a differ-ential diagnosis of the behavior changes. For instance, if a 45-year-old woman without a previous psychiatric history is brought into the emergency room by her family because of an altercation with her neighbor and is found to be suspicious, distrustful, and has ideas of reference, the differential diagnosis would include:
1) paranoid schizophrenia
2) affective illness with paranoid features
3) paranoid state

4) paranoid personality
5) amphetamine and other sympathomimetic psychoses
6) other organic states—chronic and acute
  Simple verbal intervention with the family is not always sufficient to manage a patient in crisis.

Reduction of Patient Drop Out Rate

  Repeated users of the emergency room often are individuals who,
if they were seen in a long-term therapy arrangment, would not use
the emergency room service. If a clinician arranges a follow-up visit
to see if the patient is in treatment, or in some cases just calls a week
later, the referral drop out rate can be reduced.

Definitive Treatment

  Sometimes definitive treatment may be given in the emergency
room. For instance, a drug induced psychosis secondary to LSD
(lysergic acid diethylamide) ingestion may be adequately treated
with oral or intramuscular chlorpromazine in the emergency room.
Even in such a case, however, a follow-up visit is usually indicated to
determine how a patient is doing a week or two later. Comparably, a
chronic schizophrenic patient who has an acute exacerbation of
symptoms may be treated in the emergency room and not have to
enter a hospital.

Ability of the Clinicians to Handle Their Own Anxiety

  Crisis intervention involves many quick decisions. For instance,
what is the diagnosis? What type of treatment should be given? Does
the patient need to be on long-term medication? Who should be called in to participate in the treatment process? Is hospitalization necessary?
  Arriving at a decision is always somewhat anxiety provoking;
however, it is even more so when the data base and time are limited.
But psychiatric clinicians who are adept at techniques of crisis intervention can often take a quick hold of an electric situation. They help
to readjust the family equilibrium and overcome interpersonal impasses. They do not hesitate to employ medication to relieve intrapsychic pain. Given the time frame, they solicit information from as
many sources as possible, with care for accuracy. They use the information, obtained discriminatively, avoiding the common pitfall of
being forced into a position they do not want. Social supports are

rallied by phone, including the support that can be afforded by a patient's own therapist. The clinician's eye is always alert for a suggestion of potential violence, either self-destructive or other-oriented. Finally, they see the patient as frequently as needed to bring about a perceptable reduction in the tension of the crisis. Only after the crisis has resolved do questions of long-term therapy to offset future acute decompensations become relevant.

PATIENT POPULATION

Psychiatric clinicians, not infrequently, have catastrophic fantasies about the types of patients that they are going to be confronted with on an emergency service. While some very bizarre patients do at times present, the usual lot is of a much more mundane nature. One can generally expect to see many schizophrenics, alcoholics, depressives and individuals in acute situational crises.

Taubman, et al. (unpublished data). The Yale-New Haven Hospital Emergency Psychiatric Service in 1974, analyzed the characteristics of the patient population seen and found that 42% of the total number of patients seen were hospitalized. The number of patients who were found to have a "positive suicide factor" defined by Taubman as any recent or current indication of suicidal intent written on the record of the emergency room admission (e.g. recent suicidal ideation, gesture, or threat; present ideation, threat or overdose) was 19.1% and 8.98% were described as violent or threatening. About an equal number of men and women were seen (47.1% vs 52.9% respectively). The groups of patients with the highest hospitalization rates were the alcoholics and schizophrenics who constituted 65.4% of all the patients hospitalized. Taubman and others (Robins, et al., 1974) have found that patients with affective disorders, alcoholism and antisocial personality are the diagnostic groups most frequently seen. Another study, Zonana (1973), contrasting utilization of services in 1969/1970 to utilization in 1960/1961 revealed that:

1) A slightly larger predominance of women used the emergency room in 1969/1970 than in 1960/1961.

2) There was a sixfold increase in appearance in the emergency room of individuals in the 15-21 age group in 1969/1970.

3) A greater number of "never-married" patients were seen in 1969/1970 (reflecting use by the younger age group).

4) There was a greater use of emergency room facilities by non-white members of the community in 1969/1970.

5) Utilization of emergency room services is inversely proportional to socioeconomic status (although more middle class pa-

tients were using the emergency room services in 1969/1970).
6) Utilization of psychiatric services is inversely proportional to the distance from the hospital.
7) There was an increase, over the decade, in the number of patients seen for depression and drug addiction and a decrease in the number of patients diagnosed as schizophrenic.
8) There was a decreased, over the decade, in the number of patients hospitalized.
9) Psychiatric admissions to the emergency room did not differ significantly from month to month, nor did they vary in terms of days of the week. (This finding held true even in separate diagnostic categories).
10) There was a rise, over the decade, in general use of emergency psychiatric services, out of proportion to the use of surgical and medical services.

Slaby and Perry (1979) found that factors associated with social isolation and poverty are linked both with having multiple episodes and disposition to public facilities. Individuals who are in the age range 50 to 94, are male or black, are divorced, separated or widowed, have less than a high school education, or the diagnosis of alcoholism, are more likely to be hospitalized in a public inpatient facility. Those who are in the age range 16 to 39, who are female, white, married or single and who have at least a high school education, or have diagnoses of neuroses, personality disorders or transient situational disturbances are more likely to be referred to an outpatient or inpatient facility in the community.

MEETING THE PATIENT

Introduction

1) As obvious as it may seem to introduce oneself to a patient, many busy clinicians overlook the importance that is attached to the initial introduction of the doctor to the patient. A typical introduction: "Good evening, Mr. Smith. I am Dr. Stevens, the psychiatrist. What brings you to the emergency room to see me this evening?"

2) Emergency room psychiatric residents and team leaders should devise mechanisms whereby they can be alerted intermittently to the number of patients waiting to see them and their ostensible complaints. Close liaison with the admission personnel and the emergency room nursing staff and orderlies can be of great help in this regard. A few minutes spent with such personnel, prior to on call

duty can be of inestimable advantage later on. They should be requested to inform the clinician if a patient seems to be in great distress. A few minutes spent with such individuals shortly after they have registered can help them organize their fantasies and get their anxiety under control.

Triage

A preliminary assessment of a patient should be made on his arrival to ascertain whether the patient must be seen immediately or can wait until others registered ahead are seen. This serves several purposes:

1) It reduces patient's anxiety. The presence of a grossly psychotic, delusional, violent, or hallucinating patient often renders other patients apprehensive, especially if inappropriate comments are made by a psychotic patient about other patients' misfortunes.

2) It reduces staff anxiety. Ill feelings among other emergency room staff often arise when chronic psychiatric patients, who are well known to the emergency room, present time and time again with loud or violent behavior without the clinician immediately providing orders for appropriate psychopharmacological agents which will reduce the particular patient's distress. Early brief assessment allows prompt initiation of an acute management program.

3) Finally, it is just a common courtesy to acknowledge to fellow human beings in pain that you are aware of their need and will see them at the first available moment.

Initial Observations

The patient's response to a simple introduction can provide a wealth of data that may prove useful in the evaluation. How does he comport himself? How does he walk? Is he guarded or do his eyes gaze about furtively as he talks? How does he dress and speak? Does he seem to be responding to voices or visual phenomena that don't exist? Psychiatric clinicians can create a sense of competence as they carefully and conscientiously watch the patient approach their office. Seasoned clinicians often find that they tend to develop preliminary ideas as to diagnosis in the first few minutes of an interview, and that in fact the data found later only serves to corroborate the initial diagnostic impression.

PSYCHIATRIC HISTORY AND MENTAL STATUS EXAMINATION

By necessity, an evaluation of a disturbance of mood, thought or behavior undertaken in the emergency room cannot be as comprehensive as an extended evaluation in a private therapist's office, an outpatient clinic or in an inpatient hospital setting. There are, however, certain basic questions that should be asked in every emergency evaluation. If a patient is unable to provide the answer to these, a perusal of old charts or an interview with a relative or a friend may yield the required information. This information is needed to provide the best assessment of a patient's problem from a medical, social and psychological perspective. Should hospital records or a psychiatrist's private files be subpoenaed for legal reasons or be studied as part of a PSRO review, it also demonstrates that the evaluation was complete, how a diagnosis was arrived at, and for what reasons certain therapeutic interventions, including hospitalization with or without medical certification, were performed.

Chief Complaint

The chief complaint should be stated in the patient's own words, e.g. "I feel my head is exploding." If the patient is unable to provide a chief complaint, the reason why the patient was brought to the emergency room should be stated, e.g. "The patient was brought in because he was walking naked down Main Street."

History of Present Illness

1) When did the patient's symptoms begin? Have they been constant? Increased? Decreased? Fluctuated in intensity?

2) How does the patient describe the symptoms (e.g., the patient states he feels "worthless," "sinful," and "dirty")?

3) Has there been any change in somatic functioning? Sleep disturbance? Weight changes? Appetite change? Change in sexual interest or performance? Constipation and other gastrointestinal difficulty? Headache or other pain? Palpitations and other cardiovascular symptoms? Respiratory, excretory, or neurological changes?

4) What were the circumstances when the symptoms began? Recent death or loss? Job loss or advancement? Divorce or separation? Impending jail sentence? Menopause or loss of potency? Injury?

Diagnosis of severe illness or impending surgery? First or difficult sexual experience? Pregnancy? Change of residence or job? Impending retirement? Financial reversal? Beginning or ending school? Marital reconciliation? Mortgage due? Loss of friend through death or separation? Other difficulty at home, work or play? Does the problem that precipitated the difficulty persist?

5) During the evaluation of the illness, has there been a change in the patient's mental status? Has he had auditory, visual, gustatory, olfactory, or other hallucinations? Ideas of reference? Paranoid ideation? Delusions of grandeur, persecution, etc.? Racing thoughts? Feeling his head is going to explode? Obsessions? Compulsions? Ritualistic behavior? Hypochondriasis? Somatic delusions? Overwhelming anxiety? Free floating anxiety? Depression? Feelings of elevated mood? Intense anger or fear? Derealization? Depersonalization? Identity or sexual confusions? Homicidal or suicidal ideation or attempts? Phobias?

6) What is the patient's past psychiatric history? If he has been hospitalized, how long and where? Has he been or is he on any medication? What and how much? Has he been taking it? Has he ever had electroconvulsive therapy? Who is or was his therapist? How frequently and for how long was he seen? Has he had any difficulty with the law? Has the patient ever been incarcerated? Where, for what, and for how long? Does the patient know what his diagnosis was?

7) If the patient is suicidal or homicidal, does he have a plan of action, a weapon or other lethal means of ending his own or another's life? Has he attempted before? If so, how many times? With what and where? Did he leave a note or tell someone, or would he have died if he were not found? Does he have religious or other reasons not to commit suicide? Does he see people looking at him as dead? Has he given away any possessions, especially prized ones? Does he have command hallucinations, i.e. voices telling him to kill himself or others?

Past Personal History

1) Where was the patient born? Was there any difficulty around his birth? What was his birth order? How many brothers and sisters does he have? Are they alive? What are their ages? Where do they live? What do they do? Are they married? Are his parents alive? When has he seen them last? If they are dead, when and of what did they die? How old were they or any sibling or spouse when they died? How old was the patient when they died?

2) Where did the patient go to school? How many years did he

complete? What were his grades like? Has there been any change in his academic performance? Was there any discipline problem at school? What was his major?

3) What role does sex play in the patient's life? How did a woman respond to her menarche and/or menopause? When was her last period? How does she feel about her menses? Did the patient engage in sexual play as a child? Does he/she masturbate? Has the frequency changed recently, and how does he/she feel about masturbating? What is the theme of any sexual fantasies? How old was the patient when he first began to neck? Pet? Have intercourse? If unmarried, how frequently does he date? Has he had any homosexual experiences? How frequently, and how does he feel about them? Does he reach orgasm? How many people has he had intercourse with? How old was he when he became engaged? Married? How old is his spouse? How is their sexual relationship (i.e. mutual satisfaction)? Frequency? Orgasm? How many children does the patient have? If patient is female, have there been induced or spontaneous abortions? Miscarriages? How did she respond to the birth of her children? Any post-partum depression? How do patient and spouse get on? Any physical violence? Extra-marital affairs? Talk of divorce? If divorced, what were the grounds? Does he/she still see his/her ex-spouse? How many subsequent marriages were there? If subsequent divorce, what were the grounds? Does the patient live with anyone? Any plans for marriage? Feeling about lack of commitment? Birth control? Desire for or not to have children?

Social History

1) Where and with whom does the patient live? What are the living conditions (e.g. crowded, rats, no heat, dangerous neighborhood)?

2) How much does the patient earn? Does he earn enough for food, housing, etc.? How many meals a day does he eat and what does he eat? Does he get along with the person(s) with whom he lives?

3) Did the patient have any close friends growing up? How many? Has he withdrawn from people? When? How many close friends does he have now? How frequently does he see them? Do they offer support? Are the relationships characterized by mutual satisfaction and warmth?

4) Does the patient belong to any clubs or organizations? Is he religious? If female, does she belong to a woman's group (e.g. Women's Liberation). Is this supportive? What other clubs, organizations, or social activities does the patient engage in?

Occupational History

1) Where does the patient work? How long has he been at the job? How does he get on with his employer and fellow employees? Does he enjoy the work? The working conditions? The hours? The other employees? The employer?

2) How many jobs has the patient held in his life? For how long? Why did he quit? Are jobs being held less long? Is his performance at work decreasing? Is he holding jobs below his level of competence or professional training?

3) What is his current salary? Is it sufficient to meet his expenses? What are his expenses? Does he have any outstanding debts?

Medical History

1) What medical illnesses and operations has the patient had? Does he have any chronic illness? Could this illness explain his present symptoms? Is he in treatment presently? Are his symptoms worse presently? Has he ever been hospitalized for any serious illness? How long?

2) Has he ever had a serious accident? Is he accident prone? Are the number of accidents he has increasing?

3) Does he have any medical or neurological symptoms presently? (These may give clues to an organic illness that may be at the basis of his present symptom picture.)

Drug History

1) What medications is the patient presently on and at what dosage? Has he ever been on any medications previously for a long period of time? Could these explain his present symptoms?

2) Has he ever smoked marijuana? Taken LSD? DMT? STP? PCP? Amphetamines? Mescaline? Psilocybin? Other hallucinogens? Cocaine? How many times and for how long? Have they ever caused him difficulty? Is he taking drugs? Could this explain his symptoms? What is the route of drugs taken?

3) Does he drink alcohol? How much? How many days a week? Alone? In the morning? Is it needed to perform a task (e.g. go to work?) Has he ever had delirium tremens? When and how is it treated? Does he belong to Alcoholics Anonymous? Has he ever been hospitalized for alcoholism? Where and for how long? Has it interfered with his performance at work or home?

4) Does the patient take any sedatives (e.g. barbiturates) or tranquilizers regularly? If so, how much? Has this increased? Is he dependent? Does he get withdrawal symptoms?

5) Has the patient ever been or is he presently addicted to heroin? How much? For how long? Has he ever been in a treatment program? Where? Did he get off the drug at the time? Is he withdrawn? When was his last dose? Does he use other drugs in addition?

6) Is he allergic to any medication? If so, which and what was his response?

Previous Psychiatric Treatment

1) Has the patient ever seen a psychotherapist or counselor before? For what and for how long? Does he know the diagnosis? Was he given medication or ECT? Who was or were the therapists? When is the last time he sought psychiatric help?

2) Has he ever been hospitalized for psychiatric reasons? How many times? Where? For how long? What modes of therapy were used? Does he know the diagnoses? What precipitated the hospitalization?

Family History

1) Is there any history of comparable problems in the patient's family? If so, what? At what ages were they treated? What drugs did they receive? Were they hospitalized? For how long? What are their relationships to the family?

2) Is there a family history of suicide? Dementia? Depression? Mania? Bankruptcy (as an indicant of mania)? Schizophrenia? Epilepsy? Any nervous or mental disease? Are there any particularly strange or bizarre relatives?

Mental Status Examination

1) *Thought:* Does the patient have racing thoughts? Feel his head is exploding? Does he feel people are after him? Talking about him as he walks down the street (ideas of reference)? Does he have auditory, visual, olfactory, gustatory, tactile or other hallucinations? Does he feel unreal (derealization)? Feel apart from himself like an actor on the stage (depersonalization)? Are his associations loose? Is he tangential? Circumstantial? Does he have clang associations? Déjà vu? Déjà entendu? Verbigeration? Word salad? Does he have nihilistic, somatic, or other delusions? Ambivalent? Does he have obsessive thoughts or phobias? Does he respond slowly or not at all?

2) *Mood:* Is he depressed? Euphoric? Manic? Anxious? Fearful? Does he feel worthless? Guilty? Dirty? Bad? Is his affect flat? Inappropriate? Does he have emotional incontinence?

3) *Behavior:* Is he autistic? Negativistic? Catatonic (waxy flexibility or excited)? What is his appearance like? Facial expression, dress and behavior? Is he affected? Angry? Pompous? Retarded or agitated? Is he engaging? Warm? Affable? Fearful? Seductive? Does he have compulsions? Tics? Unusual mannerisms? Tremors? Unusual posturing? Is he relaxed or tense? Does he pace the floor?

4) *Organicity:* Does he know who he is? Who the examiner is? Where he is? What the date is? What does his level of intelligence appear to be? What is his fund of knowledge like? Can he name the past three presidents beginning with the most recent? Does he know something current in the news? What is his recent and past memory like? (Clues to this come when taking the history.) Can he remember three objects after five minutes? What is his arithmetic ability like? Can he subtract 7 from 100 and continually go down (e.g. 100, 93, 86, 79, 72 etc.)? How many numbers can he repeat backward and forward? (Most can do 7 forward and 5 backward.) Can he perform simple mathematics (e.g. 70-30, 50×3, 10÷2)? Is he concrete or abstract? Can he interpret proverbs correctly (e.g. People who live in glass houses shouldn't throw stones; A stitch in time saves nine)? Can he tell how an apple and a pear are alike? Is his judgement good? What would he do if he were in a movie theatre and smelled smoke? Can he identify a simple object (e.g. a pen) and its purpose? Is there evidence of a catastrophic reaction during the interview? Confabulation? Occupational delirium?

Physical Examination

Vital signs should be taken on all emergency psychiatric patients and if there is any suggestion of organicity by history or mental status examination, a complete physical and neurological examination should be performed.

EMERGENCY PSYCHIATRIC EVALUATION FORMS

Forms used to direct the taking of a psychiatric history, the performance of a mental status examination and the development of treatment plans vary from institution to institution. Apart from the obvious teaching and research significance, these forms are helpful both in assuring quality in evaluation and in providing a vehicle by which clinicians on a team can easily work together and exchange information. The form used at the Rhode Island Hospital of the Brown Program in Medicine is a three part form. The same form is used on the emergency service that is used in all other parts of the hospital, i.e., the inpatient psychiatric service, the psychiatric consultation-liaison service, the child and family psychiatric service, the outpatient psychiatric clinic and the behavioral medicine unit. Pages 2 and 3 have modified versions for use with children. This facilitates flow between units and negates the need for gathering redundant information. Clinicians working on the inpatient unit supplement the three-page form with a two-page addendum which provides the rationale for hospitalization and an outline of the treatment plan. The treatment plan is developed by all members of the treatment team: the physician, the psychologist, the primary nurse clinician and the social worker.

Facsimilies of the three-page evaluation form and two-page addendum for patients admitted to the inpatient unit are given on the following pages.

USE OF RESTRAINTS

Acutely agitated patients and those who are at imminent risk of harm to themselves or others may need to be restrained in an emergency situation. In every instance, the least restrictive and most humane option given the circumstances should be chosen. Chemical restraints (e.g. chlorpromazine, haloperidol and thiothixene) are preferable to the use of physical restraints. They are both more humane and less restrictive than physical modes of retention. Careful titration of the minimum dose of medication necessary to control patient's violent or agitated behavior will allow patients to participate more fully in the development of a treatment program as well as allow them some freedom to return to their more usual activities such as eating, toilet care and dressing.

Chemical restraints may be contraindicated or insufficient to calm a patient with considerable self or other destructive potential in a number of instances. These include:

1) The violent behavior is part of an underlying organic process which is undiagnosed. Medication may confuse a clinical picture. For instance, phenothiazines, thioxanthenes and butyrophenones cause generalized slowing on the electroencephalogram. If a cause of

RHODE ISLAND HOSPITAL
DEPARTMENT OF PSYCHIATRY
PSYCHIATRIC CONSULTATION
(Page 1 of 3 pages)

NAME _____ | UNIT # _____

ADDRESS _____

BIRTH DATE _____   S.S.# _____   # YEARS SCHOOL:

REFERRED BY _____   REFERRAL PROBLEM:

PRIMARY CLINICIAN _____   OCCUPATION: RACE: B   W   S   ORIENTAL
AMER. INDIAN   OTHER

INSURANCE STATUS _____   SEX: F   M   RELIGION: J   P   RC   OTHER:

MARITAL STATUS: _____ S   M   D   W   SEP.   NO. OF CHILDREN: OCCUPATION OF PARENT IF SINGLE
OR SPOUSE IF MARRIED:

RESPONSIBLE PERSON: _____   RELATIONSHIP TO PATIENT:

ADDRESS: _____   PHONE:

VITAL SIGNS: BP _____   PULSE _____   TEMPERATURE _____   RR _____

PATIENT'S CHIEF COMPLAINT: _____

HISTORY OF PRESENT ILLNESS: _____   INFORMANT: _____

_____

_____

_____

_____

_____

_____

_____

_____

_____

_____

_____

PAST PSYCHIATRIC HISTORY (Outpatient, hospitalization, medication responses, etc.) _____

_____

_____

M-309 CAT. #2984771 REV. 3/80   **1**

CHART COPY

RHODE ISLAND HOSPITAL
DEPARTMENT OF PSYCHIATRY

(Page 2 of 3 pages)

DEVELOPMENTAL AND SOCIAL HISTORY:

Perinatal Complications: _____

Milestones: _____

MBD (Learning disability, hyperactivity): _____

Anti-social Behavior: _____

School Phobia: _____

Significant Recent Life Events: _____

Is there a problem in: _____

Self-care: _____

Daily Activity: _____

Social Support: _____

Living Conditions: _____

HABITS: (Alcohol; Drugs; Tobacco; Caffeine; Eating): _____

Is Drug/Alcohol Detox indicated: Yes ☐ No ☐   Is there an alcohol problem? Yes ☐ No ☐

MILITARY HISTORY: _____

FAMILY HISTORY: (Include psychiatric hospitalization, dementia, depression, mania, suicide, alcoholism, anti-social behavior, seizures, major medical illnesses): _____

Is there a family issue pertinent to evaluation or treatment? Yes ☐ No ☐

MEDICATIONS PATIENT IS ON: (Specify: doses, duration, and recently discontinued): _____

MEDICAL HISTORY:

Allergies: Surgery:

Head Injuries: When next period is expected:

Chronic Medical Problems   Active Medical Problems:

PERTINENT NEUROLOGIC AND MEDICAL FINDINGS ON EXAMINATION: _____

M-309 CAT. #2984771 REV. 3/80

CHART COPY

RHODE ISLAND HOSPITAL
DEPARTMENT OF PSYCHIATRY

(Page 3 of 3 pages)

MENTAL STATUS EXAMINATION:

Appearance:	Interview Participation:
Orientation:	Suicidal:
Memory:	Homicidal:
Judgement:	Sensory Distortions:
Intellect:	Hallucinations:
Affect:	Delusions:
Libido:	Ideas of Reference:
Mood:	Phobias:
Sleep:	Anxiety Attacks:
Appetite (weight change):	Aphasia Screen:

DIFFERENTIAL DIAGNOSIS: _____

_____

_____

DIAGNOSTIC IMPRESSIONS AND DSM III CODE: _____

_____

_____

DISPOSITION AND TREATMENT PLAN: _____

_____

_____

Social Work ☐ _____   Behavioral Medicine ☐ _____

Psychology Testing ☐ _____   Psychiatry ☐ _____

Medical-Neurology-Surgery ☐ _____   Outside Referral ☐ _____

Need collateral information ☐ _____

SIGNATURE: _____

DATE: _____   TIME: _____

M-309 CAT. #2984771 REV. 3/80 **1**

CHART COPY

RHODE ISLAND HOSPITAL
DEPARTMENT OF PSYCHIATRY

ADDENDUM TO PSYCHIATRIC HISTORY FOR AN INPATIENT ADMISSION

1. REASON FOR ADMISSION (Please check and comment)

a. Treatment cannot be initiated or continued unless in a supervised setting _____

b. Destructive or suicidal behavior is an imminent possibility _____

c. Magnitude of deviant behavior is no longer tolerable to family or society _____

d. Ambulatory treatment has not been successful in management of patient illness _____

e. Previous hospitalizations do not use approach available here _____

f. Initiation of psychotherapy or social rehabilitation cannot be commenced on an outpatient basis _____

g. Condition other than psychiatric disorder required hospital care but psychological components cannot optimally be handled in another setting _____

COMMENT: _____
_____
_____
_____
_____
_____
_____
_____

2. IMMEDIATE TREATMENT PLAN ON INPATIENT UNIT

a. Psychopharmacotherapy _____
_____
_____
_____

b. Psychotherapy (Include problems to focus on) _____
_____
_____
_____

c. Sociotherapy (Include family, vocational, etc., issues) _____
_____
_____
_____

M-312 CAT. NO. 2984862 REV. 3/80 (FRONT) **1**

ADDENDUM TO PSYCHIATRIC HISTORY FOR AN INPATIENT ADMISSION — 2

d. Other (ECT, Sodium Amytal Interview, EEG, Neuropsychological Testing, CAT Scan, etc.) _____

_____

_____

_____

_____

_____

e. Consultations Requested (Neurological, Endocrine, etc.) with reason or purpose of request: _____

_____

_____

_____

_____

f. Is Patient Violent or Suicidal   ☐ Yes   ☐ No.   If Yes, plan of management of violent behavior _____

_____

_____

_____

_____

g. Management Plan for Other Medico-Surgical Problems Present (Specific Medications, dosage schedule, etc., Tests, Consults): _____

_____

_____

_____

_____

_____

_____   _____   _____
        Interviewer   Attending Physician   Date

M-312 CAT. NO. 2984862 REV. 3/80 (BACK)

a patient's agitation is inflammation of the brain or its meninges, the examining clinician may discount the significance of the generalized slowing of the electroencephalogram as due to medication if a patient has been given one of the major tranquillizers.

2) Use of significant amounts of medication may be contraindicated. A person who is acutely agitated or self-destructive following a closed head injury in an automobile crash may be vomiting. Patients regurgitating in a sedated state may aspirate and die or develop aspiration pneumonia.

3) Medication takes time to act. Staff may be unable to manage the patient in the interim or may be insufficient in number given the size of a patient or the magnitude of the disturbance.

4) Medication chosen or the amount that can be safely used may be insufficient to calm the patient. Side effects or the medical state of the patient may dictate that physical rather than chemical restraints be used. An older person may have a cardiac condition. Many of the drugs used for acutely agitated patients have strong anticholinergic side effects such as hypotension or increase cardiac irritability. Haloperidol (Haldol) is remarkable for its relative safety at high dose levels.

In all of the above mentioned instances, physical rather than chemical restraints may be indicated.

When physical restraints are necessary, the following guidelines should be adhered to:

1) Leather restraints are considered the safest, most effective and preferred mode of control.

2) If leather restraints are unavailable, heavy webbing may be used with precaution. If a jacket binder is used, leather restraints should be used in addition to prevent a patient from becoming entangled in the restraint.

3) Rope, wire, chain, elasticized bandages, gauze and cloth should not be used. These are either inhumane (e.g. chains, rope and wire) or entail risk of strangulation of an extremity which may lead to ischemia of a limb.

4) Staff members should be educated in the indications and use of physical restraints.

5) Regular patient checks should be made (a) to assure that a patient is not unduly restrained, (b) to reevaluate the possibility of substitution of chemical for physical restraints, (c) to assure that a patient is not being injured by the restraints, and (d) to maintain the restraining devices.

6) Seclusion rooms, where present, should be considered. If used with good clinical judgement, these are more humane than physical restraints. Patients who have concommitant medical or surgical

problems are seldom appropriate for management in a seclusion room (e.g. an acutely suicidal patient who has sustained several fractures when jumping from a building).

7) Patients who are restrained should be so placed as to allow frequent observation by staff.

8) Records should be kept of the rationale for restraint and a notation why physical restraints rather than other modes of restraint have been used. All such cases should be reviewed.

9) The responsible physician should always be kept alert to changes in a patient's status so that restraints may be removed as soon as possible.

10) Ward structure should minimize the need of both chemical and physical restraints. A staff ratio of at least 1:4 (Staff-Patient) is preferred but not always possible. The use of name tags and regular patient-staff meetings are factors which facilitate management of patients with minimum use of restraints.

11) If there exists an undue number of instances of use of physical restraints, attempts should be made to examine what is happening on the ward. Severely ill psychiatric patients are particularly sensitive to tensions among staff members or between patients or staff and act out more at times of conflict.

REFUSAL OF MEDICATION

Patients sometimes refuse to take medication despite the fact that the attending psychiatrist feels that psychopharmacotherapy is a necessary part of management. In most instances, it is possible to obtain cooperation of the patients, but effort and time is required. An understanding of the reasons for refusal is the first step in obtaining patient cooperation.

REASONS FOR REFUSAL OF MEDICATION

1) A lack of understanding of what the etiology of their illness is thought to be and the role of medication in the management of it.

2) Patients', relatives' and friends' fears of medication and its side effects.

3) Patients' fear that medication is being used to "control" them (which, of course, to some degree is true).

4) Lack of rapport between patient and clinician medicating the patient.

5) Feeling that medication is being provided in lieu of, rather than as an adjunct to, psychotherapy and sociotherapy.

6) Patient's struggle with the clinician over medication reinacts earlier struggles with parents centering around feeding or toilet training.

7) Fear of real and/or fantasized side effects of medication. (e.g. Fear of becoming a zombie).

8) Fear of becoming dependent on medication.

9) Previous bad experience with medication (e.g. Patient had several extrapyramidal reactions such as occologyric crises).

Management

1) Attempt to develop a relationship with the patient and his or her family and friends. No one likes to be impersonally dealt with. A few moments with a patient and his significant others is time well spent and may obviate problems over taking medication in the emergency situation as well as regarding hospitalization and follow-through on outpatient therapy.

2) Explain to the patient the assumed etiology of their difficulty and the role and probable mechanism of action of medication in the management of symptoms.

3) Be direct, frank and authoritative in a discussion of the cost-benefit ratio of the use of medication in a given situation. Every drug has potential side effects. Some relatively minor but a few potentially quite harmful. Comparably severe psychiatric illness has some minor and several major consequences such as job loss, loss of relationships, and self- and other-destructive behavior. A patient and family must weigh options.

4) Avoid complicated schedules of drug administration for ambivalent patients and use the route of intake that is most acceptable. Some patients will refuse oral but accept intramuscular medication. The psychodynamic interpretation at that moment is less important than the need that the patient have the medication. If it is possible to give all the medication as a single pill, capsule, liquid or injection without serious side effects, do so.

5) If a patient requiring antipsychotics is recurrently reluctant to take oral medication (such as a paranoid schizophrenic) use long-acting fluphenazine decanoate or enanthate. If given an appropriate schedule, this will usually hold patient's symptoms in check.

6) Minimize unnecessary medication.

7) Use psychotropic drugs with minimum side effects. Patients who are ambivalent about taking medication to start with may use side effects as an excuse to discontinue the drug.

8) If a patient is particularly sensitive to a particular side effect

of a drug, choose another member of the same class of drugs with the least risk of that effect.

9) Elicit the help of the individuals with the best relationships with patients to encourage them to take medication. This may be a family member, friend, clergy, primary care clinician or therapist.

State laws vary concerning administration of medication to involuntary or incompetent patients. The general rule of thumb is that, if required in an emergency situation, medication may be given against a patient's will. Incompetent patients usually may be treated if the next of kin provide written consent until such a time that the patient may provide it. Certification of commitment alone in some states is not sufficient license for the physician to provide chemotherapy without consent of a patient (Malmquist, 1979).

TRANSPORTATION OF ACUTELY PSYCHOTIC PATIENTS

Management

1) Patients should be appropriately medicated. There are a variety of methods available to sedate agitated patients and a number of side effects which the clinician must be alert to. If patients receive intramuscular doses of medication and are sent off without allowing some time for observation, they may arrive dystonic (especially after haloperidol). Therefore, some time should be allowed to lapse to assess the possible extent of any adverse side effects to medication.

2) Ambulance drivers should be informed of possible difficulties. If patients are potentially homicidal, they should be humanely but adequately restrained. If suicidal or homicidal, they should be searched after commitment for concealed weapons (e.g. loaded gun, knife) or concealed drugs (e.g. supply of barbiturates).

3) Unless there is evidence that patients are currently overtly violent, they should be given an opportunity to cooperate before they are labeled dangerous. Patience, understanding, and calm reassurance are valuable tools in managing potentially dangerous patients. If there is concern on the part of the clinician, or concern voiced by patients that they may erupt, oral medication should be given to calm them. Patients' ability to recognize the need for the volitionally take more oral medication makes them feel they have some control over what is happening to them.

4) Patients who are not committed cannot be forced against their will to be taken to or from a hospital. Unless a patient has been

committed, they must be assumed to be within their legal rights to protest against hospitalization and transportation to or from a hospital against their will could constitute liability for a suit.

5) Patients should never be deceived about their destination. Families may have told patients that they were gong to see a nonpsychiatric physician. The psychiatrist should not collude with this deception as it undermines further faith in the doctor's word.

6) An ambulance service may require that even patients with no potential for violence be restrained. If patients are to be restrained they should be told they will be, or that it is ambulance policy. If they are violent and it is necessary for both their protection and that of the ambulance crew to restrain them, it should not be undertaken until adequate personnel are available to help. Family members and the patients' friends may be of great value in calming them. Once in restraints, many patients feel more comfortable and secure, resting assured that they are controlled and their violent behavior in check.

7) A woman should always accompany a female patient in the ambulance. A delusional patient may fantasize that she was sexually abused, and the presence of the female attendant as witness assures protection for both patient and male crew.

8) Seldom are psychiatric patients a dire emergency; that is, rarely do they require speedy arrival at a hospital, particularly if properly restrained and medicated by the evaluating physician. Rapidly blinking lights and a loud siren may serve to aggravate the patient's already decompensated condition. Driving at the usual speed with calm, mature attendants is usually the best transportation that can be provided for a disturbed patient.

9) If there is any question of a serious nonpsychiatric medical problem, the patient should always be medically and surgically cleared before being transported over a great distance to a receiving psychiatric hospital from an emergency room. Neither ambulance personnel nor the staff of a large psychiatric hospital, public or private, are equipped to handle medical emergencies as is a well staffed city emergency room. Sometimes nonpsychiatric medical staff are unaware of the limitations of psychiatric hospitals in dealing with medical and surgical problems. If they are reluctant to examine a psychiatric patient or perform only a cursory exam, they should be tactfully reminded that just as they are not experts in the evaluation and treatment of psychiatric patients, neither are psychiatrists expert surgeons and internists.

10) We would like to emphasize again the importance of maintaining good rapport with nonmedical members of the community who work with acutely disturbed patients. Included in this genre are

ambulance drivers, clergy, police officers and firemen. High quality care at a time of crisis requires smooth communication between a number of concerned care-givers. One way to achieve this is the participation of emergency room staff in educational programs for the community. Seminars provide excellent opportunities for exchange of information about frequently encountered problems, and as a forum to develop ways in which all members of care-giving teams can better work together at times of crisis.

PSYCHIATRIC EMERGENCY AREA REQUIREMENTS

Effective evaluation and management of individuals presenting with psychiatric emergencies is best achieved in a setting that meets the following standards:

1) There should be an interviewing room that is both sufficiently soundproof so that a patient and his or her family and friends may talk confidentially with the evaluating clinician as well as secure so that violent or potentially self-destructive patients do not harm themselves or others.

2) There should be no large glassed areas, medication stores, or sharp objects such as surgical blades in the area where patients are evaluated.

3) Security guards should be readily available and (ideally) alertable by an alarm button that is readily accessible to the evaluating clinician if attacked.

4) The door to the interviewing room should not be able to be locked from either the inside or the outside.

5) The interviewing room should be so located that other staff can easily get to it if needed.

6) Parenteral and oral psychotropic medications should be available if required for the use in the emergency situation.

7) A pharmacy should be available to provide the patient the amount of medication he or she may need to take in the interim between the visit to the emergency room and such a time that the patient or a friend or relative can reasonably have the prescription filled and/or have a follow-up visit.

8) The ambiance and furniture should sufficient that the patient and significant others (which may include attending police officer(s), spouse, lover, children, friend, etc.) can be seen at the same time if deemed necessary by the evaluating clinician.

9) Restraints should be available for use that are humane if management of the patient requires.

Ideally, community mental health centers, general medical hospitals, health maintenance organizations and other institutions providing emergency psychiatric services should have holding beds so that patient's treatment response may be evaluated over the course of one to three days. Some acutely psychotic or other patients and individuals with potential to harm themselves or others recompensate quickly with a combination of crisis oriented psychotherapeutic techniques and appropriate doses of psychotropic medication. These beds should be available for use at the discretion of the emergency psychiatric clinicians and in an area appropriate for brief treatment so that the need for further hospitalization in an inpatient setting is minimized.

II

PSYCHOPHARMACOLOGY

BASIC PRINCIPLES OF PSYCHOPHARMACOLOGY IN THE EMERGENCY PSYCHIATRIC SITUATION

Side Effects

Identification, management, and treatment of side effects play significant roles in drug management. Misidentification of side effects may have deleterious consequences, e.g. the akinesia secondary to neuroleptic drugs may be diagnosed as depression and treated with an antidepressant rather than with an anti-Parkinsonian drug. Hypertensive headaches secondary to monoamine oxidase inhibitors may lead to unnecessary discontinuation of a MAOI when blood pressure checks have not been instituted and the risk of hypertensive headaches has not been explained. There are a number of references which can and should be utilized in investigating established or potential side effects. These resources include the *Physician's Desk Reference*, the Monthly Index of Medical Specialties, the Medical Letter, and the Adverse Drug Effect Bulletin. Many hospitals now have drug information centers to assist clinicians in drug selection, dosage, side effect recognition, and management. The emerging role of clinical pharmacists will be an added resource in the management and prevention of side effects.

Psychosocial Issues

Over 50% of ingestions in Great Britain in 1974 occurred with medicines that were prescribed for someone other than the ingestor. Inquiry should always be made as to who in the patient's social circle might gain access to his medicines.

47

Two or more members of the same household may be taking psychoactive medication. What are the risks if a child accidentally takes one of his mother's tablets instead of his own? The outcome could be fatal if a child was taking dextroamphetamine for hyperkinesis and his mother a MAOI for depression.

The relationship between the patient, his family, and the pharmacist may be in harmony with what the physician intends, may serve a monitoring purpose to prevent physician errors or oversights, or may work at cross-purposes with the physician. The pharmacist can be viewed as a powerful figure who brings reassurance or raises fears.

Compliance

Each patient will already have been primed by previous experience and behavior with medicines. Positive previous responses to medication will enhance compliance. However, a patient who needs to control treatment will often not comply. Poor compliers usually remain poor compliers unless the physician undertakes active intervention to bring about change.

Patients often become alarmed on learning of the dosage of medicine that they are to take. Patients accustomed to the low milligram doses of some phenothiazines or antianxiety drugs may become alarmed to learn that lithium carbonate is generally prescribed in a daily dosage range of 600-1800 mg. Patients frequently know of someone else who received the same medication, and may lament that they have to take such a big dose when a friend "only had to take three of these capsules a day." Conversely, patients may complain about what they consider to be low doses: "My cousin used to take ten of them a day; do you really think I'm going to get well on just two?"

Many patients have an inherent bias against taking medicines, often expressed in terms of feeling a loss of autonomy or an implied weakness or failure. While some patients insist that their illness has nothing to do with developmental experiences and are happy to take medicines, others insist that they became ill because of earlier experiences and fear that the medication will prevent the emotional resolution of traumatic childhood events.

Personal attributes may determine response to side effects. Patients who are highly concerned about appearance may stop phenothiazines, tricyclic antidepressants, or lithium treatment after weight gain has occurred, whereas underweight patients will often welcome the weight gain. Patients who need constant accurate vision (e.g. students) may not tolerate blurry vision, just as a lawyer would object to a constant dry mouth. Thioridazine may bring a welcome slowing in premature ejaculation for one patient, while worsening a potency problem for another.

Cost of treatment, including the cost of medicine, may be a significant factor. Compliance may improve when patients are informed of the estimated cost of the medicine. In this country, outpatient prescriptions have a built-in dispensing fee, and it is generally cheaper to have one prescription for 100 tablets filled than two prescriptions for 50 tablets each. Weighted against this is the hazard of dispensing a large number of tablets to a patient who is at risk for a suicide attempt.

The physician's instructions to the pharmacist are conveyed in the form of a written prescription to confirm a verbal (usually telephone) order.

It is important that the patient understand and follow the directions for use. Preferably, the patient knows exactly what it is that he is taking, what the dose is, and so on. The physician must be assured that the patient clearly understands the instructions. If there is insufficient space on the prescription blank for clear instructions, a separate note can be sent to the pharmacist. The physician may also compile a detailed list of instructions and go over it with the patient or the patient's family until he is satisfied that the patient understands the instructions and can follow them.

NEUROLEPTIC DRUGS

Neuroleptic drugs should be used with extreme caution because of the risk of tardive dyskinesia. Great care should be used in arriving at the decision to prescribe a neuroleptic drug, and then only in doses and for a treatment time that is realistically tailored to outcome expectations. The key factor then becomes careful surveillance; the more frequently a patient is evaluated the less likely it is he will be allowed to drift through endless prescribing rituals which often more serve to keep a clinician comfortable than the patient well. The introduction of a neuroleptic should always be a medical decision made by a physician. Every patient on maintenance neuroleptic treatment should be reevaluated every three months by an experienced physician to be checked for early signs of tardive dyskinesia and whether the benefits of continuing the drug outweigh the risk of tardive dyskinesia.

Neuroleptic drugs are effective in controlling the symptoms of acute and chronic psychosis, the psychoses associated with old age, some organic mental syndromes, and miscellaneous conditions such as hemiballismus (haloperidol), Gilles de la Tourette syndrome (haloperidol), anorexia nervosa, and agitated states associated with drug addiction and alcoholism.

The Phenothiazines

The phenothiazines are subdivided into three groups according to the basic chemical structure:

1) The *aliphatic phenothiazines* include chlorpromazine (Thorazine) promazine (Sparine), and triflupromazine (Vesprin) and are characterized by:

    a) A greater sedating effect than the other two subgroups.

    b) High milligram dosages.

    c) A greater hypnotic effect than other two subgroups.

    d) Motor and mood inhibition.

    e) A greater tendency to produce hypotensive, autonomic, hemotologic, hepatotoxic, and photosensitive reactions than the piperazine subgroup.

2) The *piperidine phenothiazines* include thioridazine (Mellaril) which is sedating and especially helpful in the management of agitated and excited patients. Side effects include:

    a) Occasional severe hypotensive reactions.

    b) Pigmentary changes in the eyes (including the lens, the anterior cornea, the posterior cornea, the retina and the conjunctiva).

    c) Skin pigmentary changes ranging from slate gray to purple (also seen with chlorpromazine) is a rare side effect.

3) The *piperazine phenothiazines* include fluphenazine (Prolixin), trifluoperazine (Stelazine), perphenazine (Trilafon), and acetophenazine (Tindal) and are characterized by:

    a) High potency low milligram doses.

    b) Rarely causing hypotension.

    c) Frequently causing extrapyramidal side effects. Prolixin Decanoate and Prolixin Enanthate are long-acting preparations which are given intramuscularly when a patient is unreliable in taking drugs orally.

The Thioxanthenes

The thioxanthenes include chlorprothixene (Taractan) and thiothixine (Navane) and are somewhat comparable in side effects to the phenothiazines.

The Butyrophenones

The only butyrophenone in clinical psychiatric use in the United States is haloperidol (Haldol). It is characterized by a greater tendency than some of the other neuroleptics to induce extrapyramidal side effects and by a very low reported incidence of blood dyscrasias and liver damage.

The Dihydroindolones

Molindone (Moban, Lidone) and other dihydroindolone compounds resemble the piperazine derivatives in action and dosage requirements.

Choice of Drug

There are no established criteria for the selection of one neuroleptic over another on the basis of presenting symptoms and signs. Consideration of potential side effects is a major concern, such as anticipating anticholinergic effects from thioridazine in elderly patients, or the knowledge that haloperidol is rarely associated with hepatic damage. A hallucinating man with a history of premature ejaculation might especially profit from thioridazine while a hallucinating woman who has long fought a battle with obesity might be a particularly good candidate for molindone.

Past history of drug response is significant. Haloperidol appears to be an especially effective agent for the management of acute mania or hypomania. A piperazine phenothiazine or haloperidol should be used when hypotensive medications are or will be taken, e.g. tranylcypromine or diuretics.

Dosage

Treatment is usually initiated with divided doses. Intramuscular preparations may be necessary for faster benefit and to ensure compliance. Once an effective daily maintenance regimen is achieved, doses can be transferred from a daytime to a bedtime schedule so that sleep is ensured.

Neuroleptics have wide therapeutic margins and a corresponding range of doses. No specific maximum dose has been established for any neuroleptics, with the exception of thioridazine where doses above 800 mg a day significantly increase the risk of pigmentary retinopathy.

Usual daily dosage range of commonly used neuroleptics:
1) Phenothiazines
   a) Chlorpromazine (Thorazine) — 300-800 mg
   b) Acetophenazine (Tindal) — 40-120 mg
   c) Thioridazine (Mellaril) — 200-800 mg
   d) Perphenazine (Trilafon) — 24-80 mg
   e) Trifluoperazine (Stelazine) — 15-40 mg
   f) Fluphenazine (Prolixin) — 5-20 mg
2) Thioxanthenes
   a) Chlorprothixene (Taractan) — 75-200mg
   b) Thiothixene (Navane) — 10-40 mg
3) Butyrophenones
   Haloperidol (Haldol) — 2-40 mg
4) Dihydroindolenes
   Molindone (Moban, Lidone) — 50-75 mg

LITHIUM CARBONATE

Lithium carbonate can be singularly effective in treating agitated or excited states. Patients who present with mild to moderate hypomania or agitation can occasionally be started on lithium on an emergency basis. Hospitalization is indicated if the symptoms do not remit within a short while, if agitation or inappropriate behavior worsen, or if there is a potential for violence. Patients who have previously been treated with lithium and have shown a favorable response are good candidates for urgent reinitiation of lithium treatment if there are no medical contraindications and if other indications for hospitalization are absent, e.g. suicidality.

Lithium is administered orally in tablet, capsule, or liquid form. Lithium tablets are scored, which allows for a finer titration of dosage. The usual daily dosage range of lithium carbonate is 600-1800 mg.

Prior to initiating lithium a complete medical history should be obtained with special emphasis on cardio-pulmonary disease, thyroid disease, or kidney disease. Patients with neurological illnesses appear to be particularly prone to lithium toxicity. Hypertensive patients who are taking diuretics and are salt restricted are prime candidates for lithium toxicity.

The pre-treatment lithium workup includes thyroid function studies, serum creatinine, serum electrolytes, a urinalysis, and a complete blood count. Patients over the age of 45 should have a cardiogram before starting on lithium.

Adverse Reactions to Lithium

Side effects of lithium treatment include:
1) Renal Side Effects
   (Polyuria and polydipsia; possible development of interstitial fibrosis with long-term lithium treatment)
2) Endocrine Side Effects
   (Goiterous hypothyroidism; weight gain; hypercalcemia and hyperparathyroidism; possible provocation of diabetic keto-acidosis)
3) Cardiovascular Side Effects
   (Arrhythmias; benign, reversible T wave changes)
4) Dermatological Side Effects
   (Dermatitis; exacerbation of psoriasis)
5) Gastrointestinal Side Effects
   (Anorexia; nausea; vomiting; loose stools; diarrhea; abdominal cramps or pain)
6) Hematologic Side Effects
   (Reversible mild leucocytosis; aplastic anemia)
7) Metabolic Side Effects
   (Edema; hypokalemia)
8) Neurological Side Effects
   (Tremor; cogwheeling; convulsions)

Severe Lithium Intoxication

Lithium poisoning may occur as a consequence of faulty management (e.g. not warning a patient about the necessity of salt intake), by accident (e.g. a patient takes 1800 mg in one dose rather than in divided doses because he ran out of lithium and is trying to catch up), or as a consequence of a deliberate overdose.

Medical causes contributing to toxicity include salt restriction, use of diuretics, dehydration, illness, or childbirth. Severe toxicity rarely develops at levels under 2.0 mEq/1 , but toxicity can occur in susceptible individuals at ordinary therapeutic or even sub-thera-peutic levels. The symptoms of toxicity usually develop gradually and initially include anorexia, nausea, vomiting, diarrhea, weak-ness, fatigue, difficulty concentrating, ataxia, dysarthria, a coarse tremor, and muscle twitching. As toxicity advances, central nervous system symptoms become more pronounced. Neuromuscular irrita-bility, muscular flaccidity, confusion, somnolence, delirium, hallu-cinations, seizures, and coma are the major symptoms. Fluid and electrolyte imbalance, arrhythmias, hypotension, shock, oliguria, and anemia may occur. Death may supervene from intercurrent infection, cardiovascular collapse, or central nervous system depression.

Management

The patient should be admitted to an intensive care facility. A toxicology screen should be obtained to rule out ingestion of other drugs when an overdose is suspected.

The severity of intoxication is related to the serum lithium concentration and the duration of the toxic level. Removal of unabsorbed lithium can be accomplished, provided the patient is conscious, by inducing emesis or by endotracheal intubation and gastric lavage when the patient's level of consciousness has been compromised.

Renal clearance of lithium is often reduced in cases of toxicity. If this is due to a negative sodium balance, sodium chloride should provide improvement. If lithium clearance has not been reduced, sodium chloride will not induce a significant increase in lithium excretion and may further aggravate fluid and electrolyte overload. This differentiation cannot be assessed in advance and all patients should receive approximately 150-300 mEq of sodium chloride over the first 6 hours.

Peritoneal and hemodialysis are helpful in promoting lithium loss.

Dialysis should be instituted based on clinical condition, duration of poisoning, lithium level, and rate of renal lithium excretion.

The following schedule for dialysis has been recommended:
1) Dialyze immediately if the serum lithium level is above 4.0 mEq/l.
2) Dialyze immediately if the serum lithium level is between 2.0 and 4.0 mEq/l and the clinical condition is poor.
3) In other patients the rate of renal excretion should be monitored along with the clinical condition and the decision to dialyze made on these grounds.

Osmotic diuretics, aminophylline, acetazolamide, and sodium bicarbonate may be of benefit when dialysis facilities are not available. Correction of fluid and electrolyte balance is of vital importance. General measures include monitoring vital signs, cardiac and pulmonary support, and prevention of infection and seizures.

THE MONOAMINE OXIDASE INHIBITORS

The monoamine oxidase inhibitors are valuable antidepressants. They can be dramatically effective in remitting severe depression, suicidality, phobia, and anxiety. They are a neglected modality in the pharmacotherapeutic armamentarium, basically because of insufficient studies demonstrating their effectiveness and because of the concern about hypertensive reactions. Severe hypertensive reactions occur when a dietary infraction is made, and properly informed, cooperative and responsible patients are unlikely to infract.

The MAOI's increase the concentration of endogenous amines such as dopamine, norepinephrine, and serotonin, and exogenous amines such as tyramine. MAO activity must be inhibited by at least 80-90% for amine turnover to increase to a point where clinical improvement occurs.

The metabolic degradation of barbiturates, aminopyrine, cocaine, acetanilid, and meperidine is altered by some MAOI's. MAOI's also potentiate the action of amphetamine-like compounds, sympathomimetic amines, and anticholinergics. The mechanism of MAOI's may be related to their inhibition of MAO, since the many chemical compounds called MAO inhibitors have in common only the properties of MAO inhibition and antidepressant activity.

Risk of a hypertensive episode can be minimized by detailed patient education and by instituting several precautions:

1) Patients should be given a complete list of foods, beverages, and medications that can interact with MAOI's to cause hypertensive reactions. The symptoms of a hypertensive reaction should be described to every patient taking an MAOI. The symptoms generally begin within a half an hour of a dietary infraction and include palpitations, apprehension, a throbbing or pounding generalized headache, nausea, photophobia, and a painful, stiff neck.

2) Patients should own and be instructed in the use of a blood pressure kit. Pretreatment supine and erect blood pressure readings and pulse rate should be recorded and the patient should keep a record of readings.

3) Patients should wear an engraved bracelet or pendant stating that they are taking a MAOI.

4) If an offending food or medicine is ingested an immediate effort should be made to induce vomiting, either by tickling the back of the throat or by taking 30 cc of syrup of ipecac.

5) Patients on MAOI's should be advised to alert food preparers about the restriction. Restaurant food may contain red wine or cheese, which are easily camouflaged in sauces or gravy. Travelling

overseas may be especially hazardous, particularly in countries where one's language is not properly comprehended or the proper treatment of a MAOI/hypertensive reaction is not known, or both.

6) Phentolamine (Regitine), and alpha-adrenergic blocker, is an effective treatment for a hypertensive reaction. It should be administered by slow intravenous injection at a rate of about 1 mg per minute. The drop in blood pressure is usually instantaneous. Thorazine and Mellaril have alpha-blocking properties and may be useful when a patient cannot get to a hospital quickly. However, it is easy for a patient to misinterpret a hypotensive reaction for a hypertensive one, as both cause headache, and an alpha blocker taken in this condition can cause an abrupt and potentially dangerous further drop in pressure.

The MAOI Diet

Any protein-containing food that has undergone degradation can present a hazard to patients taking MAOI's. This probably results from the fact that tyramine is produced by decarboxylation of tyrosine, which is derived from protein by proteolysis, or hydrolysis. Foods to avoid therefore include those which are naturally fermented, e.g., ripened cheese, red wine, beer, yeast, pickled herring; also to be avoided are spoiled or "gamy" foods, and only fresh food or freshly prepared frozen or canned food should be eaten.

Drugs that interact harmfully with MAOI's include:

1) *Amphetamines* (hypertensive reactions, hyperthermia, cardiac arrhythmias, death)
2) *Tricyclic Antidepressants* (excitation, hyperpyrexia, convulsions, death)
3) *Dextromethorphan*
   One patient receiving phenelzine developed nausea, coma, hypotension, and hypopyrexia following ingestion of 2 oz. of a cough syrup containing dextromethorphan.
4) *Ephedrine*
   Severe hypertensive reactions may occur and one death has been attributed to ephedrine in a patient receiving a MAOI. Ephedrine administration results in the liberation of norepinephrine stored in increased amounts in storage sites of adrenergic neurons of patients on MAOI's.
5) *Levodopa* (hypertension, facial flushing, palpitations, lightheadedness)
   Levodopa probably induces increased storage and release of dopamine and norepinephrine in patients on MAOI's.

6) *Meperidine* (Demerol, Pethidine) (excitation, sweating, rigidity, hypertension, and death have been reported)

7) *Metaraminol* (Aramine)
Metaraminol is an indirect sympathomimetic which produces its pressor effects by releasing norepinephrine. On theoretical grounds it is advisable to avoid metaraminol.

8) *Methylphenidate* (Ritalin)
It is advisable to avoid Ritalin use in patients on MAOI's for the same reason as avoidance of amphetamines.

9) *Phenothiazines and Butyrophenones*
These drugs have been safely used concommitantly with MAOI's in a large number of patients. The major risk is of hypotensive reactions, particularly when drugs with strong alpha-blocking properties are used, e.g. thioridazine, chlorpromazine. When phenothiazine/MAOI combinations are indicated, it is preferable to use high potency phenothiazines and to monitor blood pressure carefully.

10) *Phenylephrine*
Phenylephrine is capable of inducing significant hypertensive reactions in patients on MAOI's. Phenylephrine acts directly on the adrenergic receptor but is metabolized by MAOI in the intestine and liver and its effects are therefore enhanced by MAOI's.

11) *Phenylpropanolamine* (headache, vomiting, elevated blood pressure) Phenylpropanolamine, like ephedrine, causes release of stored epinephrine in adrenergic neurons and is therefore contraindicated with MAOI's.

12) *Monoamine Oxidase Inhibitors*
Hypertensive reactions may occur when two MAOI's are administered concurrently or sequentially where a washout period was not allowed for.

Monoamine Oxidase Inhibitor Overdose

Manifestations of MAOI overdose are essentially those of beta-adrenergic stimulation and a beta blocker such as propranolol may be effective.

Common Side Effects of Monoamine Oxidase Inhibitors

These include significant postural hypotension, fatigue, mild anticholinergic effects, change in temperature regulation, and insomnia. Less common side effects include nausea, diarrhea, nonhypertensive headaches, retarded ejaculation, and painful abdominal cramps.

TRICYCLIC ANTIDEPRESSANTS (TCA'S)

Poisoning with Tricylic Antidepressants

The widespread use of TCA's has led to an increasing number of overdoses with these agents, sometimes with fatal consequences. Although concern about patient access to these agents is justified, drug stores and supermarkets have shelves filled with over-the-counter drugs which are available to the patient wishing to overdose. Salicylates, in particular, are freely available, alone or combined with other pharmacological agents.

A relatively high percentage of TCA overdose subjects have a QRS duration of 100 milliseconds or more, abnormal deep tendon reflexes, unconsciousness, or require supportive respiration. Less frequent are grand mal seizures, and cardiac arrest is a relatively infrequent occurence.

Hypotension occurs in approximately 15% of overdoses. A number of arrhythmias have been reported. These include right bundle branch block, atrial premature contractions, ventricular premature contractions, junctional arrhythmias, and idioventricular arrhythmias. Plasma TCA levels predict major adverse effects more accurately than the amount of drug ingested. A major TCA overdose has been defined as that which occurs with plasma TCA levels above 1,000 mg/ml (four to ten times the optimal therapeutic level for tricyclic antidepressants). When plasma levels are not available, a QRS duration on routine EKG of 100 milliseconds or greater within the first 24 hours following the overdose is the most reliable indication of a major overdose.

The most frequently encountered manifestations of tricyclic antidepressant overdose are due to the anticholinergic actions: dry mouth, retention of urine, absence of bowel sounds, mydriasis, blurring of vision, and sinus tachycardia. Toxic doses affect the central nervous system and produce agitation, restlessness, and characteristic pressure of speech, loss of consciousness, increased tendon reflexes, and extensive plantar reflexes, twitching, and convulsions. In extreme cases of toxicity prolonged flaccid coma is seen.

With a major TCA overdose the plasma levels may be elevated for several days, particularly when the poisoning has been with a tertiary amine TCA such as amitriptyline. In such instances, patients should have continuous cardiac monitoring for 5 to 6 days, particularly as death up to 6 days after TCA overdose has been attributed to arrhythmias.

Physostigmine salicylate, a specific cholinesterase inhibitor that readily penetrates the blood-brain barrier, may reverse TCA-induced comas, choreoathetosis, and myoclonus, and may also reverse cardiac arrhythmias. However, physostigmine has a short duration of action and may cause severe cholinergic manifestations such as hypersalivation and bradycardia, as well as generalized convulsions.

Forced diuresis, hemodialysis, and peritoneal dialysis are ineffective for poisoning by TCA's. Charcoal hemoperfusion does not remove significant amounts of TCA's from the body. Some authorities recommend the use of supportive measures alone.

Withdrawal from Tricyclic Antidepressant

A withdrawal reaction to TCA's may occur, sometimes despite gradual tapering. The symptoms consist of nausea, vomiting, headache, fatigue, nightmares, and rarely, akathisia. Symptomatic management includes antiemetics and analgesics. Akathisia abates following reintroduction of the TCA.

THE BENZODIAZEPINES

The benzodiazepines are widely prescribed drugs. The most common side effects are drowsiness and ataxia.

Chlordiazepoxide (Librium)

The half life of Librium is between 6 and 30 hours. Active metabolites are synthesized so that repeated doses can produce a cumulative effect. A number of patients will therefore respond well to once or twice daily dosages.

Diazepam (Valium)

Diazepam (Valium) has a potency two to five times that of chlordiazepoxide and a half life of 20 to 50 hours. The production of metabolites requires the same precautions as with Librium.

Oxazepam (Serax)

This is a metabolite of diazepam which does not have any known metabolites in humans. The half life is 3 to 21 hours so that more frequent dosing is required such as three to four times a day.

Chlorazepate (Tranxene)

This drug is an intermediate in potency between diazepam and chlordiazepoxide. Daily or twice daily dosing is successful for a number of patients.

USE OF PSYCHOACTIVE MEDICATIONS IN THE EMERGENCY ROOM

General Information

1) Adverse drug reactions appear more frequently in the geriatric patient population.
2) Drugs appear to be metabolized at different rates by different individuals. This means that the effective serum level of two patients on the same oral dose of a tricyclic antidepressant may be remarkably different.
3) Barbiturates may induce liver microsomal enzymes thereby increasing the rate at which other drugs are degraded.
4) The degradation of alcohol, barbiturates, and narcotics is inhibited by MAOI's.
5) The CNS depressant effects of alcohol and barbiturates is enhanced by the use of phenothiazines.
6) There is a paradoxical rise in blood pressure when neuroleptics are taken with epinephrine.
7) A syndrome similar to atropine poisoning, characterized by delirium, convulsions, and excitation may occur when certain tricyclic antidepressants are taken along with an MAOI.
8) Neuroleptics may enhance the hypotensive effectiveness of the antihypertensive agents.
9) The atropine-like side effects of the anticholinergics, antihistamines, antiparkinsonian drugs, and phenothiazines are enhanced by the tricyclic antidepressants.
10) Both the thioxanthenes and phenothiazines lower the convulsive threshold in susceptible individuals so that it may be necessary to increase the amount of anticonvulsant medication taken.

11) Physostigmine may be effective in the treatment of an atropine psychosis.
12) An amicable interview may be helpful in the diagnosis and treatment of a conversion reaction.

Commonly Used Pharmacologic Agents on a Psychiatric Emergency Service

1) For the acute management of acute psychotic symptomatology, 5–10 mg of intramuscular Trilafon, or 5–10 mg of intramuscular Haldol, or 50–75 mg of intramuscular Thorazine (beware of hypotensive reactions) may be used.
2) For the acute management of moderate psychotic symptoms liquid Haldol, Thorazine, Mellaril, or Trilafon may be given orally.
3) For symptoms of a chronic organic mental syndrome, Prolixin 1 mg po tid, or Mellaril 25 mg po tid, or Trilafon 2–4 mg po tid or qid may be prescribed. Mellaril tends not to cause extrapyramidal side effects or to lower the seizure threshold.

SIDE EFFECTS OF PSYCHOACTIVE MEDICATION

Every medication can cause side effects of some kind. In some cases, such as with the extrapyramidal effects or sedative qualities of the phenothiazines, these may diminish with time. In other instances it may be necessary to lower the dose of medication, to stop the medication, or to stop the medication and institute immediate treatment (e.g. acute agranulocytosis with a phenothiazine), or to continue the medication but add another medication to counteract the side effects.

Management of the Side Effects of the Psychoactive Medications

Postural Hypotension

Postural hypotension is a frequent concomitant of neuroleptic and antidepressant treatment, and blood pressure may drop to dangerously low levels, particularly in patients with artherosclerotic disease or peripheral neuropathy. The adverse sequelae of orthostatic hypotension include chronic fatigue and dizziness, myocardial infarction, cerebrovascular occlusion, and injuries sustained after fainting. The latter may have grave consequences, especially in the elderly who are prone to fractures of the femoral neck with its attendant risks (e.g. pulmonary embolism from immobility, adverse reaction to anesthesia).

A predictor of orthostatic hypotension secondary to treatment with imipramine is a significant drop in pressure in the vertical compared to the supine position, and this predictor probably holds true for the neuroleptics. Patients should have their blood pressure measured after lying at rest for 5 minutes, and a pressure reading should then be taken with the patient standing. A prominent drop in pressure would suggest a neuroleptic with small hypotensive risk, such as haloperidol.

Prevention of orthostatic hypotension includes the above measures and warning the patient not to change posture abruptly. When arising in the morning the patient should swing both legs over the side of the bed and sit there for a few minutes. Hot baths are to be avoided, and patients should kneel before standing in the bath. Similar cautions are to be exercised when getting out of a car, particularly following a long drive. Taking the medication after meals may slow its absorption so that pressure does not drop abruptly. Increasing fluid and salt intake and wearing tight-fitting elastic stockings may be of benefit.

Orthostatic hypotension can produce frightening symptoms. Careful monitoring combined with gradual increments of neuroleptic dosage may prevent it. In some circumstances it may be wise to advise hospitalization to stabilize the blood pressure.

Emergency measures include bed rest with the head positioned below the pelvis and administering supplementary fluids and salt. Severe hypotension can be treated with norepinephrine which combats the alpha adrenergic blocking effects of neuroleptics. Epinephrine should be avoided as it cause vasodilation.

Decreased Visual Acuity and Blindness

A decrease in visual acuity and, in some instances, blindness may be associated with the maintenance use of some phenothiazines. Therefore, a patient on a drug like thioridazine should ideally have regular ophthalmological examinations. Improvement in visual acuity after drug discontinuation may occur rapidly in some cases. Subjectively, patients may report reduced visual acuity or an amber hue in vision when ocular pathology is present. If continued medication is required, primary prevention of these changes involves:
1) Keeping the dosage relatively low
2) Using drug holidays

3) Switching to a drug other than chlorpromazine or thioridazine
4) The concurrent use of a relatively low dose of thioridazine with another phenothiazine such as trifluoperazine
5) The use of dark glasses
6) Protection from sunlight
7) The use of special window glass that transmits a minimal amount of ultraviolet light

Dry Mouth

The dry mouth that occurs with the use of a number of psychoactive agents may be somewhat relieved by chewing dietetic gum or sucking a dietetic candy, or by frequently rinsing the mouth out with water.

Drowsiness

Most patients become tolerant to the drowsiness that occurs with some drugs early in treatment and do not complain of it after the first few weeks. If they do, the medication should be reduced temporarily. Patients should be warned not to drive or to operate heavy machinery if drowsiness occurs.

Constipation

A serious side effect of some medications is constipation. Fecal impaction may occur and will necessitate the use of an enema or digital disimpaction. Hardening of stools, which may be accompanied by abdominal cramping, may be treated by:
1) Dioctyl sodium sulfosuccinate (Colace)
2) If this is not effective, Milk of Magnesia 30 cc qhs or bisacodyl (Dulcolax)
3) If symptoms persist, the patient should be instructed to insert a glycerine or a bisacodyl suppository in the morning.

Excess Appetite

Some drugs may cause an increase in appetite with a weight gain far in excess of that desired by the patient. Some tricyclic antidepressants may cause a craving for candy and chocolates.

Blurred Vision

An especially annoying side effect, blurred vision may be handled in a variety of ways:
1) Reduction of medication if possible
2) The use of "Trilafon Glasses" for close reading
3) Instructing the patient to avoid driving if possible, or at least to be very careful when driving
4) Instructing the patient to avoid operating heavy machinery

In a number of cases blurred vision subsides with time alone.

Extrapyramidal Symptoms

A variety of extrapyramidal symptoms may occur with psychoactive medications. The butyrophenones and the thioxanthenes frequently induce extrapyramidal side effects such as akinesia, tremor, and rigidity. The phenothiazines vary in their production of such symptoms. The aliphatic phenothiazine chlorpromazine (Thorazine) appears less likely to produce such symptoms than the piperazine phenothiazines, perphenazine (Trilafon), trifluoperazine (Stelazine) or fluphenazine (Prolixin). The piperidine phenothiazine thiroidazine (Mellaril) seldom causes such disorders. Therefore, one way to treat an extrapyramidal effect is to convert to a drug with less tendency to cause such difficulty. Specific extrapyramidal side effects include:
1) *Parkinsonism*. This syndrome includes akinesia, muscular rigidity, tremor, masklike facies, alterations of posture, drooling and hypersalivation, and loss of associated movements. It usually develops within 5 to 20 days after initiation of treatment with phenothiazines. It occurs more frequently in females than males. An antiparkinsonian drug such as Cogentin 0.5–1.0 mg bid or qid or Artane 2–5 mg po bid or tid may be helpful.
2) *Akathisia*. An inability to sit still, tendency to pace constantly, motor restlessness and fidgeting (frequently misdiagnosed as psychotic exacerbation or tension) may occur. Akathisia generally develops with 5 to 40 days after commencement of phenothiazine medication and occurs more frequently in females than in males. Treatment involves the use of antiparkinsonian agents in the dosages mentioned above or diphenyldramine 50 mg po bid or tid may be tried.
3) *Dystonia*. Paticularly distressing, this symptom may occur from 1 hour to 5 days after commencement of phenothiazine treat-

ment. It consists of uncoordinated spasmodic movements of the limbs and body such as torticollis, retrocollis, opisthotonos and oculogyric crises. Coordinated steretoyped involuntary movements may also occur (dyskinesia). Men are more prone to develop these symptoms. Fortunately, the antiparkinsonian agents are quite effective, e.g. 2–4 mg of benztropine mesylate (Cogentin) daily. With acute and particularly distressing symptoms, Cogentin or Benadryl may be given intramuscularly or intravenously. The intramuscular dosage of Benadryl is 50–100 mg and of Cogentin 1–2 mg. These symptoms are sometimes misdiagnosed as catatonia, tetany, or hysteria.

4) *Tardive Dyskinesia.* This unfortunate result of neuroleptic treatment may persist indefinitely. It is very resistant to treatment, and sometimes appears after a phenothiazine has been discontinued. It generally occurs late in the course of treatment with a phenothiazine.

Tardive dyskinesia consists of buccolingual or buccofaciomandibular movements such as sucking or smacking movements of the lips, rhythmical forward, backward or lateral movements of the tongue, and lateral jaw movements. These may be accompanied by athetoid movements of the ankles, toes and fingers. These movements may interfere with swallowing and the respiratory rate may be disturbed. The symptoms subside during sleep. They are often irreversible and resistant to all known treatment, but preventive measures may be employed such as drug holidays, discontinuing medication unless it is absolutely necessary, or switching to another drug.

Tardive dyskinetic symptoms are sometimes deceptively decreased when the dose of phenothiazine is elevated. These symptoms do not respond to antiparkinsonian agents nor to switching to another phenothiazine. Sadly, the tardive dyskinesia appears to limit the patient's chance of survival outside a hospital, as family and friends find the abnormal movements generally discomforting. Therefore, it is the physician's duty to explain to any patient who requires long-term neuroleptic medication that these symptoms may develop.

Convulsions

These have been reported with the use of both phenothiazine and tricyclic medications. Anticonvulsant medication may have to be increased if the patient is epileptic.

Phototoxicity

Phenothiazines such as chlorpromazine may produce a phototoxicity so that painful sunburn occurs after only a few minutes of exposure. Patients should be warned of this hazard and advised to use lotions and creams containing PABA (e.g. Uval or Presun).

Agranulocytosis

This rare side effect occurs so suddenly and dramatically that serial CBC's do not protect against it. Suggestive symptoms are sore throat and fever. Treatment includes immediate discontinuation of the offending drug, isolation, use of antibiotics, and possible transfusion of blood.

Jaundice

This rare side effect is treated by immediate discontinuation of the offending drug, bedrest, and initiation of a high protein, high carbohydrate diet.

Gastrointestinal Upset

Heartburn and nausea may occur with some phenothiazines. This is minimized by taking the medication with milk or after meals.

Cardiovascular Effects

The tricyclic antidepressants can cause tachycardia and changes in cardiac conduction. The EKG may show prolonged Q-T intervals, depressed S-T segments, and flattened T waves, which may be the forerunner of ventricular arrhythmias. TCA's exhibit a quinidine-like effect manifested on the EKG by signs of first degree atrioventricular block. Extreme caution is therefore required in administering TCA's to patients with bundle branch disease.

The propensity of TCA's to inhibit the activity of antihypertensive drugs such as guanethidine and clonidine may complicate the treatment of older patients who have both hypertension and depression. Combined use of a TCA and a thiazide diuretic may produce profound hypotension.

Concentrations of imipramine routinely obtained in the treatment of severe depression may markedly suppress spontaneously occuring atrial ventricular premature contractions.

CNS Effects

A number of CNS reactions have been reported with TCA's. These include hypomania and mania, insomnia, and a toxic psychosis primarily occuring in older patients. A fine tremor is occasionally seen, and TCA's may induce generalized seizures in patients with a predisposition to epilepsy. Untoward aggressiveness has also been attributed to TCA's.

Other Side Effects

Hepatitis is a rare but definite side effect of tricyclic antidepressant therapy. An allergic skin reaction has been reported with TCA's. Flushing and sweating of upper face and scalp is occasionally encountered, particularly in women.

III

PSYCHIATRIC EMERGENCIES

ADOLESCENTS IN CRISIS

A crisis in adolescence may be indicated by a number of behavioral changes such as drug use, promiscuity, decline in school performance, difficulty with the law, truancy, difficulty with peer relationships, pregnancy, venereal disease, abortion, alcoholism, and running away.

History

1) Children and adolescents are very sensitive barometers of the state of their parents' marriage; therefore, a careful history should be taken as to how the parents get on. Have they discussed divorce or separation? Is one or are both having an extramarital affair?

2) If an adolescent appears psychotic, remember that not all psychoses in adolescence are schizophrenic. Is there a family history of affective disorder?

3) Did the patient have a childhood history of phobias? Bed wetting? Fire setting? Sleep walking? Head banging?

4) Has there been any recent conflict with parents or siblings? Are the parents—one or both—drinking? Has there been any recent loss for the patient or his parents (e.g. job, money, death)?

5) Was there a recent newcomer to the family such as new siblings, returned divorced sibling or grandparent?

6) Has there been a recent change in thinking, mood, or behavior? Has the patient chronically been withdrawn or behaved idiosyncratically?

7) Is there a change in school, the structure of school, or a conflict in the school hierarchy?

Management

1) The clinician should be aware of state regulations regarding the treatment of adolescents. These vary as to need to contact parents, age allowed to sign into hospital, and age at which a patient may have an abortion without parental consent.

2) Is the adolescent psychotic? Does he need hospitalization because of homicidal or suicidal potential? Does he need an alternate living arrangement? Where is he living presently and what is available to him?

3) It may be necessary to call the parents in to evaluate them and the family situation. School counselors and clergyman may be another source of further historical elaboration, as well as possibly providing a viable disposition.

4) Allow the adolescent to ventilate in a supportive psychotherapeutic situation. In some instances, all that may be needed is an evaluation with a couple of follow-up visits, if the problem is not serious and adequate social and family supports are available.

5) Medicate the patient as indicated.

6) If the crisis appears symptomatic of a more deeply rooted disturbance, referral to long-term psychotherapy may be indicated.

7) An effort should always be made to manage an adolescent outside of a hospital or other institutional setting. This serves several purposes. It avoids the labeling of the patient by peers, teachers and others in the community as "crazy". The patient does not feel he is tainted or in some way inferior to those with a "better" capacity to cope and finally, it prevents the parents from seeing the problem in one of their children as solely their adolescent's problem. Families can create atmospheres of tension which make adolescents' adjustment difficult. They (the family) must work together with the therapist to reduce intrafamilial tension so that the adolescent who is so open to feeling external pressures may move more freely along the path of growth and self-actualization.

AFFECTIVE ILLNESS

The essential feature of affective illness is mood disturbance. The prolonged emotional disturbance colors all aspects of the individual's life. The alteration in mood may be episodic (i.e. last for days or months) or chronic (i.e. last for years). It may appear alone or be part of another psychological or medical disorder. The principle disturbances of mood are depression and mania.

DEPRESSION

The essential feature of any disorder with depression is depressive mood coupled with a pervasive loss of interest and pleasure.

History

1) Depression as a mood is not in itself a disease entity. We all become depressed at one time or another and only a fraction of these depressions will cause an individual to seek psychiatric consultation.

2) Of those depressions seen by physicians, there will be a number of underlying etiologies with various degrees of social, biological and psychological causations. Some may be entirely due to physiological changes and history will give clues to causation, such as use of diuretics resulting in hypokalemia or the use of reserpine as antihypertensive therapy. There may be a previous history of hypothyroidism with a recent cessation of thyroid replacement. Other depressions will follow a clearly defined stress or major life event such as death, divorce, or job advancement or loss.

3) Depression may be subdivided into those depressive syndromes of nonpsychotic proportions and those of psychotic proportions. Some of these depressions will have primarily medical bases (e.g. hepatitis) or surgical bases (e.g. carcinoma of the pancreas). Others will be what is traditionally labeled psychogenic and appear in some instances to follow a life event, and may present with a strong family history of recurrent affective disorder, suicide or both.

4) Depressions of nonpsychotic proportions are distinguished from those of psychotic proportions qualitatively by the presence in the latter case of certain symptoms not seen in the former, such as delusions and hallucinations. The depression of a nonpsychotic person may in fact in selected cases be of greater intensity and the risk of suicide higher. In both instances, there may be a family history of affective disorders, the presence of a recent life event which might have been a precipitant, and a past personal history of depressions of nonpsychotic proportions, hypomania or mania. Both types may be recurrent or occur only once in a patient's life.

5) A carefully taken history may provide clues to appropriate treatment both during emergency consultation as well as for long-term therapy. One important part of the evaluation is to determine whether the change in mood can be viewed as posture assumed by the patient in order to obtain some gain, or as having a strong biological basis with neurovegetative signs. In the former instance, clinicians should try to identify the secondary gain. In the latter, they should

document the chronology of sleep loss, appetite loss, weight loss, social dysfunction, etc. Clinicians should obtain some understanding of the degree of guilt and how realistic it is as well as of denied guilt. If guilt is denied by the patient but should be present, what are the reasons for the patient's failure to acknowledge its presence?

6) Try to identify what brought the patient to seek psychiatric help at this time. Some people are somewhat depressed all their lives and the help-seeking behavior is more of an indicant of a life stress than the presence of depression per se. Was there a recent major life event? Was there a recent loss, be it real such as the death of a loved one or divorce, or a psychologic one such as a loss of self-esteem? Depression may also follow a gain such as a job promotion. While this may signal an increase in status and money it also means the addition of personal responsibility, loss of a relatively more dependent relationship, or moving to a position of social status for which the patient has had no preparation from his past personal life experiences.

7) Some patients who present with the symptom picture of anorexia nervosa have underlying affective illness and respond to antidepressant medication (Cantwell, et al. 1977)

Symptoms

1) Depressed mood
2) Hopelessness
3) Sadness
4) Neurasthenia
5) Negative self-image
6) Feeling "blue"
7) Apathy
8) Preoccupation with thoughts of death, suicide and wishing to be dead
9) Decreased sexual drive
10) Loneliness
11) Despondency
12) Self-blame
13) Worry
14) Constipation
15) Fearfulness
16) Discouragement
17) Desire to escape or hide
18) Irritability

19) Anhedonia
20) Sleep disturbance (difficulty falling asleep, awakening during the night, early morning awakening, or hypersomnia)
21) Hyperphagia
22) Feeling worse in the morning
23) Loss of energy
24) Tiredness
25) Slowness of thinking
26) Decreased interest in usual activities
27) Mixed-up thoughts
28) Fatigability
29) Pessimism
30) Guilt
31) Diminished ability to concentrate or think
32) Increasing use of alcohol and other drugs
33) Psychomotor retardation
34) Hypochondriasis
35) Depressive equivalent (e.g. chronic headache, atypical pain)

Signs

1) Weight loss or gain
2) Reduced animation of facies
3) Psychomotor retardation or agitation
4) Decreased salivation

Differential Diagnosis

1) Reactive depression
2) Depressive character style
3) Schizoaffective schizophrenia
4) Chronic schizophrenia
5) Acute schizophrenic episode
6) Manic-depressive illness, depressed type
7) Borderline schizophrenia
8) Unipolar affective illness
9) Hypokalemia
10) Antihypertensive (e.g. reserpine, Aldomet, propranolol) toxicity
11) Steroid psychosis
12) Hypothyroidism
13) Cerebral neoplasia
14) General paresis
15) Cessation of amphetamine or cocaine use

16) Carcinoma of pancreas
17) Hepatitis
18) Post-viral infection syndrome
19) Degenerative diseases of the nervous system (e.g. Huntington's chorea, Alzheimer's disease, Pick's disease)
20) Cirrhosis of the liver
21) Arteriosclerosis
22) Infectious mononucleosis
23) Hyperthyroidism
24) Occult malignancy (Solomon and Solomon, 1978)

Management

Assess the suicidability along with other parameters. In addition to all those factors delineated in the section on suicide assessment (e.g. mental status, living situation, family history, previous attempts) overt hostility is highly correlated with suicide. Depressed patients who are argumentative, hostile, and irritable are at higher risk. If a patient is not psychotically depressed but grossly suicidal and impulsive, he or she will need hospitalization to protect him during the crisis.

2) If a patient is without any of the major neurovegatative signs of depression (indicating that an antidepressant may be appropriate) and without any evidence of a cyclic mood disturbance (suggesting that lithium carbonate may be efficacious), all that may be needed may be supportive psychotherapy around the crisis precipitating the depression, be it loss of self-esteem, job, lover, or something else. The task of the therapist in such instances would be to help identify the loss and empathize with the patient around its significance for him. In an emergency room situation, some encouragement and perhaps direct advice may need to be given. A follow-up appointment should be scheduled to discuss what, if any, further treatment may be necessary as well as the desire on the part of the patient to pursue it.

3) If the patient has sleep loss and is seen in the emergency room, a medication to guarantee sleep should be written. Diphenhydramine (Benadryl) 50 mg–100 mg or flurazepam (Dalmane) 15 mg–30 mg usually will suffice for the night. A more definite plan can be worked out when the patient begins therapy where his clinician can monitor symptom response to medication.

4) As a general rule, antidepressant drugs should not be dispensed in the emergency room. They take several days to weeks to

have any effect and if taken as an overdose can cause serious medical problems. Antidepressants, like lithium carbonate, should be commenced after physical examination and appropriate laboratory examination including an electrocardiogram. Patients on tricyclics, monoamine oxidase inhibitors, and lithium carbonate should always be under a physician's supervision.

5) The crisis intervention model of treatment is often applicable to the management of patients with depressive symptoms of a nonpsychotic nature in the emergency room setting. Patients may be significantly helped in a single interview in the resolution of a conflict and finding more choices available than they previously thought. This may entail social engineering such as referral to an abortion clinic if that is a patient's desire, or in other cases, referral to a variety of other social agencies which may assist the patient in financial, religious, or legal problems. All the patient may want is a homemaker to help out during a particularly rough time, a clergyman, or a lawyer to initiate divorce proceedings.

6) Once the need for hospitalization has been ruled out, the essential goals in the emergency room management of a patient with a depressive syndrome of nonpsychotic proportions is assurance of sleep, the instillation of hope that things will get better, and the sense that benefit can come from the psychiatric care the patient has or plans to seek.

7) Combined psychopharmacotherapy and psychotherapy has been found to be more effective in the treatment of endogenous depressions than either treatment alone and to delay the return of symptoms (Weissman, et al. 1979).

PSYCHOTIC DEPRESSION

History

1) Psychotic depressions are distinguishable from nonpsychotic depressions by the presence of symptoms normally associated with psychosis such as auditory or olfactory hallucinations and delusions. The content of the delusions may be paranoid, nihilistic, somatic, religious or otherwise.

2) While suicidal behavior may be seen with nonpsychotic depressions, it is generally more of a risk in patients who have a history of psychotic thinking which impedes their reality testing. Patients who are delusional, or have hallucinations which are of a command or imperative nature, are alcoholic, physically ill, homosexual or

have a personal history of previous attempts or a family history of suicide, are especially at risk. A middle-aged divorced alcoholic who is manifestly depressed has high self-destructive potential.

3) Patients who are psychotically depressed are particularly adept at hiding certain telltale symptoms such as hallucinations, ideas of reference and paranoid ideation. It sometimes takes exceptional skill to extract a reliable history.

4) Assessment of solid supports is the key in the evaluation of patients who are psychotically depressed. In many instances, the presence or absence of a viable social matrix may be the crucial factor in determining whether a patient should be hospitalized or not.

5) History and clinical evaluation of a depressed patient usually does not quantitatively distinguish a psychotically depressed patient from a nonpsychotic one. The nosological difference is qualitative, based on the presence of delusions and hallucinations or other evidence of psychotic thinking. A nonpsychotic patient may be profoundly depressed with marked weight loss and sleep disturbance but not hallucinate or be delusional. In instances of the latter (i.e. nonpsychotic depression), the patient may be more of a suicide risk than some psychotic patients.

6) Depression sometimes follows initiation of treatment of a psychosis. When this occurs, the depression is referred to as postpsychotic depression. In some instances, the observed depression may be due to a toxic effect of the antipsychotic medication. Treatment of akinesia with appropriate antiparkinson medication has been found to bring about improvement in depression, anxiety, blunted affect, somatic concern, motor retardation and emotional withdrawal in several of these instances. (Van Putten and May, 1978).

Symptoms

The symptoms of a nonpsychotic depression are also found in patients who are psychotically depressed. In addition, however, depressed patients who are psychotic may show:
1) Somatic delusions (e.g. brain being eaten by worms)
2) Hallucinations (particularly auditory and olfactory)
2) Illusions
4) Ideas of reference
5) Paranoid delusions
6) Delusions of guilt and self-reproach (e.g. accusing oneself of sins never committed)

Differential Diagnosis

The differential diagnosis of a psychotic depression is the same as that for a nonpsychotic depression.

Management

1) The mere fact that patients are psychotically depressed does not mean that they must automatically be hospitalized. Suicide risk and strength of social supports coupled with ego strength, previous history and previous response to outpatient antidepressant therapy, psychotherapy and sociotherapy are important factors in determining the need for inpatient treatment.

2) Some patients become psychotically depressed in a matter of days to weeks and this group tends to respond quickly to antidepressants. When there is a history of rapid onset without risk of suicide, the patient should be begun on an antidepressant coupled with psychotherapy and sociotherapy. Response to a particular antidepressant may be somewhat predicted by a patient's previous response to a particular medication or by the response of another member of his biological family.

3) If patients have been using barbiturates for sleep, they should be withdrawn from them. Not only are barbiturates potentially addictive and dangerous for patients to have who are at risk for suicide but, like alcohol, barbiturates also increase the amount of tricyclic antidepressant needed to achieve a clinical response.

4) If there is a history of a cyclic mood disturbance with either recurrent episodes of depression, or of depression and mania or hypomania, lithium carbonate maintenance therapy should be initiated. Like commencement of antidepressants, this is not an emergency room procedure. Before either is begun, the appropriate laboratory tests should be obtained such as an electrocardiogram, BUN, T3, T7, creatinine, urinalysis and serum electrolytes.

5) If the depression is part of manic-depressive illness, the patient may respond better on a monoamine oxidase inhibitor such as phenelzine (Nardil) or tranylcypromine (Parnate) in appropriate doses. A number of foods and medications must not be taken by patients on these drugs (e.g. sherry, beer, pickled herring, amphetamines, tricyclic antidepressants). The patient will require careful medical supervision, particularly when phenelzine is used in daily doses in excess of 75 mg/day or tranylcypromine in doses in excess of 30 mg/day.

6) If there is evidence of paranoid ideation, if the level of anxiety is high, or hallucinations or agitation are evident, an antipsychotic

medication such as phenothiazine should be used in conjunction with the antidepressant. Patients with delusional unipolar disease have been found to respond better to combined antipsychotic-antidepressant pharmacotherapy that antidepressant therapy alone (Nelson and Bowers, 1978). In fact, delusional thinking may be worsened by tricyclic medication even in the absence of a schizophrenia or manic process (Nelson, et al. 1979).

7) Indications for hospitalization include high suicide risk, lack of viable social supports, previous history of a long illness and lack of response to antidepressant medication as an outpatient.

8) Some patients who are psychotically depressed, particularly the elderly, are labile and respond to adjustment of social support. In such instances, social engineering may be more important than psychopharmacotherapy or psychotherapy. This may entail something as simple as calling a depressed widow's children in to make them alert to her depression, and/or contacting her clergyman so that other members of the parish who have some free time may engage her in social activities.

9) A number of pharmacologic agents either increase (e.g. methylphenidate and phenothiazines) or decrease (e.g. barbiturates) plasma levels of tricyclic antidepressants (Garbutt, et al. 1979).

10) Patients who appear nonresponsive to tricyclics may be at inadequate levels and require serum tricyclic level assay. A significant relationship has been documented between plasma levels of imipramine and its metabolite desipramine hydrochloride (desmethylimipramine) and clinical responsiveness. (Glassman, et al. 1977). Older depressed patients treated with amitriptyline or imipramine develop higher steady-state plasma levels of amitriptyline and imipramine and desimpramine associated with a decreased rate of elimination from the plasma. This in part may explain the heightened susceptibility of older patients to side effects of these drugs. Smaller doses, therefore, are often required in the management of older depressed patients (Nies, et al. 1977).

11) The side effects of blurred vision, decreased salivation, constipation, dryness of pulmonary secretions, and urinary retention seen with antidepressant medication are dose related. Bladder and bowel function must be observed and recorded. Preexisting partial bladder obstruction as seen with prostatic hypertrophy increases risk. Laxatives, stool softeners and a high bulk diet reduces the likelihood of impaction. (Dunn and Gross, 1977). Desipramine causes significantly less reduction in salivation and less sedation than amitriptyline (Blackwell, et al. 1978).

12) The potentially most dangerous side effects of the tricyclic

antidepressants is in the cardiovascular area. Congestive heart failure and tachyarrythmias observed in older patients is felt to result from the combined effects of dose-related anticholinergic activity, inhibited norepinephrine uptake, and direct myocardial toxicity. Orthostatic hypotension is common and can lead to decreased cerebral perfusion with syncope and risk of both cerebrovascular accidents and myocardial infarction (Dunn and Gross, 1977).

13) Clouding of consciousness, impaired memory, paranoia, disorientation, increased agitation and hallucinations of all senses may occur in patients on tricyclic antidepressants and are considered part of the toxic encephalopathy due to the central anticholinergic effects (Dunn and Gross, 1977).

14) Imipramine has a mildly respiratory depressant effect at therapeutic levels and, therefore, must be used cautiously in patients with pulmonary disease. Active pulmonary toilet may be required to avoid small airway obstructions and loss of critical ventillary space because of the drying of lung secretion (Dunn and Gross, 1977).

15) Electroshock is indicated for acutely suicidal and severely depressed patients not responsive to antidepressant medication (Greenblatt, 1977). Electroshock is still considered the treatment of choice for severe depression when monoamine oxidase inhibitors and tricyclic medication is not successful. In both psychotic and neurotic depression electroshock has been found superior to monoamine oxidase inhibitors and tricyclic therapy in resistant depressants but has little or no effect when depression is accompanied by a character disorder (Davidson, et al. 1978). Right unilateral electroshock is deemed preferable to bilateral electroshock because the risk of anterograde memory loss is less (Squire, 1977).

16) Severe head, chest and abdominal pain presenting as a depressive equivalent is sometimes responsive to high doses of desipramine (Brown, et al. 1978).

MANIA

The advent of lithium carbonate in the adjunctive treatment of manic and hypomanic episodes and in the maintenance prophylaxis of manic-depressive symptomatology, has made it imperative that evaluating clinicians keep this diagnosis in mind when interviewing acutely disturbed patients. In the past, psychiatrists in this country have had a tendency to underdiagnose manic-depressive illness in contrast to psychiatrists in European countries. A history of phasic disturbance in mood or behavior and a positive family history for affective disorder should make the clinician strongly suspect manic-depressive illness even if the presenting symptomatology is floridly psychotic. Manic-depressive psychoses occur in childhood and adolescence. Clinicians should be very careful not to automatically diagnose schizophrenia in a young person with florid, psychotic symptoms. (Carlson, et al. 1977).

History

1) Manic-depressive illness may present with mania or depression or an admixture of both and will usually follow a course of recurrent episodes of either mood elevation or depression or both.

2) Interepisodic functioning of patients with this disorder is usually quite good and these patients often maintain employment in high standing and are responsible members of a family.

3) Lithium carbonate in most instances can sufficiently regulate the fluctuations in mood so that hospitalization may be avoided at times where, in the past, there would be no alternative.

4) The depressions that occur in patients with this illness are characteristically of the hypersomic, hyperlethargic, and hyperphagic type.

5) Many patients with manic-depressive illness abuse alcohol or sedative medications such as barbiturates or benzodiazepines. Intoxication with these agents or withdrawal from them will frequently cloud the clinical presentation.

6) Morbidity risk for bipolar and unipolar affective illness in first degree relatives has been reported as high as 30%. Probands with a positive family history, in addition, have a greater risk for alcoholism in first degree relatives (Johnson and Leeman, 1977).

7) In one study (Loranger and Levine, 1978), one-third of a population of individuals with bipolar illness were hospitalized before their twenty-fifth birthday with the early twenties as the peak age of onset. Onset after age 60 was rare.

8) Many individuals who suffer a severe episode of mania do not go on to have a second. Others go on to have recurrent episodes of mania or are found on follow-up to have bipolar affective illness with episodes of both pronounced mania and depression.

9) There is no fixed pattern, and a patient, after a series of manic episodes, may become depressed. A mild depression may, in fact, precede a manic episode. These periods may not always be remembered by a patient, but their relatives may remark that the patient seemed "blue" or "down" just before he became manic.

10) Family studies have revealed a strong genetic component, and when attempting to distinguish a schizophrenic episode with a

strong affective component from an episode of mania or depression, a history of either schizophrenia or manic-depressive illness in the family should incline the therapist toward the disorder suggested by family inheritance.

11) It was once felt that precipitants were needed to set off a manic or depressive episode, but vigorously controlled studies have not always been able to unequivocally support this hypothesis.

12) When mania occurs in association with organic dysfunction, such as infection or metabolic disturbances, it is referred to as secondary mania (Krauthamner and Klerman, 1978).

13) Juvenile manic-depressive illness is often associated with an early tendency for a cyclothymic mood with increasing severity and length of mood swings and delirious manic or depressive outbursts during febrile illness. Environment appears to have a minimal influence on the symptoms (White and O'Shanick, 1977).

14) Amitriptyline, chormipramine and other antidepressant pharmacotherapy may be associated with a switch into mania in unipolar depressed patients felt to be due to the psychopharmacologic effect of the drugs on the activity of central dopamine and serotonin systems (Van Scheyen and Van Kammen, 1977).

15) Comparably, maintenance of tricyclic antidepressant therapy can induce rapid cycling between mania and depression in bipolar patients even while on lithium carbonate. In these instances, it is felt that the tricyclics accelerate the natural cyclic course of the illness in all its phases (Wehr and Goodwin, 1979).

Symptoms

1) Flight of ideas
2) Hyperactivity
3) Racing thoughts
4) Euphoria
5) Grandiosity
6) Insomnia
7) Irritability
8) Hypersexuality

The patient may feel that the world is at his command, and he often appears to have boundless energy. His demandingness, egocentricity, and inability to tolerate criticism sometimes serve to alienate those about him. Although uncommon, hallucinations may occur secondary to sleep deprivation. There is frequently a festive air about the patient and an infectiousness about his enthusiasm. Clinicians usually feel that they can empathize more with manic patients than with those who have schizoaffective psychoses. Delusions, when present, are often fascinatingly grandiose in nature. Not infrequently, a premonitory symptom or the predominant presenting symptom is paranoia. Other warning symptoms are: increase in social and motor activity, grandiose ideas and plans, extravagant spending, increased use of the telephone, an increase in letter writing, litigiousness, and increased sexual drive, decreased appetite and decreased need for sleep. Some patients with manic-depressive illness will begin to use or increase their intake of alcohol or sedatives in an attempt to calm themselves or get some sleep. Occasionally there are no ostensible premonitory symptoms and the manic or hypomanic episode occurs precipitously. Catatonia has been reported as part of and as great as 28% of patients presenting with mania and when present, does not of itself forbode poor treatment response (Taylor and Abrams, 1979).

Signs

Physical examination is important to rule out organic states such as drug toxicity or encephalitis which may be accompanied by motor hyperactivity.

Differential Diagnosis

1) Bipolar affective disorder (manic episode)
2) Manic disorder (single episode or recurrent)
3) Schizoaffective schizophrenia
4) Alcoholic excited states
5) Catatonic excitement
6) Delirium secondary to cerebral infection
7) Hyperthyroidism
8) Postencephalitic syndrome (Wiesert and Hendrie, 1977)
9) Drug-induced mania (e.g. steroid-induced, amphetamine-induced, cocaine-induced and phencyclidine-induced mania) (Rosen, 1979)

Management

1) When patients present with mania or hypomania, the first question that should be asked if patients are known to be manic-depressive is: Is the patient on lithium carbonate? If so, has he been taking his medication and what was the most recent serum lithium

level? Patients who had been well-maintained at a serum level of 1.1 mEq/liter may report that their recent level was 0.6 mEq/liter and that they have been faithfully taking their medication. A temporary increment in dosage plus a few weeks of closer surveillance with family support may be all that is necessary. Adjunctive treatment with haloperidol may also be required. Some social engineering may be necessary.

2) If the patient has not been on lithium carbonate, then the first task becomes that of management of the acute episode. If the patient is truly manic, his judgement may be so impaired and he may be so sleep deprived that hospitalization will be necessary for management with the appropriate psychotropic agents and lithium carbonate. If they are only hypomanic, it may be possible to control the derangement of mood with a drug such as haloperidol 2 mg to 20 mg daily and to arrange a work up for the institution of lithium carbonate maintenance. Adequate sleep is essential in bringing about a resolution of the acute symptomatology and sufficient antipsychotic medication should be given during the evening to insure restful sleep. A cooperative and knowledgeable family member can be of great help in establishing a viable treatment plan.

3) A careful history should be taken to determine if there are any clear precipitants such as recent loss, an anniversary, etc. which may be responsible for the change in mood occurring at this time. Often, none can be identified.

4) Family members may need some support and guidance, particularly if it is decided that it may be possible to manage the patient as an outpatient. Firm limit setting and some restriction of activities is usually necessary during the acute phase when judgement may be impaired.

5) Patients in a manic or hypomanic exacerbation are particularly sensitive to external and internal stimuli. Every effort should be made to interview the patient and begin medication in a quiet and controlled setting and to insure that extraneous stimuli (e.g. television, radio, telephone) are kept to a minimum once the patient returns home.

6) Well conducted lithium maintenance treatment has a favorable morbidity suppressive effect in patients suffering from a number of cyclic behavioral disorders in addition to clinical bipolar or recurrent manic illness (Perris, 1978).

SCHIZOAFFECTIVE SCHIZOPHRENIA

1) Patients with schizoaffective schizophrenia frequently present

with symptoms of both a mood disorder and a thought disorder.

2) In some cases, it is extremely difficult to differentiate manic-depressive illness from schizoaffective schizophrenia. The bizare character of a patient's thoughts help to identify a schizophrenic with a mood disturbance.

3) Family history of affective disorders and alcoholism as opposed to a family history of schizophrenia is a further point of distinction.

4) Patients with a primary affective disorder are less frequently found to have the severe interpersonal and employment derangements found with schizophrenics.

5) The premorbid personality is more often cyclothymic.

Symptoms

1) Disturbance of mood—this may be in the direction of elation or depression.

2) Suicidal preoccupation. The risk of self-destructive behavior, in particular, suicide, is often considerable in patients who are schizoaffective. Suicide may be unpredictable, and a clinician should be particularly alert to this possibility.

3) Paranoid ideation. These patients frequently are paranoid in addition to being depressed, with both ideas of reference and paranoid thinking.

4) Auditory hallucinations. Particularly dangerous if imperative or command in nature, auditory hallucinations may be present and may be particularly distressing to some patients.

5) Bizarre behavior and thought. The grossly bizarre character of the patient's thoughts and behavior leave the clinician with the impression that the patient "really must be crazy". This contrasts with the empathy that one feels for a patient with a depressive syndrome. Comparably, there is often an infectious air in a person with a circular mood disorder who presents with mania. The excited schizophrenic seldom is able to draw a clinician into a "party" mood. Paralogical thinking is another characteristic of schizoaffective schizophrenia.

Signs

1) Physical examination, as with other forms of schizophrenia, serves primarily to rule out symptomatic schizophrenia.

2) Because of the bizarre somatic delusions and hypochondriasis sometimes seen with these patients, there is always the danger that a real somatic illness may be misdiagnosed as having a psychological origin.

Differential Diagnosis

The differential diagnosis is the same as for acute schizophrenic episodes. In addition to the sometimes difficult differential involving the affective disorders, it should be remembered that the superimposition of a disease such as hypothyroidism or a drug such as reserpine may make a person with a thought disorder appear schizoaffective or primarily affective. Treatment of the hypothyroidism or discontinuation of the reserpine would result in a accentuation of the thought disorder.

Management

Treatment generally follows the approach outlined under acute schizophrenic episode. However, there are a few points which should be particularly remembered while treating these patients:

1) Patients with schizoaffective schizophrenia, like some depressed borderline patients, may become psychotic when given and antidepressant medication.

2) Since suicide is unpredictable in schizoaffective schizophrenics, the presence of depression or suicidal ideation, especially in a patient who has attempted suicide previously warrants immediate hospitalization.

3) If a viable social matrix exists in the form of family, friends, or a psychotherapist who is following the patient, outpatient management may be possible. In fact, if the patient has been followed in therapy for some time, his therapist may be able to suggest those interventions that have been successful in the past.

4) The combination of neuroleptics and antidepressants tends to work better than either drug alone in schizoaffective patients who are depressed (Prusoff, et al. 1979). Lithium carbonate may be helpful in modulating the mood swings of these patients but alone is inferior to the combination of neuroleptics and antidepressants as indicated (Biederman, et al. 1979).

ALCOHOL USE PROBLEMS

ALCOHOLISM

There is growing evidence that there is a genetic or biological predisposition to the development of alcoholism. Alcoholism alone may run in families, or it may be seen together with a family history of suicide or manic-depressive disease. In some instances, alcohol may, in fact, be used to self-medicate anxiety, an affective disorder, or a schizophrenic disorder.

History

1) It is difficult to obtain an accurate history of alcohol intake, and the amount stated by the patient frequently represents a conservative minimum. Relatives and friends may be needed to obtain a more realistic estimate of a patient's intake. Early in an individual's career as an alcoholic, his drinking is generally limited to evenings and weekends. As tolerance increases, these individuals may begin to experience periods of memory loss without loss of consciousness referred to as "blackouts." When these occur frequently on moderate amounts of alcohol, alcohol addiction is probably near. An individual at this time begins to sneak drinks and at times has episodes of losing control. Eventually the individual imbibes to intoxication each evening and awakens the next morning with a hangover. Drinking alone may begin at this stage. Alibis are developed to excuse the individual from social events and work. He begins to miss more and more work at this stage and eventually quits his job or is fired. Drinking begins to occur in the morning, and it may continue for periods of days. As the individuals's tolerance increases, drinking becomes nearly constant, and he progressively deteriorates. Sudden cessation of alcohol may result in delirium tremens; and with the passing years, the physical stigmata of chronic alcohol abuse appears. In the absence of drinking the individual notices that tremor, an indefinable fear, and difficulty performing simple motor tasks appear. Taking a drink relieves these symptoms.

2) Symptoms of abuse and dependence are generally seen within five years of the onset of regular drinking. A history of heavy drinking in adolescence is associated with a high incidence of alcohol related problems in adult life.

3) Alcoholism is a rising problem among career women and the elderly who live alone. Fixed budgets with rising inflation results in decreased amounts of money to spend on food. Alcohol may be delivered to an apartment gratis, whereas, an infirm older person may have to pay someone to purchase groceries for him.

4) Drinking may be continuously heavy, restricted to weekends with lighter drinking during the week or may be limited to binges (heavy daily drinking that lasts for weeks). All are associated with increased psychological and medical morbidity and mortality.

5) Long-term use of alcohol leads to a number of medical complications which associated with alterations in mood, thought and

behavior may further complicate the picture. These include vitamin deficiency, neurological diseases and liver disease.

6) Suicide risk is greater among alcohol dependent people and may occur in either the sober or intoxicated state.

7) Alcohol dependence is said to occur when there is a compelling desire to use alcohol with an inability to reduce or stop drinking. Continuous or episodic use should have occurred for at least one month and be associated with social complications such as decreased functioning at work, arguments with family members or friends over excessive use of alcohol or legal difficulties such as arrests for driving while intoxicated. The individual should be tolerant (i.e. require increasing amounts of alcohol to achieve the desired effect) or have experienced malaise or "shakes" that are relieved by drinking.

The syndromes associated with excess alcohol rise and their management are discussed in the following sections.

ALCOHOLIC INTOXICATION

History

1) The patient or his friends will usually report that the patient drank to excess. Usually there is a history of several such previous episodes.

2) The clinical effects of alcohol are usually seen when the blood alcohol level is above 150 mg percent. Above 400–500 mg percent, coma usually sets in and levels above 600 mg percent to 800 mg percent are usually fatal. Unconsciousness usually occurs before an individual can drink enough to die.

3) The initial effects of alcohol are usually disinhibitory but as a person continues to drink inhibition predominates.

4) Duration of intoxication varies depending on the amount of alcohol consumed; ranging from several hours to as long as 12 hours after cessation of drinking.

5) Alcohol is metabolized at the rate of one ounce of drinking alcohol per hour. Symptoms of intoxication usually appear more obvious as blood levels of alcohol rise than when they are falling.

6) Alcohol intoxication is associated with a marked increase in automobile accidents, household accidents, industrial accidents, drownings and airplane crashes. Obviously, an unconscious or conscious self-destructive dynamic is often operant when one drinks and has an accident.

7) Medical complications include fractures, subdural hematomas, frostbite and sunburn.

8) More than one-quarter of suicides occur after one has been drinking and more than one-half of murders and victims of homicides are intoxicated at the time of the act. Incest, rape and spouse abuse are also associated frequently with alcohol intoxication.

9) Schuckit and Morrissey (1979) found that misuse of prescription drugs was more prevalent among alcoholics. Misuse is found to be greater among young alcoholics and older middle socioeconomic status female alcoholics. The drugs most frequently abused are depressants, usually obtained from physicians by prescription.

10) When death occurs, it is usually either from respiratory paralysis or aspiration of vomitus.

Symptoms

1) Thinking is slowed down
2. Decreased self-control
3) Distractibility
4) Decreased sensory perception
5) Decreased retention
6) Decreased muscular control
7) Euphoria or depression
8) Memory for recent events is patchy
9) Labile emotion with weeping or laughter
10) Exaggeration of underlying personality traits
11) Rage
12) Self and other directed violence
13) Emergence of repressed and suppressed desires
14) Irritability
15) Loquacity
16) Interference with social or occupational function
17) Failure to meet responsibilities
18) Exaggeration or muting of personality traits
19) Amnesia for events while the individual was intoxicated but fully alert (blackouts)

Signs

1) Smell of alcohol on breath
2) Incoordination
3) Slurred speech

4) Vertigo
5) Vomiting
6) Tremors
7) Unconsciousness
8) Unsteady gait

   Alcoholic coma represents a medical emergency and a medical consultant should be immediately called in to manage the treatment. Alcoholic coma is characterized by:
1) Subnormal body temperature
2) Decreased respiratory rate
3) Stertorous breathing
4) Weakened pulse
5) Contraction or dilation of the pupils
6) Decreased or absent reflexes
7) Pale or cyanotic skin
8) Incontinence or retention of urine

   A blood alcohol level should be obtained and monitored.

Differential Diagnosis

1) Alcoholic intoxication
2) Hypomania
3) Hypoglycemia
4) Subdural hematoma
5) Gastrointestinal bleeding with severe blood loss
6) Hepatic failure
7) Other cerebral trauma
8) Epilepsy
9) Toxic psychosis of other etiologies, such as that seen with barbiturates, amphetamines or cocaine
10) Carbon monoxide poisoning
11) Hypothyroidism
12) Meningitis
13) Diabetic acidosis and other metabolic disorders
14) Postictal and postconcussion states

Management

   1) Alcoholic intoxication may be accompanied by a number of other medical conditions which may contribute to the clinical picture or be primarily responsible for it; these should be treated. Physical

examination and history may reveal bleeding from one of the body orifices, cardiac arrythmia, pneumonitis, or one of the alcoholic syndromes, such as Korsakov's psychoses or Wernicke's encephalopathy.

2) If necessary, 50–100 mg of chlordiazepoxide (Librium) or 10–20 mg of diazepam (Valium) may be given orally or intramuscularly to sedate the patient.

3) The patient should be placed in a room with a minimal distraction where he may be calmed and prevented from bringing harm to himself or others. Soft physical restraints may be needed.

4) Some patients, both occasional drinkers and chronic alcoholics, when acutely intoxicated, may respond to coffee and support and become sober.

5) The best disposition after an acute episode of alcohol intoxication is usually home with supportive relatives or friends, who will watch the patient until he has entirely recovered. If this is impossible or for medical reasons he needs to be observed further, he should spend the night in a bed in the emergency room, or be hospitalized. Other dispositions would include religious or otherwise privately supported hostels for people without a place to go for the night, the local YMCA or YWCA, the Salvation Army, and some inexpensive hotels. If the patient has physically harmed a person or property and has no acute medical problems, jail is a real alternative that must be considered, especially if the patient is a repeated threat to the well-being of the community.

ALCOHOL AMNESTIC SYNDROME (KORSAKOFF'S SYNDROME)

History

1) The alcohol amnestic syndrome may develop insidiously, or it may follow an episode of delirium tremens.

2) It is most frequently seen with alcoholic polyneuritis, but may also occur in other disorders such as the polyneuritis of pregnancy.

3) The age range of presentation is the same as that for alcoholic polyneuritis. Since prolonged use of alcohol is necessary to develop the syndrome, it is seldom seen before age 35.

4) Men are affected with the disorder more commonly than women.

5) Generally, the patients have a history of several years of alcohol dependence with poor dietary intake.

6) The amount of peripheral nerve involvement may be minimal to quite severe, with the occurrence of convulsions not uncommon.

7) The core feature is short-term memory disturbance due to prolonged heavy use of alcohol. Immediate memory is not disturbed. The individual has a normal digit span but cannot remember the name of three objects after 20 minutes.

8) The irreversible memory defect usually follows an episode of Wernicke's encephalopathy and may be avoided if Wernicke's is treated in the early stages with large doses of thiamine before the short-term memory defect becomes permanent.

9) Impairment is often severe requiring custodial care.

10) Both Wernicke's encephalopathy and Korsakoff's syndrome are believed due to thiamine deficiency. Prolonged heavy alcohol use leads to a malabsorption syndrome even if dietary intake is sufficient. Malnutrition, however, alone predisposes the individual to this disorder.

11) This condition is rare, and has become even rarer because of the prophylactic use of parenteral thiamine whenever individuals with a history of alcohol dependence are seen in the health care system.

Symptoms

1) Short-term but not immediate memory disturbance.
2) Confabulation.
3) The patient's sensorium should be clear.

Management

1) The patient should be given thiamine 50 mg p.o. TID or QID as well as high potency vitamin B complex preparation.

2) The patient should be withdrawn from alcohol.

3) If a polyneuritis is present, the affected muscles should be supported and massage exercises prescribed as tenderness subsides.

ALCOHOL IDIOSYNCRATIC INTOXICATION (PATHOLOGICAL INTOXICATION)

History

1) Alcohol idiosyncratic intoxication is a term used for an uncommon condition seen in a group of patients who, after drinking

only a small amount of alcohol, act as if they had consumed much more.

2) The onset is usually rather sudden and quite dramatic with subsequent amnesia for the behavioral change.

3) Alcohol idiosyncratic intoxication may last a few minutes or as long as 24 hours or more.

4) Some authors feel it occurs in people with an epileptic predisposition and that alcohol serves as the trigger mechanism.

5) The usual behavioral change consists of aggressive or assaultive behavior that is atypical of the person when not drinking. During the episode the individual appears out of contact with others.

6) The usual age of onset is early in life.

7) A small number of individuals with this disorder are found to have temporal lobe spiked on the electroencephalogam after receiving just small amounts of alcohol.

8) The usual brain injuries associated with this disorder are encephalitis and trauma and the loss of tolerance may be permanent or temporary.

9) Use of tranquilizers and sedative hypnotics that have additive effects with alcohol, fatigue and debilitating medical illness are felt to contribute to a lower tolerance to alcohol with a tendency to respond inappropriately to small amounts.

Symptoms

1) Uninhibited behavior
2) Illusions
3) Assaultive, irrational, combative and destructive behavior
4) Transitory delusions
5) Hallucinations
6) Increased activity
7) Impulsivity
8) Anxiety
9) Rage
10) Depression
11) Suicidal behavior

Signs

1) Impairment of consciousness
2) Confusion
3) Disorientation

Serum alcohol level helps to corroborate the diagnosis; however, the clinician should always be aware of superimposed conditions, such as temporal lobe epilepsy, that may be set off by drinking and be present in addition to acute alcohol intoxication.

Management

1) If untreated, these episodes usually terminate in a long sleep, with amnesia for the episode on wakening.

2) If violent or aggressive, the patient should be protected from injuring himself or others. This may require sedation and physical restraints.

3) Sedation can be provided by intramuscular or oral Librium or Haldol.

ALCOHOLIC JEALOUSY

History

1) Patients who present with alcoholic jealousy usually have a long history of alcoholic use. In some instances, this may be denied by the patient, and the clinician will need to get corroboration of his diagnosis from the patient's friends or relatives.

2) The premorbid history of these patients often revels the absence of any mature heterosexual relationships.

3) The paranoid delusions have been interpreted by some psychiatrists as a defense against unconscious homosexual desires.

4) Since delusions of jealousy can occur in both alcoholic and nonalcoholic states, some authors feel that alcohol may just serve as a precipitant and that alcohol jealousy does not exist as a separate entity but rather is a paranoid state associated with alcohol use.

Symptoms

1) Anger
2) Suspicion
3) Resentment
4) Ideas of reference
5) Delusions of jealousy
6) Distrust
7) Assaultive behavior with homicidal risk
8) Self-destructive behavior with suicidal risk
9) Accusations that wife is having illicit sexual affairs with friends, strangers, children, or relatives

10) Accusations that wife has insatiable sexual desires
11) Claiming to find seminal stains of other men about the house
12) Suspecting wife of changing underwear in preparation for an affair
13) Accusing wife of being colder than usual

Differential Diagnosis

1) Alcoholic jealousy
2) Paranoid schizophrenia
3) Paranoid states
4) Paranoid personality
5) Other forms of schizophrenia with paranoid symptoms
6) Depressive syndrome of psychotic proportions with paranoid symptoms
7) Amphetamine psychosis
8) Cocaine psychosis
9) Organic brain syndromes with paranoia

Management

1) The prognosis of these patients is guarded.

2) The symptoms of alcoholic jealousy are usually controllable in a hospital with appropriate psychopharmacotherapy. Unfortunately, paranoid patients are especially prone to discontinuation of medication because of their delusions of persecution. Soon after a patient stops medication, the symptoms usually return.

ALCOHOL WITHDRAWAL DELIRIUM (DELIRIUM TREMENS)

History

1) The probability that alcohol withdrawal will occur relates to the amount and duration of drinking before withdrawal. The onset of symptoms usually occurs 2 to 10 days after cessation or reduction of heavy alcohol ingestion.

2) The duration of the delirium, once it begins, may be several days or only a period of hours. The mortality rate due to such complications as hyperthermia or circulatory collapse is quoted in various textbooks as between 4 to 20%.

3) The clinical presentation and course may be complicated by a number of medical problems, including infections such as pneumonitis, profound dehydration with electrolyte imbalance,

hyperthermia, vascular collapse, malnutrition, meningitis, cerebral laceration, anemia, gastritis with hematemesis, and cirrhosis.

4) Because of their great proneness to head trauma, due to falls, muggings, and seizures, the possibility of an epidural or subdural hematoma complicating the picture should always be entertained, and, when suspected, investigated by careful neurological examination, skull films, lumbar puncture and echoencephalogram.

5) Concurrent physical illness predisposes the individual to alcohol withdrawal delirium.

6) Only about 5% of patients being treated for alcohol withdrawal develop delirium.

Symptoms

Symptoms seen early in the course of delirium tremens include:
1) Nightmares
2) Anxiety attacks while attempting to fall asleep and insomnia
3) Panic
4) Illusions
5) Vivid hallucinations

As the illness progresses, there may be seen:

1) Agitation
2) Delirium
3) Increasing psychosis
4) Disorientation
5) Hallucinations, either of rapidly moving small animals such as snakes or Lilliputian hallucinations. (Auditory hallucinations are rare).
6) Suggestibility
7) Restlessness
8) Dizziness

Signs

1) Coarse persistent hand tremor
2) Diaphoresis
3) Tachycardia
4) Dilated pupils
5) Increase in temperature
6) Seizures
7) Restlessness

8) Hyperactivity
9) Ataxia
10) Clouding of consciousness
11) Disturbance of speech with slurring, thickness, and word distortion
12) Elevated blood pressure
13) Coated tongue
14) Dry lips
15) Stigmata of chronic alcohol abuse such as hepatomegaly and peripheral neuropathies

Differential Diagnosis

The differential diagnosis includes all other causes of delirium tremens such as fever and central nervous system depressant withdrawal (e.g. barbiturate or meprobamate withdrawal).

Management

1) The patient should be placed in a well-lit room. As procedures are performed (i.g. blood drawing), they should be explained simply. If available, a family member should be present to help calm the patient. The patient's location on a service should be where his delirium will cause minimal disturbance to other people.

2) Mechanical restraints may be needed, in addition to medication, to help calm the patient.

3) Of extreme importance in the treatment is maintenance of fluid and electrolyte intake. As much as 6000 ml of fluid may be needed per day of which 1500 should be normal saline, to counter the extreme loss through profuse perspiration and agitation. Serum electrolytes and BUN should be monitored to guide the treatment.

4) Sedation should be liberally used to reduce agitation, to prevent exhaustion, to make the patient more comfortable, and to produce rest and sleep. Many different methods have been tried, and currently, diazepam and chlordiazepoxide are quite popular. The dose of chlordiazepoxide would be 50–100 mg every 4 hours, up to 300–400 mg/day or more in cases of severe agitation. Paraldehyde is another frequently used agent with up to 10 ml given orally, or in an oil retention enema every 2 hours. Chloral hydrate may be given in doses of up to 1 g every four hours. The physician should be aware of the danger of oversedation, as such may mask symptoms of an epidural or subdural hematoma. This can be minimized if the physician reassesses the situation before each new dose of medication is

ordered and then writes a new order at that time. The intramuscular route for paraldehyde should be avoided to prevent sterile abscesses and damage to nerves.

5) The patient's temperature should be monitored. The physician should always be alert to the possibility of a superimposed infection, such as pneumonitis. In the absence of any infection, sponge baths, cooling blankets and aspirin can be used to keep the temperature down. Obviously, if there is an infection superimposed, appropriate antibiotics should be employed.

6) Chronic alcoholic patients are usually vitamin deficient. Therefore 50–200 mg of thiamine should be given intramuscularly, followed by 100 mg of thiamine b.i.d.

7) Ideally, pulse, blood pressure and temperatures should be recorded at half-hour intervals at the height of the illness, in order to minimize the occurrence of the lethal complications and alcohol withdrawal delirium, circulatory collapse and hyperthermia. If these occur, they must be immediately treated with the appropriate measures. Whole blood transfusions, fluids and vasopressors may be used to combat shock and ice packs and a cooling mattress to treat hyperthermia.

8) Prophylactic anticonvulsant medication is usually not needed for simple alcohol withdrawal. If convulsions or status epilepticus occur, these must be appropriately treated.

9) If hypoglycemia accompanies the alcohol withdrawal, glucose must be administered.

10) Other medical problems, such as cirrhosis and gastritis, should be attended to. Skull and chest films and a lumber puncture should be routinely performed.

All the drugs used in the management of alcohol withdrawal delirium have their limitations. Some authors feel the benzodiazepines (chlordiazepoxide and diazepam) are not effective in severe cases. Paraldehyde is addicting, and sudden death may follow its use. Hepatotoxicity has been reported with phenothiazines, and they lower the seizure threshold. Barbiturates are addicting and can produce paradoxical excitement.

Once it has established that a patient is in alcohol withdrawal delirium, he/she is to be considered a medical emergency and must be hospitalized.

ALCOHOL HALLUCINOSIS

1) Alcoholic hallucinosis is a syndrome in which hallucinosis

persists after an individual has recovered from the symptoms of alcohol withdrawal and is no longer drinking.

2) Some authors feel that it occurs in individuals with an underlying predisposition to schizophrenia.

3) The onset is 1 to 2 weeks or more after cessation of drinking.

4) Because many patients deny a history of alcohol abuse, especially upper middle class housewives and executives, friends, or relatives of the patient may be needed to confirm the history.

5) The patient usually is a male between the ages of 30 and 50 although the disorder may occur at any age.

6) The duration of drinking prior to the abstinence in which the hallucinosis occurs must have been sufficient so that the individual has become dependent.

7) The course varies from several weeks to years without remission.

8) The incidence of this condition is so small that the disorder is considered very rare.

Symptoms

1) Hallucinations, usually auditory, in a clear sensorium with orientation to time, place and person intact. The voices heard by men often accuse them of, or threaten them with, homosexual attack. Women are frequently accused of promiscuity. The auditory hallucinations may at times be of a command or imperative type.

2) Olfactory hallucinations

3) Delusions of persecution

4) Violent self-destructive (e.g. suicide) or other destructive (e.g. assaultive) behavior

5) Ideas of reference

6) Rarely visual hallucinations

7) Apprehension

8) Litigious behavior

9) Panic

10) Fear

11) Distractibility

12) Anger

Differential Diagnosis

1) Alcoholic hallucinosis
2) Hyperthyroidism
3) Acute toxic reactions, (e.g. amphetamine and cocaine psychoses)

4) Schizophrenia
5) Affective illness with auditory hallucinations

Management

1) The patient should be hospitalized to protect him from harming himself or others.
2) Sedation may be necessary. In some instances, 50–100 mg of intramuscular chlordiazepoxide (Librium) will suffice. In other instances, an antipsychotic agent such as perphenazine 5–10 mg IM or haloperidol 5–10 mg IM may be needed.
3) If violent and destructive, physical restraints may be needed to protect the patient and staff.
4) The patient should be medicated sufficiently so that he can sleep at night.
5) Careful attention should be given to assure that the patient's diet and vitamin intake is adequate.
6) Every attempt should be made to keep the patient oriented to reality. Procedures should be explained as they are performed, and the room should be well lit. At night, this would take the form of a night lamp.

WERNICKE'S ENCEPHALOPATHY

History

1) This syndrome presents with the onset of paralysis of the extraocular muscles, disturbances of consciousness, and ataxia.
2) While it is usually associated with chronic heavy alcoholic use, it can also be seen with nutritional deficiencies, intestinal carcinomas with vomiting, pernicious anemia, and with pernicious vomiting of pregnancy.
3) It is usually seen in young or middle-aged males.
4) It is due to a deficiency of thiamine.

Symptoms

1) Loss of appetite
2) Nausea
3) Vomiting
4) Delirium
5) Excitement
6) Insomnia

7) Giddiness
8) Confabulation
9) Apathy
10) Apprehension
11) Diplopia
12) Photophobia
13) Tremor
14) Memory loss for recent events
15) Intellectual deterioration
16) Mild confusion
17) Disorientation
18) Hallucinations

A classical alcohol amnesic syndrome may be seen with this syndrome.

Signs

1) Ophthalmoplegia
2) Clouding of consciousness
3) Nystagmus
4) Ataxia
5) External rectus palsy
6) Loss of visual acuity
7) Coma
8) Ptosis
9) Spasticity
10) Pupillary abnormalities
11) Polyneuritis
12) Papilledema
13) Seizures
14) Hypotension
15) Other signs of chronic heavy alcohol use, such as evidence of liver damage and anemia

Management

1) The cerebral changes seen with thiamine deficiency can rapidly become irreversible. Therefore, 100 mg of thiamine should be given intramuscularly in the emergency room to all alcoholic patients.

2) The patient should be placed at bed rest and withdrawn from alcohol.

3) He should receive a high caloric diet with vitamin supplements.

4) A rehabilitation program should be started to maximize remaining potential.

CHRONIC ALCOHOLISM

History

1) The long-term side effects of chronic alcohol use include Korsakov's psychosis, Wernicke's encephalopathy, delirium tremens, alcoholic hallucinosis, alcoholic jealousy, cerebellar degeneration, dementia, and peripheral neuropathies.

2) It is extremely difficult to obtain an accurate history of the exact amount of alcohol used, but it is generally quite high and the diet is usually poor.

3) Alcoholics are prone to develop several medical and surgical problems. Falls while intoxicated or head injuries incurred in muggings or during a seizure may result in a subdural hematoma. Alcoholics are prone to infections such as pneumonia and tuberculosis. Pancreatitis is not uncommon, and gastrointestinal bleeding is a frequent problem.

4) When evaluating a patient who chronically uses alcohol, the clinician should carefully look for evidence of another disorder which the patient may be self-medicating, such as schizophrenia, an affective disorder, or recurrent anxiety attacks.

5) Examination of a patient's relationship to his family may reveal much stress with markedly ambivalent feelings towards several family members. In other cases, the patient may not be the only family member who is drinking.

6) Drinking may cause a patient to neglect chronic health problems, as well as contribute to the development of new ones. Family members should be utilized in helping assure that the patient receives a thorough medical evaluation, including a proper physical examination, blood chemistries, and a chest x-ray.

7) Even if a patient's family history is riddled with alcoholism, suggesting a strong genetic predisposition, a careful longitudinal history should be obtained to see what factors increase or decrease the intake of alcohol.

Symptoms and Signs

The symptoms and signs of chronic alcohol abuse are those of the various psychiatric and medical syndromes which occur in these patients.

Differential Diagnosis

Alcohol may be taken to self-medicate a number of conditions. These should be sought out and treated to improve the prognosis. Common disorders of which alcoholism may be a symptom include.

1) Schizophrenia
2) Borderline schizophrenia
3) Manic-depressive syndromes (both manic and depressed phases)
4) Other depressive syndromes of various etiologies
5) Arteriosclerosis
6) General paresis
7) Other causes of dementia

Management

1) Any acute medical problem, including delirium tremens, must be treated first.

2) The patient should be withdrawn from alcohol, using the usual precautions.

3) An adequate diet with vitamin supplements, including thiamine 50 mg t.i.d. or q.i.d. should be provided.

4) The patient should receive the best medical attention that can be provided. Good personal hygiene should be encouraged, and special attention paid to both minor medical problems (e.g skin infections, bunions) and major problems. Regular physical examinations are a necessary part of good medical follow-up of an alcoholic.

5) Sleep should be assured. Appropriate medications such as flurazepam (Dalmane) 15–30 mg should be prescribed.

6) If alcohol has been used to medicate an underlying psychiatric disorder such as schizophrenia, recurrent anxiety attacks or an affective disorder, an antipsychotic agent, an antianxiety agent, lithium carbonate or an antidepressant will be needed for long-term management.

7) Place the patient in an appropriate psychotherapeutic or sociotherapeutic modality. In many instances, this may be Alcoholics Anonymous (AA) alone, with family members referred to the appropriate groups for spouses and teenage children. In other instances, a different form of treatment may be indicated, alone or together with AA. Some alcoholics may need educative and supportive individual psychotherapy. For others, a group may be appro-

priate, especially for those who have difficulty asserting themselves, for those who can't get on with peers, and for those who suffer from an inability to relate to authority figures.

8) Employment is important. Every effort should be made to encourage a patient to secure and maintain a job within his realistic potential and one which contributes to a sense of self-esteem.

9) Some patients may be candidates for disulfiram (Antabuse) therapy or aversion therapy. The psychiatrist should provide these treatments if he is skilled at them, or refer appropriate patients to those who have had experience with them.

10) Relatives, friends, clergymen and other close associates of the patient, and organizations which are available in the community are potentially part of a complete treatment program. This may demand that a psychiatrist serve, with the patient's permission, as a consultant to clergy, social workers, or general practitioners about the problems of treating alcoholics in general and the patient in particular.

11) When there appears to be no viable social matrix to support the patient it may be necessary to refer him to a halfway house, therapeutic farm, or other live-in program to help him get off and stay off alcohol during the critical early period.

AMPHETAMINE AND OTHER SYMPATHOMIMETIC INTOXICATION, DELIRIUM AND DELUSIONAL STATES

The oral or intravenous use of amphetamine and similar acting sympathomimetic substances may lead to states of intoxication, delirium and delusion. Cessation of use may lead to profound depression in which risk of suicide is considerable. If an individual presents with the physiological, psychological, and behavioral effects of the use of such substances and evidence of delirium or delusion, the syndrome is referred to as *intoxication*. If signs of delirium such as fragmented thinking, dysattention, confusion and difficulty in goal-directed behavior develop within 24 hours of taking the substance, the clinical picture is referred to as *delirium*.

Paranoia and other evidence of delusional thinking may follow prolonged use of moderate to high doses of sympathomimetic substance; this state is referred to as amphetamine or other sympathomimetic *delusional syndrome*.

History

1) Patients who develop sympathomimetic intoxication,

delirium or delusional syndromes have a history of recent use of sympathomimetic substances. These include amphetamine, dextroamphetamine, and methamphetamine and substances differing from substituted phenylethylamine that have amphetamine-like actions such as methylphenidate and a variety of diet pills.

2) Popular names for sympathometic substances taken for recreational use are "bennies," "dexies," "speed," and "crank."

3) Sympathomimetic substances may be taken orally or intravenously.

4) Signs of intoxication usually begin within one hour of use. Delirium, when it occurs, develops within 24 hours of intake. Prolonged intake of moderate or high dose sympathometic substances are required for development of a delusional state. If the substance is taken intravenously, symptoms may begin nearly immediately. Delusions should not develop after a single dose unless preceded by prolonged use. If delusions are seen after a single dose the clinician should think of the possibility of the presence of other underlying psychopathology such as paranoid schizophrenia.

5) Symptoms of psychoses are common in individuals who have taken more than 90–100 mg of amphetamines a day. An hallucinating panic state may occur after a single dose in a predisposed person.

6) The degree of paranoia seen may vacillate in a chronic user dependent on the amount taken on any given day.

7) It is common for individuals in the drug culture as well as for professional people with access to a number of euphorogenic and sedating substances to mix drugs. This practice confuses the clinical picture and increases the risk of unattended withdrawal as withdrawal from a number of "downers" can lead to delirium tremens with its risk of mortality. The use of heroin in combination with cocaine or amphetamines is known as a "speedball." Heroin may be used alone to bring an individual down from an amphetamine binge.

8) Amphetamine, cocaine and other sympathomimetic delusional states are sometimes virtually indistinguishable from paranoid schizophrenia. In addition, sympathomimetic substance delusional states may complicate the course of schizophrenia or other major psychiatric disorders and contaminate the clinical presentation.

The characteristics of cocaine intoxication are identical to that of amphetamine and other sympathomimetic psychoses with the exception that when the symptoms are due to the latter, they may persist long beyond the time of substance use. Delusions and hallucinations seen with cocaine use are always transient unless there is some underlying psychopathology.

9) The symptoms of a sympathomimetic delusional state develop rapidly with paranoia the predominant feature.

10) The clinical picture of sympathomimetic intoxication, delirium or delusional state always represents an interaction of a patient's premorbid psychological and physical condition, the dose and duration of sympathomimetic intake, the environment in which it is taken, and the number and the quantity of other drugs taken. One individual may look like an emotionally labile hypomanic with paranoid features; another may look like a paranoid schizophrenic.

11) The symptoms of intoxication and delirium when present usually are over within 6 hours of cessation of drug intake whereas the delusional symptoms may last for as long as a year.

12) The usual course of a sympathomimetic delusional syndrome is a week or less. Delusional syndromes are seen more frequently than delirium.

13) Patients who are toxic or delusional from sympathomimetic substances usually remain oriented.

14) Corroboration of the diagnosis of amphetamine intoxication can be made by urinary or serum tests for amphetamines.

Symptoms of Sympathomimetic Intoxication

1) Euphoria
2) Hyperarousal
3) Grandiosity
4) Irritability
5) Loquacity sometimes to the extent of pressured speech
6) Emotional lability
7) Hypervigilance
8) Anorexia
9) Aggressiveness and hostility
10) Anxiety
11) Panic
12) Resistance to fatigue
13) Restless wakefulness (Insomnia)
14) Changes in body image
15) Chronic muscular tension
16) Severe abdominal pain sometimes mimicking an acute abdomen
17) Impaired judgment
18) Interference with social and occupational functioning
19) Chest pain

Signs of Sympathomimetic Intoxication

1) Dilated but reactive pupils
2) Tachycardia
3) Elevated temperature
4) Elevated blood pressure (Both tachycardia and elevated blood pressure may be absent in chronic users.)
5) Dry mouth
6) Perspiration or chills
7) Nausea and vomiting
8) Psychomotor excitement
9) Tremulousness
10) Hyperactive reflexes
11) Furtive glancing about the room
12) Malnutrition (especially apparent after prolonged intravenous use of large doses)
13) Repetitious compulsive behavior
14) Biting stereotypies may cause ulcers on the tongue and lips
15) Teeth may be worn from bruxism
16) Needle marks on the arm if the drug is taken intravenously
17) Cardiac arrhythmias and subdural and subarachnoid hemorrhage are occasional complications of the elevated blood pressure and tachycardia
18) Skin flushing
19) Cutaneous abscesses and excoriation

Symptoms of Sympathomimetic Delusional Syndromes

In additon to the symptoms and physical signs seen with sympathomimetic intoxication, individuals with an amphetamine or similar acting sympathomimetic delusional syndrome have:
1) Thought disorder
2) Ideas of reference
3) Auditory hallucinations frequently of voices commenting, criticizing and accusing the patient of misconduct. (They may threaten the patient with violence or have an imperative or command quality necessitating hospitalization.)
4) Paranoid ideation with delusions of persecution with a clear sensorium
5) Visual hallucinations sometimes with distortion of faces and disturbances of body image
6) Formication (hallucination of bugs or vermin crawling under

the skin sometimes leading the individual to scratch himself with resultant excoriations of the skin)

Sympathomimetic Delirium

In addition to the other symptoms and physical signs seen with sympathomimetic intoxication or delusional syndrome, an individual with an amphetamine or similar acting sympathomimetic delirium, shows the usual symptoms of delirium such as dysattention, fragmented thinking and fluctuating levels of consciousness. Affect is labile and both olfactory and tactile hallucinations may be seen. Individuals with a sympathomimetic delirium may become so violent that restraints may be required.

Differential Diagnosis

1) Amphetamine psychosis
2) Cocaine psychosis
3) Other sympathomimetic psychoses
4) Paranoid schizophrenia
5) Alcoholic hallucinosis
6) Acute schizophrenia episode
7) Hypomania
8) Catatonic schizophrenia (excited phase)
9) Obsessive compulsive neurosis

Management

1) Symptoms of psychoses usually subside 2 to 3 days after cessation of amphetamines. Visual hallucinations usually remain 24 to 48 hours while delusions when present last for a week to 10 days. Rarely delusions in an attenuated form may remain as long as a year.

2) Within 24 hours of the final dose, a patient may be found to be spending increasing amounts of time in sleep. In some instances, this may be as much as 18 to 20 hours for up to 3 days with considerable dreaming. "Crashing"—depression sometimes accompanied by suicidal ideation—may occur and increase over the weeks following discontinuation of use. Without treatment this depression may last a considerable period of time. Characteristically such individuals show a greater amount of fatigue, apathy and flattening of affect than in the usual depression.

3) Clinicians evaluating individuals with sympathomimetic

intoxication should always be aware of the patients' potential to act out violently and be prepared to protect themselves. It is recommended that these patients be treated on an inpatient service where appropriate sedation and restraints can be provided if necessary.

4) Patients should be placed in a quiet room, reassured and kept as calm as possible during the acute stages of intoxication. Two-five mg of haloperidol intramuscularly followed by 2–4 mg t.i.d. is usually sufficient to handle even delusional patients. Frequently no medication is required after a day.

5) Amphetamine intake is discontinued immediately; gradual reduction of dosage is not necessary.

6) Phenothiazines and the other antipsychotic drugs including haloperidol should not be given if it is known the patient has ingested significant amounts of antipsychotic drugs with strong anticholinergic properties in addition to the sympathomimetics. Diazepam 10 mg–20 mg p.o. or I.M. or another similarly acting benzodiazepine is a satisfactory alternative.

7) In rare instances life support measures may be necessary. In such instances transfer to a medical ward may be necessary where ice packs, gastric lavage and other needed measures may be instituted.

AMPHETAMINE AND SIMILAR ACTING SYMPATHOMIMETIC WITHDRAWAL

The symptoms and physical signs of withdrawal from amphetamines or similar acting substances generally commence within 3 days of cessation of use and peak within 2 to 4 days. Depression and irritability may persist, however, for months and, in fact, necessitate the use of antidepressants, medication or electroshock because of the risk of suicide.

Symptoms and Physical Signs of Sympathomimetic Withdrawal

1) Depression
2) Increased dreaming
3) Fatigue
4) Disturbed sleep (with increased REM activity on the electroencephalogram)
5) Agitation
6) Suicidal ideation
7) Irritability
8) Apathy

Management

1) The most critical aspect of managing patients who are withdrawing from amphetamines is a heightened sensitivity to their capacity to attempt to take their lives. Suicide precautions and in some instances of profound depression hospitalization with appropriate safeguards may be required.

2) Individuals who present intoxicated on amphetamine or another sympathomimetic substance should be given haloperidal 2–5 mg p.o. t.i.d. or q.i.d., or an equivalent dosage of a similar acting phenothiazine. A benzodiazepine (e.g. diazepam or chlordiazepoxide) should be used if the individual is also using drugs with strong anticholinergic side effects.

3) Dosage of the haloperidol or similar acting drug is gradually reduced over days or weeks as the patient's symptoms subside.

4) Intake of amphetamine or similar acting sympathomimetic should be discontinued immediately.

5) The depression that frequently follows the pronounced fatigue and apathy after cessation of sympathomimetic use is usually countered by administration of tricyclic antidepressants for a month or two. If suicidal risk is significant, the use of electroshock should be entertained.

6) Individuals should be allowed to sleep during the few days of hypersomnia that follows cessation of drug use.

7) Individuals should be evaluated for benefit from brief psychotherapy to explore reasons for sympathomimetic abuse if present. Patients should be alerted to the fact that the normal after effect of sympathomimetic use is a period of decreased initiative, apathy, and depression, and that these symptoms tend to pass in 2 to 4 months. These symptoms are not necessarily an indicant of intrapsychic turmoil but rather the usual sequence.

8) Remember that even individuals who have been prescribed sympathomimetic substances for narcolepsy, minimal brain damage and asthma may also develop intoxication, delusions and delirium and go through withdrawal symptoms upon cessation of use.

9) Attending physicians should not be reduced into providing a new source of amphetamine or another sympathomimetic substance at times of stress. Individuals who have abused sympathomimetic substances should continuously be evaluated for the need of long-term antidepressant therapy or psychotherapy and if indicated this treatment should commence.

10) It may be necessary with sociopathic patients to periodically obtain serum or urine samples for amphetamine content to maintain a patient free of drugs.

11) Group therapy with "speed freaks" may be of some value.

ANGEL'S TRUMPET INTOXICATION AND DELIRIUM

Angel's Trumpet (Datura sauvealens) is a poisonous plant that grows wildly in several Southeastern and Gulf states. It is readily available for individuals interested in experimenting with hallucinogens, as a legal source of a drug with atropine-like qualities. The flowers of Angel's Trumpet are either eaten directly or brewed in a tea to produce a central nervous sytem anticholinergic syndrome. Hyoscine (scopolamine) is the principal and most toxic alkaloid found. Lesser amounts of atropine and hyoscyamine are also present.

Individuals who have taken the drug because of its hallucinogenic properties or have inadvertently ingested the substance may present intoxicated or delirious to psychiatric clinicians. The following facts regarding the diagnosis and management of Angel's Trumpet intoxication and delirium should be kept in mind:

1) The clinical symptoms and physical signs of intoxication are comparable to those seen with intoxication from other strongly anticholinergic substances. Individuals present agitated, confused and hallucinating. Pulse pressure is widened and the skin is hot, dry and flushed. The sensorium is usually clouded and they have a persistent memory disturbance. Severe intoxication may result in convulsions, flaccid paralysis and death. The elevation in body temperature is the combined result of inhibition of sweating and a hyperthermic response. Scopolamine further elevates temperature by increasing the basal metabolic rate. The skin is flushed because of the dilation of the cutaneous blood vessels.

2) The treatment, in addition to supportive measures to prevent patients from harming themselves or others, is gastric lavage coupled with physostigmine to reverse the effects of the alkaloids found in Angel's Trumpet. The usual dosage is 1 to 4 mg intramuscularly.

3) Phenothiazines and other antipsychotic drugs which have strong anticholinergic properties should not be given because they potentiate the anticholinergic effects of the alkaloids. The alpha blocking effects may precipitate cardiovascular collapse and death.

ANOREXIA NERVOSA

There are few diseases in psychiatry that are fatal. Extreme manic states and catatonic excitement may be accompanied by psychomotor excitation that leads to death from exhaustion. Individuals in catatonic stupor and profound depressions may have to be tube fed so that they do not die from inanition. Homicide and suicide may accompany profound depressions, some schizophrenic disorders and a number of toxic encephalopathies such as LSD-induced or amphetamine-induced psychosis. Finally, some individuals will starve to death thinking they are overweight. This last group, patients with anorexia nervosa, is predominantly composed of young women, usually of middle class background. Some authors feel that there is no such illness as anorexia nervosa but rather the symptom complex seen in patients with anorexia nervosa is a symptom of diseases as varying as endocrinopathies, illness, and schizophrenia.

History

1) The clinical picture is usually that of profound weight loss resulting from self-imposed restriction of food intake.

2) Weight loss may be aggravated by patient's hyperactivity, self-induced vomiting and purging by strong laxatives.

Symptoms

1) Distortion of body image such that patients insist that their weight is normal or that they are fat despite their emaciation and cachexia.
2) Anorexia.
3) Loss of self-esteem.
4) Increased self-consciousness about physical appearance.
5) Unreasonable fear of eating with pride in ability to lose weight, the "anorectic attitude" (Casper and Davis, 1977).
6) Restlessness.

Signs

1) Hypothermia
2) Bradycardia
3) Hypotension
4) Amenorrhea
5) Weight loss such that weight is about 75% of that expected for height, age, sex and bone structure.
6) Anemia and leukopenia (may result from starvation induced bone marrow hypoplasia).
7) Hyperactivity

Management

1) Many of these patients have document endocrinopathies, particularly deficiencies in production of pituitary gonadotropins, which must be evaluated and treated. In some patients, a functional anterior hypothalamic defect may be etiological (Rieger et at. 1978).

2) Amitriptyline produces a modest weight gain and rarely obesity in some cases of anorexia nervosa. This response raises the question of the relationship of some cases of anorexia nervosa to affective illness (Moore, 1977; Kendler, 1978).

ANTICHOLENERGIC INTOXICATION, HALLUCINOSIS AND DELUSIONAL STATES

Anticholinergic psychoses resemble those caused by atropine and are therefore often referred to as atropine psychoses. The symptoms and signs seen are the result of parasympathetic blockade.

History

1) Atropine psychosis may develop from ingestion of a variety of drugs including atropine, hyocine, belladonna, Jimson weed pods, scopolamine, henbane, stramonium, thorn apple pods, and hyoscyamine.

2) Cogentin, the tricyclic antidepressants, phenothiazines, antihistamines, and hypnotics such as glutethimide have prominent anticholinergic properties as do some over-the-counter sedatives.

3) Some cough mixtures contain scopolamine.

4) Signs of toxicity may appear after intranasal use of solutions as well as after ingestion of plants containing belladonna alkaloids.

Symptoms

1) Dryness of mouth and other mucous membranes
2) Hoarseness
3) Urinary retention
4) Dysphagia (difficulty in swallowing)
5) Intense thirst
6) Burning of eyes and throat
7) Strangury (slow and painful urinary discharge)
8) Restlessness
9) Disorientation
10) Visual hallucinations without perceptual distortion

11) Double vision
12) Memory impairment
13) Poor concentration
14) Body image distortion

Signs

1) Talkativeness
2) Widely dilated and inactive pupils
3) Hot, dry skin
4) Flushed skin
5) Rapid and weak pulse
6) Terminal coma and circulatory collapse
7) Because of the inability to sweat, hyperthermia may occur, particularly if the weather is hot.
8) Psychomotor excitement
9) Blood pressure is normal or decreased

Scopolamine Toxicity

Scopolamine toxicity is said to differ from that of atropine by the presence of a slow pulse, lack of flushing of the skin, and central nervous system depression, with lethargy and somnolence rather than excitement. The Babinski sign may occur with scopolamine poisoning but not after atropine poisoning.

Management

1) Give the patient sips of water.
2) Use "artificial tears" to moisten the eyes, nose and other mucous membranes.
3) Gastric lavage should be performed after oral ingestion.
4) Catheterization may be necessary.
5) If sedation is necessary, proceed cautiously. Use of neuroleptics with anticholinergic side-effects will contribute to the cause of difficulty rather than help to cure it and the patient will be more confused and agitated.
6) With scopolamine toxicity, mild stimulation with caffeine or amphetamines combats depression.
7) If respiration is inadequate or appears to be failing, artificial respiration may be necessary.
8) Methacholine or pilocarpine relieves the peripheral symp-

toms. However, if there is a severe degree of block these parasym-pathomimetic drugs have little or no effect. If there is no response after the injection of 5 or 10 mg of methacholine subcutaneously, poisoning with belladonna alkaloids should be considered.

9) The anticholinergic drug-induced delirium and coma is readily reversed by the anticholinesterase physostigmine. Unlike related substances like neostigmine, this drug crosses the blood-brain barrier and thereby reverses both peripheral and central nervous system cholinergic blockade. By inhibiting the destructive action of cholinesterase, physostigmine prolongs and exaggerates the effect of acetylcholine. One–three mg of physostigmine given intramuscularly or intravenously will in most cases reverse CNS toxic effects of the tricyclic antidepressant drugs. Since there appears to be a complete breakdown of physostigmine in the body within 1½ to 2 hours, doses should be repeated at 30 minutes if symptoms persist. The usual adult dosage of physostigmine salicylate is 0.5–2.0 mg intramuscularly or intravenously. Reversal of anticholinergic effects of atropine sulfate or scopolamine hydrobromide given as a preanesthetic medication usually requires a dose of physostigmine that is twice that of the anticholinergic drug administered by injection.

Side-Effects of Physostigmine

1) Nausea
2) Vomiting
3) Excessive sweating
4) Pupillary contraction
5) Increased intestinal muscular tone
6) Salivary secretion
7) Bronchial construction

Management of Side-Effects of Physostigmine

1) Reduce the dosage of physostigmine.

ANTICONVULSANT INTOXICATION DELUSIONAL STATES AND DELIRIUM

Patients taking anticonvulsant medication may become psychotic or delirious at normal or elevated serum levels of the seizure medication. Phenytoin, primidone, carbamazepine and clonazepam, among others, have been implicated in alterations of thought, mood and behavior resembling functional psychiatric disorders, such as schizophrenia. The usual physical signs of toxicity such as lethargy, dysarthria, nystagmus and ataxia are not always present. Inappropriate affect, bizarre behavior and evidence of a thought disorder have been reported as well as clinical syndromes more organic in character with clouding of the sensorium, visual hallucinations, and decreased short-term memory. The serum level of the anticonvulsant should be obtained in an attempt to document toxicity. If the serum is within the normal range, a trial of lower drug dosage may be necessary to establish the diagnosis.

ANTIMALARIAL TOXICITY

Antimalarial drugs such as amodiaquine, chloroquine and hydroxychloroquine may cause alterations in mood, thought and behavior resembling major psychiatric disturbance (Good and Shader, 1977). Therapeutic doses of these agents have been associated with depression, psychosis, delirium and other personality changes. Patients tend, significantly, to have some insight into their condition in the early stages of the change. Moderately low doses of chloroquine can lead to state dependent overdosage, however, and death. This is an increasing danger since chloroquine is being used more commonly, as Americans travel more frequently, as well as in rheumatology.

In one study, neurotic-like changes were reported in as many as 28% of patients on chloroquine. Symptoms are usually reversible within one week of cessation of drug use and generally do not reappear after reinstitution of therapy. Age and sex do not seem to play a role in determining who develops symptoms.

ANXIETY STATES

Anxiety and depression are part of the human experience. Everyone feels anxious at one time or another during their life just as everyone is depressed at some time. The difference between the anxiety that most of us feel and that experienced by patients who present to psychiatric clinicians is either the intensity of the feeling or the fact that the family and friends of the patient cannot tolerate it.

History

1) The first task in the evaluation of the etiology of anxiety is to carefully document the circumstances associated with the first and subsequent appearances of anxiety. What was happening in the patient's life at the time? Since its first appearance has it gotten worse, better, or remained the same in intensity? What is the duration and frequency of the anxiety attacks? Does it vacillate in intensity? If it does, what makes it better or worse? What other psychological (e.g. phobias) or physical symptoms (e.g. tachycardia, headaches) are associated with it? Is the patient's appetite, sleep or sexual potency affected by the anxiety attacks?

2) Medical conditions such as hyperthyroidism, pheochromocytoma and temporal lobe epilepsy may present with constant or episodic anxiety. A careful medical history and physical examination may be needed to ascertain if significant medical disease is present.

3) Fear should be distinguished from anxiety. Fear is an emotional response to something in the environment perceived as dangerous. This may be a person, a place or an activity. Anxiety is subjective fear. The cause is not as often readily apparent.

4) Anxiety has many forms. It may always be vaguely present and free floating. There may be times when it is nearly of panic proportions. Anxiety may be combined with phobias and depersonalization. It may accompany depression or be part of the clinical picture of an acute or chronic psychosis.

5) At times, no precipitant may be found or there may be a clear link to a life event such as divorce, job promotion, impending graduation, death, or first sexual experience.

6) Individuals vary in their ability to tolerate anxiety. Social and personal historical factors to some degree determine how an individual may handle anxiety.

7) Family studies (Noyes, et al. 1978) indicate that risk for anxiety neurosis is significantly greater for first degree relatives of neurotics than for controls. Relatives of anxiety neurotics are also at higher risk for the development of alcoholism. Female relatives are at greater risk for anxiety neuroses than male relatives.

Symptoms

1) Feeling of panic
2) Feeling of impending danger

3) Phobias
4) Apprehension
5) Loss of interest
6) Difficulty concentrating
7) Dryness of mouth
8) Nausea
9) Vomiting
10) Tenseness
11) Vague sinking feeling in abdomen
12) Diarrhea
13) Constipation
14) Urinary frequency
15) Light-headedness
16) Sense of fullness in stomach
17) Palpitations
18) Unceasing worry
19) Amenorrhea
20) Sleep disturbance
21) Lack of pleasure
22) Dyspepsia
23) Irritability
24) Sense of pressure in the chest
25) Impotence
26) Nightmares
27) Incapacity to relax
28) Sense of choking or suffocating
29) Decreased appetite
30) Shortness of temper
31) Episodic panic attacks
32) Restlessness
33) Impatience

Signs

1) Hyperactivity
2) Hyperventilation
3) Sweaty palms
4) Dry mouth
5) Tremor
6) Tachycardia
7) Increased muscle tone
8) Fidgety movements of the hands
9) Respiratory irregularity

10) Facial tics or grimacing

Differential Diagnosis

1) Normal anxiety
2) Anxiety neurosis
3) Insipient psychosis
4) Depressive illness
5) Thyrotoxicosis
6) Hyperthyroidism
7) Hypoglycemia
8) Pheochromocytoma
9) Caffeinism
10) Borderline schizophrenia
11) Chronic schizophrenia
12) Phobic-anxiety-depersonalization syndrome
13) Psychomotor epilepsy
14) Other temporal lobe disease
15) Paroxysmal atrial tachycardia and other cardiac arrhythmias
16) Internal hemorrhage
17) Impending myocardial infarction
18) Post-concussion syndrome
19) Manic-depressive illness
20) Alcohol withdrawal
21) Barbiturate and other drug withdrawal
22) Essential hypertension
23) Cerebral arteriosclerosis
24) Phobias
25) Amphetamine and other sympathomimetic psychoses
26) Cocaine psychosis
27) Homosexual panic
28) Hypocalcemia
29) Hypokalemia
30) Mitral valve prolapse
31) Hyperventilation syndrome
32) Encephalitis
33) Pulmonary embolism
34) Subacute bacterial endaortitis

Management

1) The first step in management is identification of the underly-

ing etiology of the anxiety states. History, physical examination and laboratory tests are generally required.

2) If the etiology is felt to be psychological in origin:

a) Allow the patient to ventilate in a supportive psychotherapeutic setting.

b) If the anxiety seems overwhelming, and ventilation fails to bring about sufficient amelioration of the symptoms, an antianxiety agent may be given and prescribed as needed. Chlordiazepoxide (Librium) 10 mg p.o. or diazepam (Valium) 2 mg p.o. q.i.d. prn is usually sufficient.

c) Some engineering may be required to minimize the precipitant stresses in the environment.

d) The disposition of the patient depends on the intensity of symptoms and response to a crisis psychotherapeutic intervention and antianxiety agents, given either orally or intramuscularly. If there is a reduction of tension and a patient is obviously more relaxed, he or she may return home. If the anxiety appears to be unresponsive to crisis therapy or seems to be escalating, hospitalization may be necessary to get patients away from intolerable situations and allow some rest and relaxation.

e) If the problem is one of long standing, the patient should be placed in long-term supportive psychotherapy. The patient should explore with the therapist those situations which are the most overwhelming and look at which alternatives may be available.

f) If the anxiety is part of an affective or schizophrenic illness, antidepressants and antipsychotics are needed in addition to or in lieu of benzodiazepines. Benzodiazepines are primarily anxiolytic (Schatzberg and Cole, 1978). They may be useful, however, in the anticipatory anxiety that accompanies some affective and schizophrenic disorders. Anticipatory anxiety should be distinguished from psychotic anxiety. Antipsychotic medication is required for the management of the latter.

g) Monoamine oxidase inhibitors, beta-blocking agents and tricyclic antidepressants have been used with some success in the treatment of panic attacks and certain phobic disorders. (Pariser et al. 1978). Patients with panic attacks usually respond to 60–120 mg of propranolol when used. If propranolol is used, care should be given to the usual contraindications such as asthma and congestive heart failure.

3) If the etiology is a medical disorder such as hyperthyroidism, the appropriate medical intervention is indicated. Psychotherapy or

sociotherapy may be needed if a life event or interpersonal stress has precipitated the medical or surgical condition.

BARBITURATE OR SIMILAR ACTING SEDATIVE–HYPNOTIC AMNESTIC SYNDROME

Heavy use of barbiturates or similar acting sedative-hyponotics may lead to a disturbance in short-term, but not immediate memory. Digit span on testing is normal but the individual cannot recall the name of three objects after a lapse of 15 minutes. Prolonged use of barbiturates or a similar acting sedative-hypnotic substance is necessary to develop the amnestic syndrome. Onset is usually in the twenties. Unlike with the alcohol amnestic syndrome, recovery is often complete.

BARBITURATE AND SIMILIAR ACTING HYPNOTIC OR SEDATIVE MENTAL DISORDERS

Barbiturates, hypnotics and similar acting minor tranquilizers can cause alterations of mood, thought and behavior both when taken in excess through intoxication and at the time of sudden cessation from doses that were sufficient to cause addiction. More prolonged usage of the benzodiazepines is required to produce the withdrawal syndrome of barbiturates and similar acting sedative-hypnotics.

History

1) Patients will have a history, although they may deny it, of taking one of a number of long, intermediate, or shortacting barbiturates or one of the sedative-hypnotics or minor tranquilizers. The sedative-hypnotics include methoaqualone, meprobamate, ethchlorvynol, glutethimide, methyprylon, chloral hydrate, and paraldehyde. The minor tranquilizers include the benzodiazepines—diazepam, oxazepam, flurazepam, and chlordiazepoxide. These drugs are nearly always taken orally.

2) The most frequently abused barbiturates are short-acting ones such as amobarbital, pentobarbital and secobarbital. Phenobarbital abuse is rare.

3) It is generally difficult to get a good history of barbiturate abuse. A clinician may be fooled by a quite proper woman who, once

placed in a situation where barbiturates are not available (e.g. hospitalization for depression or for emergency surgery following trauma) goes into withdrawal.

4) The various barbiturates, benzodiazepines and sedative-hypnotics differ in rates of absorption, metabolism and distribution but are quite comparable in the signs and symptoms of intoxication and withdrawal. The severity of the symptoms of and the duration of withdrawal, however, depends on the particular type of drug used, individual susceptibility and the duration of use.

5) Untreated, withdrawal from several of these drugs can be fatal.

6) If a patient admits to taking 1,500 mg or more of short-acting barbiturates, one may expect *severe* withdrawal symptoms if not properly treated. Barbiturate intake equivalent to 400 mg or more of pentobarbital will result in withdrawal symptoms on cessation of the drug. About 10% of individuals who take 500 mg per day will have withdrawal seizures and psychotic symptoms whereas 80% of those who take 900 mg a day will have seizures and nearly all will appear psychotic.

7) The essential signs and symptoms of withdrawal from these drugs is similar to that of alcohol withdrawal with the exception that the coarse tremor that is always seen with alcohol withdrawal may be absent. Similarly, barbiturate intoxication resembles alcohol intoxication. It is difficult to determine clinically what symptoms are due to alcohol and due to the use of barbiturate or similar acting drugs. Serum and urine toxicology screens are often necessary. Differences sometimes attributed to the drug used, relate more to the setting or the personality of the user than to alcohol or barbiturate.

8) The initial clinical symptoms of barbiturate intoxication are those of disinhibition. Only with continued use is inhibition seen. If enough is taken, death may result due to the central nervous system depression.

9) Clinically severe intoxication from barbiturates with depression can be differentiated from opioid intoxication by parenteral administration of naloxone or another opioid antagonist. Opioid antagonists have no effect on intoxications due to other drugs.

10) Serum and urine toxicology tests usually confirm the diagnosis of barbiturate or a similar acting drug intoxication.

Symptoms of Withdrawal

1) Anxiety
2) Disturbance of sleep

   3) Nausea and vomiting
   4) Malaise
   5) Irritability
   6) Restlessness
   7) Dysattention
   8) Disturbances in goal directed thought and behavior
   9) Illusions
10) Depression
11) Visual hallucinations
12) Formication
13) Paranoid ideation
14) Confusion

Signs of Withdrawal

   1) Increased or decreased psychomotor activity
   2) Muscular weakness
   3) Tremulousness
   4) Hyperreflexia
   5) Blepharospasm
   6) Postural hypotension
   7) Hyperpyrexia
   8) Delirium
   9) Convulsions
10) Tachycardia
11) Sweating
12) Elevated blood pressure
13) Coarse tremor of tongue, eyelids and hands
14) Status epilepticus
15) Death

    Delirium, when it occurs, is seen within one week following cessation of a barbiturate or similar acting drug and resembles the delusion seen with alcohol withdrawal.

Symptoms of Intoxication

   1) Loquacity
   2) Irritability
   3) Feeling in a dreamlike state
   4) Labile mood
   5) Derealization and depersonalization
   6) Disinhibition of sexual and aggressive impulses

Signs of Intoxication

1) Slurred speech
2) Ataxia
3) Incoordination
4) Dysattention
5) Memory impairment
6) Poor judgement
7) Interference with goal directed behavior

Management

1) The amount of barbiturate a patient is taking daily is estimated from history and use of barbiturate tolerance test. The patient is then withdrawn slowly, using doses of a barbiturate that just produces toxic symptoms.

2) A short-acting barbiturate such as pentobarbital or long-acting phenobarbital may be substituted for the drug the patient is taking.

3) Those who support the use of phenobarbital for withdrawal, reason that because of its longer duration of action it produces smaller fluctuations in barbiturate blood levels, thereby producing protection against withdrawal symptoms. Furthermore, phenobarbital generally does not produce the euphoria or "high" seen with shorter-acting barbiturates.

After the daily dose is estimated in terms of short-acting barbiturates, using the patient's history of use and data from the barbiturate tolerance test, the total initial daily amount of phenobarbital to be taken is calculated by substituting 30 mg of phenobarbital for each 100 mg of the short-acting barbiturate. After 2 days on this dose, withdrawal is begun. If there has been an overestimation of the daily dose, signs of toxicity such as slurred speech and ataxia appear. If withdrawal symptoms and signs appear, 200 mg of pentobarbital can be given, and there should be an increase in the daily dose of the phenobarbital. After the patient is stabilized, this daily dose is reduced by 30 mg each day as long as there are no remarkable withdrawal symptoms. The daily amount taken should be divided into four doses to allow the nurse or physician to check each time how the withdrawal is progressing. If there is evidence of toxicity one of the daily doses (i.e. ¼ of the total daily dose) can be omitted that day.

4) Those who prefer the short-acting barbiturates for withdrawal emphasize that the action of drugs like secobarbital and pentobarbital lasts only 4 to 6 hours, making withdrawal flexible.

The initial dose to be given is estimated by history and the barbiturate tolerance test. If the addiction is mixed, consideration must be given to the other drugs taken. Approximately 3 to 4 ounces of whiskey is equivalent for withdrawal purposes to 100 mg of pentobarbital. Comparably, 400 mg of meprobamate or 500 mg of Doriden is equivalent to 100 mg of pentobarbital. After the daily intake of barbiturates is estimated, the daily dose is given in 4 divided doses. If evidence of intoxication occurs, a dose may be omitted as with the long-acting drugs, and if withdrawal symptoms appear, 100 to 200 mg of pentobarbital may be given every hour or two until intoxication occurs. The dose of pentobarbital is then reduced by 100 mg each day unless there is evidence of intoxication or withdrawal. The bedtime dose is the last to be withdrawn.

5) Because of the danger of the medical complications of barbiturate withdrawal and the hazard of the patient taking additional amounts, withdrawal from barbiturates should *always* be performed in a hospital.

6) After withdrawal is complete there should be some exploration in psychotherapy as to why the patient abused the drug.

7) Barbiturates or similar acting sedative-hypnotic drugs are frequently used in suicide attempts, quite often successfully. Management of these overdoses is discussed in handbooks of medical emergencies.

BARBITURATE TOLERANCE TEST

When a patient gives a history of barbiturate abuse, or denies it, but the clinician feels there is a strong likelihood that the patient does abuse barbiturates, he may want to conduct a barbiturate tolerance test in order to ascertain whether or not a patient must be covered for withdrawal symptoms. The test is usually performed on the morning after a patient has been admitted to an inpatient unit and is as follows:

1) A test dose of 200 mg of pentobarbital is given orally.
2) One hour later the patient is examined for signs of clinical toxicity.
3) If the patient is not tolerant at the end of one hour, he will be soundly asleep but arousable.
4) If the patient is tolerant to a dose of less than 500 mg, gross ataxia, pseudoptosis, nystagmus, somnolence and Romberg's sign are present.
5) If tolerant to 500 to 600 mg he will show mild ataxia, nystagmus, and perhaps dysarthria.

6) Nystagmus would be the only sign in a patient tolerant to 700 mg to 800 mg.

7) If a patient is tolerant to 900 mg or more of pentobarbital he should show no signs of intoxication one hour after a 200 mg test dose, then a test dose of 300 mg should be tried. For a valid interpretation of the above test it is assumed a patient is not presently withdrawing nor intoxicated. Agitation and severe anxiety may raise the tolerance. The elderly and very debilitated may require only a 100 mg dose of pentobarbital. The clinician should be certain that the patient received and took the entire test dose.

BORDERLINE PATIENTS

There are a group of patients who, much like the fabled Richard Corey, look normal to all the world and one day go up to their room and kill themselves. This group by history often talk about depression as long as they can remember, anger as the strongest felt emotion, inconstant identity and never feeling close to anyone. This phenomenon has been variously referred to as latent schizophrenia, pseudoneurotic schizophrenia (Hoch and Polatin, 1949), the "as if" personality (Deutsch, 1942), the borderline personality (Kernberg, 1967), the borderline state (Knight, 1953) and the borderline syndrome (Grinker et al. 1968). There is much disagreement among clinicians and researchers as to whether or not what is observed is a real illness or rather a psychodynamic constellation. It is true that the descriptions provided by various authors make it difficult to examine this group from an empirical basis. It is also time, however, that clinicians working in emergency settings are confronted with patients who do have these dynamics and find them as a group, as difficult, or more difficult than other patients to deal with. The crises these patients present may involve:

1) Suicidal ideation
2) Suicidal gesture
3) Serious suicide attempt
4) Homicidal ideation
5) Homicidal gesture or attempt
6) Drug abuse
7) Other impulsive behavior
8) Micropsychotic episodes
9) Major psychotic decompensations

History

1) These patients often look quite good clinically, even in a crisis. What reveals the severity of their illness is a careful history. It is these patients about whom people comment after they success- fully commit suicide that "there never was any indication that anything was wrong." This, in fact, is what is most destructive to these patients. They themselves may be very supportive to others and never given the opportunity to express how depressed and lonely they are. Never has anyone asked them if they view death as an arbitrary line to be drawn unexpectedly by them or someone else at a mo- ment's notice. They may express the fact that although they do not feel suicidal now, when they do they will do it quickly and silently. No one will be notified; and they do commit suicide, often capriciously.

2) Hoch and Polatin (1949) characterized pseudoneurotic schizophrenia by the presence of pan-anxiety, pan-sexuality, and pan-neurosis. More helpful diagnostically, however, are the charac- teristics of the core borderline discussed by Grinker's group (1968). Depression as a mood is predominant. Some of these patients, in fact, cannot remember a time when they have not been depressed. There is an absence of any consistent self-identity. Borderline pa- tients, at times, go through life taking on the predominant features of people in their environment. Therefore, a woman raised in a con- vent may be pious and devout in her adolescence, but later, as an art student in Paris, become sexually free and devoid of any religious or personal value system. The strongest felt emotion is usually anger; and history may reveal episodes of acted-out or overt expression of anger. Their interpersonal relationships tend to lack any real sense of commitment, and they tend to vacillate in their involvement with others.

3) Gunderson and Singer (1975) summarize the diagnostic literature on the subject by identifying six predominant features of the syndrome:

a) There is a history of impulsive behavior. This may be episodic in nature, such as acts of self-mutilation and overdose of drugs, or more chronic in the form of promiscuity or drug dependence. Even though the original purpose of many of these acts is not self-destructive, the end result may be.

b) Intense affect is present. This may be in terms of a depres- sed mood or strong hostility. There may be depersonalization, the absence of pleasure, or flatness of affect.

c) Brief psychotic episodes are often found to occur. Frequently these have a paranoid tinge. Unstructured situations and relationships or drug use may provoke them. Even in the absence of such experience it is felt that the potential is present.

d) Social adaptiveness. There may be a history of good achievement at work or in school. Appearance and manners may be appropriate and a certain social awareness evident. These features, however, may reflect the absence of any firm identity and be due to a form of mimicry or form of superficial and rapid identification with others.

e) Vacillation in interpersonal relationships. These characteristically reveal a vacillation between transient superficial relationships and intense dependent ones that are marred by manipulation, demandingness and devaluation.

f) Psychological testing response. While borderline patients often do quite well on the Wechsler Adult Intelligence Scale (WAIS), responses to unstructured tests such as the Rorschach are often primitive, bizarre, illogical and dereistic.

4) Alcoholism and drug dependence may mask a borderline personality constellation.

Symptoms

The symptoms of the borderline state have been covered somewhat in the above discussion. To recapitulate, however, patients often complain of being depressed for as long as they can remember. Nothing seems to help, and a decision to commit suicide is almost arbitrary. Even though they may say that at the moment they have no plans to end their lives, they cannot promise that in a moment or two they may feel differently. Often they complain of intense periods of derealization and depersonalization. They never feel they can get close to anyone and find no purpose in life. Sex is relatively unimportant to them, and they may not consistently see themselves as male or female. They may be sexually abstinent, have a seemingly traditional sex life ("without feeling") or be hetero- or homosexually promiscuous. They feel they cannot control their impulses and may abuse drugs and alcohol.

Signs

While schizophrenics, on the whole, do not present with physical signs, it is not unusual for these patients to have burn or cut marks.

They will state that they cut themselves to feel "pain" or see "blood flow," which made them feel more real. Comparably, their forays into drug use and sex also sometimes reveal an attempt to make them feel more real. Masturbation makes them "know" they really exist.

Differential Diagnosis

1) Borderline personality
2) Depressive neurosis
3) Depressive character disorder
4) Chronic schizophrenia
5) Temporal lobe epilepsy
6) Obsessive compulsive neurosis
7) Hysterical character disorder

Management

1) These patients tend to get overinvolved with their therapists and the slightest change in a clinician's affect may be a sufficient stimulus for self-destructive behavior. The best prophylaxes against the development of this "psychotic transference" is for the therapist to be real and structure the interview. All tendency to regress should be countered, and coming in with a crooked tie would not be bad now and again. After all, in reality, the therapist is not God but another real live human being with no more magical power than anyone else. These patients cannot tolerate silences, and the therapist should be willing to take an active role in the therapy. These patients have a limited capacity to accept themselves and tend to see things in black or white. They are either *all* good or *all* bad. It is unfathomable to them that most of us are neither saints nor sinners but something in between. When they feel good, it seems nothing will ever go wrong again, but when they are down, it is hell, and suicide seems the only alternative.

2) Termination is extremely difficult for these people. All past endings of relationships are conjured up and like the concrete child, they imagine that if a therapist leaves he may be dead, that they were the cause of his going, and they will not be able to survive without him. They may, in fact, feel their anger killed the therapist. To avoid this, the therapy contract should be clear when it is set up and its duration indicated. Encouragement of outside relationships allows a dilution of the transference and mollifies termination.

3) The patient's therapist should be called when the patient pre-

sents in the emergency room. This may be the single most valuable emergency psychotherapeutic ploy. A follow-up appointment soon after the emergency evaluation may negate a need for hospitalization even if the patient is mildly suicidal. They should feel that their therapists and the emergency room are readily available in times of crisis.

4) It is imperative to determine why at this point in time a patient who is recurrently suicidal presents in the emergency room. They may be having a micropsychotic episode, or some fantasy may have got out of hand. Such might be controlled by a therapist's reassurance or a phenothiazine. Marijuana or another drug may have made them feel more unreal, and a small dose of phenothiazine (e.g. 8–12 mg of perphenazine p.o.) may reduce his anxiety. He may have a temporary stress-related sleep problem and may require a hypnotic such as Dalmane 15–30 mg p.o. for the night. The emergency room psychiatrist should assess their social and personal adaptive resources (i.e. "ego strengths"). If in the past they have made a serious suicide attempt, they may require hospitalization. If the precipitant is as uncomplex as their therapist going on holiday, all that may be needed is that the emergency room psychiatrist or the therapist's backup follow the patient until the therapist returns.

5) A subgroup of patients with borderline personality constellations respond to low doses of neuroleptic drugs (Brinkley et al. 1979), either antipsychotic or antidepressants. If antidepressants are to be used, however, they should never be started in an emergency situation. The response to antidepressants is too unpredictable in them, and the potential for self-poisoning too great to use a potentially lethal medication. Antipsychotic, antianxiety or hypnotic agents will suffice in emergency situations.

6) Borderline patients tend to decompensate at times of pressure and recompensate when the pressure is reduced. A discussion of what is going on in the patient's therapy may reveal that he is drawing "dangerously" close to his therapist, and is threatened by a loss of self, of personal annihilation. Reassurance and a single dose of medication may relieve the tension.

BROMIDE INTOXICATION, AFFECTIVE AND DELUSIONAL SYNDROMES

1) Acute intoxication from bromide ingestion is rare because bromide tends to irritate the gastrointestinal tract. It is difficult to retain much without vomiting.

2) Bromide is excreted slowly by the kidneys and, therefore, tends to accumulate if taken daily.

3) The incidence of bromide psychosis is felt to be greatly underestimated because physicians do not tend to think of it and consequently fail to look for its signs, symptoms, and presence in the serum.

4) Over-the-counter sedatives that contain bromides are available to the public without prescription.

5) The diagnosis of bromism can be corroborated by obtaining a serum bromide level. Generally symptoms are slow in developing and usually will not be manifest until the serum bromide level exceeds 50 mg/100 cc. Urine bromide levels are not a reliable guide to intoxication.

6) Bromism, like tuberculosis and syphilis, was once called the great masquerader. Individuals intoxicated from bromides may present as delirious, demented, manic, depressed, schizophrenic in addition to having symptoms suggestive of a number of other clinical syndromes. Symptoms do not necessarily correlate with serum bromide levels.

7) As with all drug psychoses, the clinical course and presentation is a function of the interaction of patients premorbid physical and psychological state, the environment, the dose of and duration of bromide use, and the number of other drugs taken.

8) Bromism may be mistaken for a number of neurological disorders and should be suspected whenever a diagnosis remains unclear after a thorough history and physical examination have been performed.

9) Patients may become quite terrified and violent during the withdrawal phase and require protection from harming themselves or others.

10) The serum half-life of bromide is reported to be about 12 days (Brenner, 1978)

Symptoms

1) Delusions
2) Lethargy
3) Auditory and visual hallucinations
4) Dizziness
5) Impairment of thought and memory
6) Drowsiness
7) Emotional lability
8) Irritability

9) Photophobia
10) Loss of memory
11) Mania
12) Irrelevant speech
13) Headache
14) Decreased libido
15) Fabrication
16) Disturbance
17) Vertigo
18) Depression
19) Confusion
20) Blurred vision
21) Anorexia
22) Diplopia

Signs

1) Dermatitis (The classical bromide rash begins as an acneform eruption on the face or around the hair rods, and later spreads to the entire body. A nodular type of lesion may appear on the legs, known as nodose bromoderma)
2) Delirium
3) Coma
4) Pupillary dilation
5) Heavily furred tongue
6) Foul breath
7) Babinski's sign
8) Headache
9) Gastric distress
10) Constipation
11) Mild conjunctivitis
12) Cyanosis
13) Tremor
14) Ataxia
15) Disorientation
16) Reflex disturbances
17) Papilledema
18) Stupor
19) Vacuous facies
20) Muscular weakness
21) Motor incoordination
22) Decreased superficial reflexes
23) Sluggishness of movement
24) Thick, slurred speech

In severe cases the cerebrospinal pressure may be elevated. At high plasma levels the electroencephalogram may show a diffuse slow wave pattern. At low plasma levels there may be a pattern of sustained fast wave activity.

Differential Diagnosis

1) Bromism
2) Acute alcohol intoxication
3) Acute and chronic schizophrenia
4) Tabes dorsalis
5) General paresis
6) Uremia
7) Cerebral neoplasm
8) Multiple sclerosis
9) Encephalitis
10) Depressive syndrome of psychotic proportions
11) Depressive syndrome of nonpsychotic proportions
12) Mania
13) Other toxic syndromes

Management

1) Obtain a serum level to confirm the diagnosis. A patient is considered toxic if his level is greater than 50 mg/100 cc (Brenner, 1978).

2) Discontinue all intake of bromide.

3) Specific treatment involves the administration of large quantities (up to 6–12 g daily) in divided doses of sodium chloride orally or intravenously in the form of physiologic saline. Ammonium chloride not only provides a chloride ion but also acts as a diuretic.

4) In severe cases, hemodialysis may be used.

5) The patient's food intake should be monitored to correct the malnutrition often encountered with bromism.

6) Sedation is contraindicated unless a patient is extremely agitated. Paraldehyde and neuroleptics have been used intramuscularly or orally when required. Intramuscular administration of paraldehyde may cause sterile abesses and nerve damage and should be avoided where possible. When given, the dosage of paraldehyde is 10–15 cc orally every 4 to 6 hours or 4 cc intramuscularly in each buttock every 6 hours. Alternately, 50–75 mg I.M. of chlorpromazine, 5–10 mg of haloperidol, or 5–10 mg of

perphenazine may be given intramuscularly every 4 hours while monitoring blood pressure.

7) Following treatment of the bromide psychosis, exploratory psychotherapy may be used to get at the origins of the bromide abuse. Symptoms may last as long as 2 to 6 weeks after cessation of bromide intake because of the long serum half life.

CAFFEINE INTOXICATION (CAFFEINISM)

The cause of acute or continuing anxiety may be as mundane as the intake of excessive amounts of coffee, tea or cola drinks. In other instances, individuals who are unable to sleep because of emotional turmoil will drink cup after cup of coffee thereby adding a physiological cause of anxiety to a psychological one.

History

1) Individuals presenting with the symptoms and physical signs of caffeinism have ingested large amounts of coffee and/or other caffeine-containing compounds such as tea, hot chocolate, cola drinks, and cocoa or caffeine-containing over-the-counter cold preparations, stimulants, and analgesics or prescription drugs.

2) Individual susceptibility to caffeine varies. Fifty–250 mg of caffeine is usually needed to produce the characteristic pharmacologic action of caffeine. One cup of brewed coffee contains about 100–150 mg of caffeine.

3) Many people consume enough caffeine daily to produce symptoms without realizing it. Tea contains about half the amount of caffeine of coffee and cola contains about one-third. Instant coffee contains about 86–99 mg/cup of caffeine and APC's, 32 mg/tablet. The caffeine content of other commonly used medications are as follows:

Darvon Compound	32 mg/tablet
Excedrin	60 mg/tablet
Anacin	32 mg/tablet
Aspirin Compound	32 mg/tablet
Bromo Seltzer	32 mg/tablet

Over the counter stimulants and migraine medications contain about 100 mg/tablet.

4) Doses greater than 1,000 mg/day can result in muscle

twitchings, increased psychomotor activity, and cardiac arrhythmias. Higher doses result in ringing in the ears and doses in excess of 10 g of caffeine can result in grand mal seizures and death secondary to respiratory failure.

5) Patients failing to respond to the usual effective doses of psychopharmacologic agents or nighttime hypnotics should be suspected of caffeine intoxication. Absence of the expected effects of antidepressant medication on sleep may relate to the fact that a depressed patient is drinking a considerable quantity of coffee at night.

6) Symptoms of caffeine intoxication may be superimposed upon symptoms of mania, depression, or an anxiety, neurosis, or acute schizophrenia episode. People in emotional turmoil naively may sit up and drink coffee because they are having difficulty sleeping.

7) Excessive amounts of caffeine may endanger a patient's cardiac or gastrointestinal status. Extremely high doses of caffeine can cause hypertension, cardiac arrhythmias and circulatory failure and should therefore be avoided by patients with a history of recent myocardial infarction. Epigastric distress, nausea, vomiting and diarrhea are usual concommitants of caffeinism. Rarely, large amounts of caffeine has been implicated in the production of hematemesis or peptic ulcer.

Symptoms

 1) Restlessness
 2) Frequent sleep interruption
 3) Delayed onset of sleep
 4) Palpitations
 5) Excitement
 6) Subjective feeling of anxiety
 7) Flushing
 8) Diarrhea
 9) Irritability
10) Nervousness
11) Epigastric pain
12) Nausea
13) Vomiting
14) Rambling speech
15) Periods of inexhaustability
16) Visual flashes of light
17) Ringing in the ears

18) Diuresis
19) Sensory disturbances
20) Agitation
21) Tremulousness
22) Headaches

Signs

1) Muscle twitching
2) Cardiac arrhythmias
3) Tachypnea
4) Hyperesthesia
5) Extrasystoles
6) Tachycardia

Differential Diagnosis

1) Mania
2) Hypomania
3) Anxiety neurosis
4) Delirium
5) Depression

Management

1) Patients should be encouraged to restrict caffeine intake. This may be difficult since many people are accustomed to having several cups of coffee a day and withdrawal symptoms appear as intake is cut down or ceased.

2) Benzodiazepines may be used if indicated by symptom intensity to treat the acute effects of a single episode of caffeine excess.

3) Symptoms of caffeine withdrawal include dysphoria, inability to work effectively, restlessness, headache, lethargy, irritability and nervousness. These symptoms pass within 24 to 48 hours of cessation of caffeine intake.

CANNABIS INTOXICATION AND DELUSIONAL SYNDROME

Cannabis, most frequently referred to as marijuana, is more frequently used than alcohol in some circles.

History

1) Cannabis and its related derivatives of the cannabis plant—hashish and delta-9-tetrahydrocannabinol—may be smoked (e.g. "reefers" or "joints") or taken orally with a number of substances including food (e.g. "Alice B. Toklas brownies").

2) It is variously known as pot, MJ, Mary Jane, grass and bhang.

3) Use may range from a brief first experimental trial to chronic daily use.

4) Individual's reaction to cannabis varies and relates to:

   a) Set—expectations as to what is to happen or has in the past.

   b) Setting—(e.g. a response in a laboratory setting may be strikingly different from that in a room with incense, strobe light and acid rock).

   c) Personality—(e.g. an obsessive-compulsive person would be expected to respond differently than a hysteric).

   d) Dose—hashish is generally quite potent, but some "grass" is just that with no tetrahydrocannabinol (THC).

5) Most smokers of marijuana, like alcohol users, have mild to moderate reactions, and do not seek medical assistance. As there is no physiological dependence, there is no addiction, in the strict sense of the word, and therefore no withdrawal symptoms.

6) Intoxication occurs nearly immediately after smoking cannabis and peaks in about one-half hour. Nearly all symptoms disappear after 3 hours. Absorption of cannabis taken orally is slower with a lower peak level, but more prolonged effect. Symptoms should be entirely gone 6 hours after ingestion.

7) The individual may have the characteristic sweet smell of cannabis on his clothing.

8) Impairment of coordination may lead to automobile, airplane and motorcycle accidents, and to industrial accidents.

9) It is the psychiatric clinician's task in an emergency evaluation to ascertain from history:

   a) Whether or not the premorbid personality of the patient was stable and whether the symptoms can be presumed to be a toxic reaction of the drug.

   b) Whether the patient was having a psychotic decompensation and took the drug in an attempt to self-medicate or help organize the internal chaos, or to be part of a group which would accept him despite his bizarre behavior.

   c) Whether he was basically unstable and/or with a family history of psychiatric difficulty and marijuana was the sufficient stimulus to put him over the edge.

Symptoms

1) Sensation of slowed time and apathy
2) Heightened sensory awareness
3) Changes in thought, incoherence and impaired associations
4) Self-confidence
5) Depersonalization and derealization
6) Disinhibition
7) Impairment of immediate memory
8) Laughter, silliness and light heartedness
9) Sensation of floating
10) Disorientation
11) Altered reality testing
12) Suggestibility
13) Decreased attention and concentration span
14) Elation, euphoria and marked relaxation
15) Rapid or impaired speech
16) Feelings of detachment
17) Fear of dying
18) Delusions of persecution and paranoia
19) Paresthesias
20) Illusions
21) Changed sense of self-identity and body image
22) Anxiety and panic attacks
23) Nausea
24) Sleepiness
25) Depression
26) Suspiciousness and ideas of reference
27) Emotional lability
28) Auditory and visual hallucinations
29) Dreamy state
30) Feeling of a heavy or pressured head
31) Feeling more insightful
32) Changed sexual feeling
33) Increased appetite and thirst
34) Precordial distress
35) Feeling one is going crazy
36) Impaired judgement
37) Diarrhea
38) Light headedness
39) Confusion

Signs

1) Tremor
2) Tachycardia
3) Dry mouth
4) Increased sensitivity to touch and pain
5) Nystagmus
6) Profuse sweating
7) Restlessness
8) Conjunctival injection
9) Ataxia
10) Urinary frequency
11) Interference with social or occupational functioning

Differential Diagnosis

1) Cannabis intoxication or delusional syndrome
2) Schizophrenia
3) Adolescent adjustment reaction
4) Depressive syndrome of psychotic and nonphyschotic proportions
5) Manic-depressive illness
6) Phobic-anxiety-depersonalization state
7) Anxiety states of varying etiology
8) Alcohol intoxication or delusional syndromes
9) Hallucinogenic intoxication or delusional syndromes

Treatment

1) Assess the suicidal and homicidal potential of the patient and whether there is any psychiatric condition other than the toxic effects of marijuana. If other major psychopathology is identified, appropriate treatment should be made.

2) If the behavioral, mood and thought changes are felt primarily due to marijuana, an attempt may be made to "talk down" the patient in a supportive safe atmosphere with minimal distortion. It should be explained to the patient that what he is experiencing can be attributed to the drug and that he will get better.

3) Medication may be needed for anxiety or psychotic symptoms. Effective antianxiety agents include chlordiazepoxide (Librium) 10–15 mg or diazepam (Valium) 5–20 mg orally or intra-

muscularly. For psychotic symptoms, haloperidol (Haldol) 5–10 mg or chlorpromazine (Thorazine) 25–50 mg p.o. or I.M. may be used as well as a number of other antipsychotic agents.

4) The patient should be scheduled for a return appointment in one week to see if all symptoms have subsided. Flashbacks may occur with marijuana as with other psychotomimetic agents and are treated with the usual antianxiety and antipsychotic drugs. If reevaluation suggests that the original symptoms were due to another condition or that another condition is present, it should be treated accordingly.

5) Cannabis may be contaminated with other drugs such as phencyclidine. In such instances, it is necessary to treat the patient for the mixed drug intoxication and be alert to the complications due to the contaminants used.

CIMETIDINE PSYCHOSES

Cimetidine, a competitive histamine H_2 receptor antagonist, is widely used as an inhibitor of gastric secretion in the short term management of duodenal ulcer, and in the treatment of pathological hypersecretory syndromes such as multiple endocrine adenomas, systemic mastocytosis, and the Zollinger-Ellison syndrome. The drug is usually tolerated well. An increasing number of cases are being reported, however, of neuropsychiatric toxicity with severe acute confusional psychoses, lethargy, slurred speech, unsteadiness, disorientation, restlessness, agitation, delirium, visual impairment, incontinence and coma (Jefferson, 1979). In most of these instances, there has been coexiting psychiatric illness, a history of the concurrent use of psychotropic medication that has strong central anticholinergic effects, old age, decreased brain perfusion due to cerebrovascular disease in older people and/or overdosage. Symptoms usually disappear upon reduction or discontinuation of dosage.

COCAINE INTOXICATION AND DELUSIONAL SYNDROME

Cocaine intoxication and delusional syndromes resemble those of amphetamine and other sympathomimetic substances. Cocaine differs from amphetamines and most other sympathomimetic substances in cost and, therefore, availability. It is the recreational drug that is most frequently associated with use by people of circumstance. Professional men and women such as lawyers, physicians and business people, and those in the theater and art world will report using it. It is not addictive in the strictist sense of the word but its use is associated with a number of physicial and psychological complications.

History

1) Cocaine is sold as crystalline flakes or powder (hence it is sometimes called "snow").

2) The usual route of intake is by application to the mucous membrane of the nose ("snorting coke") and by intravenous or subcutaneous ("skin popping") administration. Nasal application may result in perforations of the nasal septum. In some instances, there may be some evidence of the white powdery substance in the nasal area. It is inactivated when taken orally.

3) The onset of symptoms and physical signs is more rapid than with amphetamine and related substances. The symptoms begin within one hour after administration and are usually entirely gone within 24 hours. Depression, fatigue, irritability, anxiety and tremulousness may appear within the hour or following the subsiding of the psychological and behavioral manifestations of use. In instances of intravenous administration of cocaine, the effects may be brief—lasting only minutes—while the effects of intravenous administration of methamphetamine may be hours.

4) As with all drug intoxication states, the clinical presentation represents an interaction of the patient's premorbid personality, the environment in which the cocaine is taken, other physical and psychiatric illnesses the individual may have, genetic constitution, the number, kind and quantity of other drugs that the individual may also have taken, the dose of cocaine and the route of administration.

5) Amphetamine and cocaine is sometimes taken with heroin and called a "speedball."

6) Cocaine, like marijuana, amphetamine and the antipsychotic agents, produces little if any physical dependence.

7) The intake of a large dose of cocaine over a brief period can lead to seizures and even death from respiratory paralysis or cardiac arrhythmias.

8) Identification of the metabolites of cocaine in a urine specimen may be the only absolute way to differentiate cocaine from amphetamine intoxication. Unfortunately, detectable amounts of cocaine remain in the urine for only 4 to 6 hours after usage.

Symptoms of Cocaine Intoxication and Delusional Syndrome

1) Loose associations

2) Euphoria and elation*
3) Decreased sleep
4) Paranoid ideation
5) Ideas of reference
6) Vivid auditory and visual hallucinations which at times may be quite frightening ("Snow lights" may be present that resemble migraine hallucinations).
7) Grandiosity
8) Feeling of mental agility
9) Insomnia
10) Loquacity
11) Heightened awareness of sensory input
12) Restlessness
13) Sense of confidence
14) Anorexia
15) Impaired judgement
16) Inability to meet social and occupational responsibility
17) Confusion
18) Anxiety and apprehension
19) Ringing in the ears
20) Sensations of seeing insects and feeling insects, small animals and other vermin crawling up the skin (formication) which may lead to picking at the skin and subsequent excoriation of the skin.
21) Hostility
22) Feeling of immunity to fatigue and great muscle power
23) Illusions
24) Dream-like states
25) Broodiness
26) Irritability
27) Hypervigilance

Physical Signs of Cocaine Intoxication and Delusional Syndrome

1) Pupillary dilation
2) Perforated nasal septum (sometimes seen with a whitish powder on it).
3) Seizures
4) Perspiration or chills

---

*The feeling of extreme well-being and confidence that frequently follows rapidly after intravenous administration is referred to as a "rush."

5) Vomiting
6) Tachycardia
7) Elevated blood pressure
8) Psychomotor excitement
9) Skin pallor
10) Haggard look
11) Elevation of body temperature
12) Tremulousness
13) Some users will show evidence of "skin popping" and/or needle marks.
14) Violent or assaultive behavior of the patient is paranoid.

Differential Diagnosis

1) Cocaine intoxication or delusional syndrome
2) Amphetamine or similar acting sympathomimetic intoxication or delusional syndrome
3) Anxiety states (see Differential Diagnosis of Anxiety States)
4) Mania
5) Acute schizophrenic episode
6) Paranoid schizophrenia
7) Chronic schizophrenia
8) Delirium tremens

Management

1) The management of cocaine intoxication and delusional syndrome is comparable to that of sympathomimetic intoxication.

2) Cocaine intoxication is usually self-limited and an individual feels fully recovered within 24 hours.

3) If medication is needed, haloperidol 2–5 mg or equivalent doses of a similar acting antipsychotic agent orally or intramuscularly is usually sufficient. If an atropine-like substance has been taken together with the cocaine, a benzodiazepine such as 10–20 mg of diazepam should be given to manage the psychomotor retardation rather than one of the antipsychotic agents that have anticholinergic properties.

4) There is no danger in immediately withdrawing the individual from cocaine.

5) An hour or so after the individual's symptoms have subsided, he or she may "crash" (i.e. feel depressed, anxious, irritable and fatigue). The desire for more cocaine is great during this period and

the individual may resort to crime to obtain the money needed to purchase the expensive drug.

6) The use of sympathomimetic substances incuding amphetamines and cocaine may precipitate a psychosis in predisposed individuals or be taken as "self-medication" as an individual is breaking down.

Cocaine Overdose

Large doses of cocaine may result in syncope, chest pains, delirium, tremulousness and seizures with a temporal lobe discharge pattern. Death may result from respiratory paralysis or cardiac arrhythmias. The treatment is basically supportive. Intravenous barbiturates or intramuscular antipsychotic agents can be employed but *only* with caution because the respiratory depression that accompanies cocaine poisoning can be aggravated by large doses of sedating agents. Anticonvulsants are not felt to be effective in preventing seizures.

DELIRIUM

The cognitive changes we associate with delirium are the result of changes in cerebral metabolism secondary to a variety of toxic, metabolic, traumatic, vascular, neoplastic and degenerative processes. The primary treatment is that of the etiologic process. Psychiatry can offer sociotherapeutic and psychopharmacologic suggestions that will contribute to the comfort of these patients and facilitate their management while they are receiving clinical diagnostic examinations and treatment. The psychiatrist, therefore, should be able to recognize the signs and symptoms of delirium, sometimes also referred to as an acute organic mental syndrome, and be prepared to make recommendations for management.

History

1) Delirium may occur at any age. It is sometimes very difficult to detect in very young children.

2) Onset is rapid, usually over hours or days. Symptoms generally first appear at night when sensory input and environmental cues are reduced.

3) The patient may have a history of infections, recreational or prescription drug use, or other contributing illness such as recent cardiac surgery or trauma.

4) Cognitive impairment tends to fluctuate unpredictably and often rapidly. Lucid intervals in which a patient is more rational are interspersed with confusional states (frequently more marked at night).

5) The duration is usually brief, lasting a few days to a week. Occassionally, it may last longer as with bromism.

6) Recovery is usually complete. Rarely the patient will go on to have more permanent cognitive deficits consistent with dementia, or will die.

7) Older people and those with preexisting brain damage are more likely to develop delirium than younger people and those without brain damage.

8) Etiological factors include a number of medical and surgical illness as well as substance intoxication and withdrawal.

9) Delirious patients present management problems both in and out of the hospital and are at risk for accidents and violent behavior including suicide.

10) Patients with delirium become worse at night when frightening dreams and hallucinations may be interpreted as actual events.

11) There is usually evidence on physical examination or laboratory tests of the etiology of the disorder.

Symptoms

1) Clouding of the sensorium
2) Fluctuating levels of consciousness
3) Insomnia, reduced wakefulness and reversal of sleepwake cycle
4) Agitation
5) Inability to sustain attention to environmental stimuli
6) Delusions
7) Disorientation
8) Anxiety, apprehension and panic
9) Vivid dreams and nightmares merging with hallucinations
10) Emotional lability
11) Lack of cooperation with medical staff
12) Hallucinations (predominantly visual)
13) Perceptual difficulty including illusions
14) Difficulty performing simple calculations
15) Outbursts of rage and anger
16) Memory changes with difficulty in retention and recall (both antegrade and retrograde amnesia occurs)
17) Incoherent speech
18) Denial of defects

19) Difficulty in goal directed behavior and thinking
20) Fragmented and disjointed thinking (may be slowing of thinking in early stages)
21) Perseveration of speech and behavior
22) Misidentification of people and places
23) Irritability
24) Euphoria
25) Apathy

Signs

1) Coarse tremor
2) Sweating
3) Tachycardia
4) Urinary and fecal frequency
5) Hyperventilation
6) Restlessness
7) Slow response to questions
8) Avoidance, denial, and inconsistent responses to questions
9) Increased or decreased psychomotor activity (with picking at bedclothes, attempting to get out of bed, and sudden changes in activity are common)
10) May appear nearly catatonic at times with speech approximating mutism
11) Flushed face
12) Elevated systolic blood pressure
13) Dilated pupils
14) Flapping tremor of extended hands (called asterixis and most common with hepatic encephalopathy but also seen with other syndromes)
15) Dysnomia
16) Dysgraphia

Differential Diagnosis

1) Cerebral and systemic infections
2) Post-operative, post-traumatic and puerperal states
3) Hyperthyroidism
4) Excessive use of alcohol
5) Substance withdrawal following dependence
6) Pernicious anemia
7) Cerebral vascular insufficiency
8) Cerebral neoplasia, especially focal lesions of the right cerebral hemisphere and undersurface of the occipital lobe

9) Adrenal insufficiency
10) Substance intoxication
11) Congestive heart failure
12) Hyperparathyroidism
13) Post-convulsive states
14) Bromism
15) Hypoxia
16) Hypercarbia
17) Uremia
18) Hepatic encephalopathy
19) Ionic imbalance
20) Hypoglycemia
21) Brain trauma
22) Seizures
23) Other organic states
24) Delirium
25) Schizophrenia
26) Other psychoses with delusions
27) Sensory deprivation
28) Disassociated disorders
29) Conversion disorders
30) Factitious illness (such as Ganser's syndrome—pseudo-stupidity, pseudodementia or pseudopsychosis)
31) Dementia

Management

1) A good physical examination and appropriate laboratory tests aimed at recovering the etiology is the first step in management.

2) The primary focus of treatment is the appropriate medical and surgical treatment of the underlying disorder causing the delusion. These patients should be kept on a medical or surgical ward with a psychiatrist acting as a consultant.

3) Until the etiology of the delirium is found and treated, fluid and electrolyte balance should be maintained. Care should be taken to provide an appropriate diet for the patient, and certainty that he eats it. Blood pressure, heart rate and temperature should be monitored. If infection, hyperthermia or circulatory collapse occurs, these must be properly treated.

4) If the patient remains somewhat alert, reassure him, and explain to him in a way he can understand what is happening.

5) Structure and simplify the patient's environment. A small night light counters nighttime confusion. Placing a calendar and family pictures in the room helps by day to orient the patient. It is best to have one familiar nurse tend the patient rather than a number of them. A relative at the bedside with restriction of less familiar visitors is helpful.

6) When a patient becomes unmanageable, low doses of antipsychotics may be helpful. Such include haloperidol (Haldol) 0.5–1 mg, perphenazine (Trilafon) 1–2 mg, fluphenazine (Prolixin) 0.5–1 mg, chlorpromazine (Thorazine) 10–20 mg, and thioridazine (Mellaril) 25 mg p.o.; Valium 5–10 mg may also be used but can further confuse some patients.

7) Central nervous system depressants such as barbiturates are contraindicated as they may increase the confusion. In addition, barbiturates are specifically contraindicated in acute intermittent porphyria, and in severe renal or pulmonary disease. Chlorpromazine tends to cause hypotension and should not be used for patients with cerebrovascular or cardiovascular disease.

DEMENTIA

Dementia, like epilepsy, is a symptom of a number of illnesses. The management of some patients with these diseases (e.g. Huntington's chorea, cerebral neoplasia) may require close collaboration between a psychiatrist and members of other medical specialties such as neurology and neurosurgery. In an emergency situation, usually all that is required is either the separation of patients with true dementia from the so-called functional psychoses, or consultation about the management of patients already identified as having a chronic organic mental syndrome who are deteriorating. At all times it must be remembered that patients who are demented are sometimes quickly cast into the genre of the "incurables." This is not always the case. Normal pressure hydrocephalus, vitamin deficiencies, cerebral infections and cerebral tumors are all examples of organic brain syndromes that present with dementia that may in some cases show remarkable improvement with appropriate therapy.

Definition

The term dementia implies a deterioration of intellectual ability as a consequence of malfunctioning cerebral cortical or subcortical cells. Symptoms of dementia include disorientation, difficulty with memory, alterations in personality, impairment of judgement and deterioration of other intellectual functions such as the ability to calculate and to abstract. The syndrome may be detectable any time after the intellectual quotient is considered stable (usually after age 3 or 4).

Symptoms

1) Disorientation (first to time, then to place and last to person)
2) Dysmnesia (with impairment of recent memory greater than for past memory)
3) Changes in personality (these relate to the premorbid personality, the stage of his illness, the part of the brain affected, the sociocultural matrix, the psychological response to the organic changes, and other pathophysiologic changes due to diet, alcohol, etc.)
4) Impairment of judgement
5) Emotional lability
6) Occupational delirium
7) Catastrophic reactions when the patient is confronted with a task he cannot perform, he may show evidence of sudden autonomic arousal
8) Difficulty calculating
9) Difficulty abstracting
10) Lack of impulse control

In the later stages:

1) Paranoia
2) Global loss of memory
3) Total disorientation
4) Motor unrest
5) Perseveration
6) Verbigeration
7) Stereotypies
8) Intellectual dullness
9) Loss of sphincter control
10) Complete apathy
11) Inability to feed and clothe oneself

Signs

1) The physical signs seen when examining a demented patient

depend upon the underlying pathology responsible for the cognitive and behavioral changes. These are as numerous and varied as the number of illnesses causing dementia. For instance, normal pressure hydrocephalus commonly presents with the triad of symptoms of dementia, fecal or urinary incontinence and ataxia. Cerebral neoplasia generally presents with focal signs and symptoms.

2) Most degenerative diseases accompanied by dementia present with a gradual progressive intellectual deterioration together with diffuse neurological signs. Sometimes a presentation may be confusing. Well-localized signs are usually indicative of a neoplasm, a cerebral abscess, a syphilitic gumma, a tuberculoma, sarcoidosis, and a cerebral aneurysm.

3) Careful neurological and physical examination is always an important part of the evaluation of these patients.

Differential Diagnosis

The differential diagnosis is complex and a variety of classifications have been devised for clinical purposes. Practically speaking, the most important step is to identify those forms of dementia which may be effectively treated with arrest or reversal of symptoms.

Treatable Forms of Dementia

 1) Addison's disease
 2) Some angiomas of the cerebral vessels
 3) Anoxia secondary to chronic cardiac or respiratory disease
 4) Cerebral abscess
 5) Some cerebral neoplasias
 6) Chronic subdural hematoma(s)
 7) Electrolyte imbalance
 8) Endogenous toxins (as with hepatic or renal failure)
 9) Exogenous toxins such as carbon monoxide
10) Hypothyroidism
11) Hypoglycemia
12) Cerebral infections such as tuberculosis, syphilis, parasites, or yeasts
13) Intracranial aneurysms
14) Normal pressure hydrocephalus
15) Pseudodementia (e.g. schizophrenia or depression)
16) Vitamin deficiencies
17) Wilson's disease

Untreatable Forms of Dementia

1) Alcoholic encephalopathy
2) Alzheimer's disease
3) Arteriosclerosis
4) Behcet's syndrome
5) Cerebral metastases
6) Some primary cerebral neoplasms
7) Creutzfeldt-Jakob's disease
8) Dementia pugilistica
9) Familial myoclonus epilepsy
10) Friedreich's ataxia
11) Huntington's chorea
12) Kuf's disease
13) Marchiafava-Bignami disease
14) Mongolism
15) Multiple myeloma
16) Multiple sclerosis
17) Collagenoses
18) Parkinsonism—dementia complex of Guam
19) Pick's disease
20) Post-concussion syndrome
21) Presenile dementia with motor neuron disease
22) Presenile glial dystrophy
23) Primary parenchymatous cerebellar atrophy with dementia
24) Primary subcortical gliosis
25) Progressive supranuclear palsy
26) Sarcoidosis
27) Schilder's disease
28) Senile dementia
29) Trauma
30) Simple presenile dementia

Management

1) The first step in the management of dementia is to separate that group of patients for whom there is a specific treatment. This will frequently require admission to an inpatient setting, where in addition to the history and mental status examination, and physical and neurological examinations, a complete battery of other tests may be ordered as indicated. such as:

a) laboratory studies (these would include a CBC, serum B_{12}

assay, gastric acidity tests, bone marrow studies, serology, erythrocyte sedimentation rate, serum albumen-globulin ratio, BUN, glucose tolerance curve, serum cholesterol, T_3, T_4, T_7, serum enzymes, serum copper and ceruloplasmin. Urinalysis should be performed for presence of red cells and the Bence-Jones protein).

b) lumbar puncture (opening and closing pressures should be recorded and samples sent off for cells, protein, serology, viral titers and appropriate cultures where indicated).

c) skull and chest films

d) echoencephalography

e) electroencephalography

f) brain scan

g) CAT scan

h) cerebral angiography (if indicated)

i) isotope encephalography (if indicated)

j) neuropsychological testing

2) When patients with a treatable form of dementia have been isolated the specific treatment should be initiated. In the instance of cerebral neoplasm this would usually mean surgical extirpation, and at times radiotherapy. Ventriculoatrical shunting is the treatment of choice for normal pressure hydrocephalus. In case of thyroid or vitamin deficiencies, replacement therapy would be indicated.

3) With patients with untreatable forms of dementia, individual and family therapy can help both patients and their families maximize their strengths as patients deteriorate. Obviously, in the later stages any individual work with a patient may be futile, but early in the course of the illness when there is only a mild memory deficit, patients can be directed to areas of activity which will allow them to maximize their strengths. Family members can use therapy both as a situation in which they can learn how to manage a patient with organic brain damage as well as an opportunity to ventilate their feelings. This is especially important when dementia occurs early in life as with Pick's or Alzheimer's disease and leaves a man or woman solely responsible for the economic welfare and child raising of the family. A therapist can help with many practical everyday problems, from helping to guide family members in taking over financial responsibility for the family to restricting any car driving by the patient. Explanations of how unfamiliar situations may result in a catastrophic reaction may help a family to minimize demands on a patient that result in confusion or intense adverse emotional responses.

4) Familiarity of environment is a key in maintaining a pa-

tient's orientation. Changes in their physical surroundings should be minimized. If hospitalization or nursing home placement is necessary, objects that are familiar to them like a favorite lamp, family picture or religious object should be placed in his new bedroom. A night lamp is important in reducing the confusion present when a demented patient awakens in a dark room.

5) Psychopharmacotherapy is often helpful in the management of demented patients but doses should be scaled down especially if there is evidence of renal or hepatic damage. Both agitation and depression specifically respond to pharmacotherapy. Thioridazine (Mellaril) 25 mg p.o. b.i.d. or q.i.d. is often helpful both for agitation and depression. Amitryptyline (Elavil) or imipramine (Tofranil) 10 mg–25 mg p.o. b.i.d. or q.i.d. are more specifically antidepressant in the elderly demented patient. For excitement, insomnia or agitation small doses of the phenothiazines may be helpful. Patients in their senior years may already have some extrapyramidal disease and the phenothiazines may aggravate this. Unfortunately, while the antiparkinsonian drugs can be used quite successfully in many cases, they can provoke an atropine psychosis.

6) In all instances, patients should be encouraged to do as much as they can for themselves. Regression is always a danger and is not only destructive to patient's continued functioning but also further frustrates, depresses and angers those close to them.

7) Food and vitamin intake should be monitored, perhaps with the help of daily weighings, and supplementary vitamins provided. Patients who are mildly demented and neglect their diet or abuse alcohol can develop additional cognitive changes.

8) There are several other considerations in the management of patients who are demented and deteriorating. These include:

    a) recommending soft diets or tube feedings in the latter stages when swallowing may be impaired

    b) physiotherapy to improve a patient's functional capacity

    c) recommending use of a writing pad to patients who are not aphasic but because of a process involving muscles find it difficult to speak

    d) supportive devices for weakness of feet, hands, neck, etc.

    e) anticonvulsants for seizures

    f) antispasmodics for muscular spasms

    g) antiparkinsonian drugs for extrapyramidal dysfunction

    h) antibiotics for infection

    i) custodial care when the family can no longer care for the patient by themselves

9) Hydergine and drugs reported to increase cerebral blood flow

and improve neuronal intermediary metabolism have been used with varying success in patients with dementia secondary to degenerative brain disease (Gaitz, et al. 1977; Yesavage, et al. 1979).

DIGITALIS TOXICITY

Digitalis preparations are one of the most widely prescribed medications and one found most frequently to be at toxic levels. Studies indicate that as many as 35% of medically hospitalized patients on the drug are at toxic levels (Shear and Sacks, 1978). Cardiac arrythmias is the most serious side effect but anorexia, nausea, vomiting, diarrhea and visual and other CNS disturbances are also frequently found. The visual disturbances include chromatopsia (i.e. objects appear to have yellow-green edges or tints), scotomas, hazy vision and flickering halos. Psychiatric complications include restlessness, agitation, malaise, fatigue, delirium, hallucinations, illusions, delusions and irritability. Distractability and labile mood have also been reported. These changes are seen more frequently in the elderly. Chronic obstructive pulmonary disease (COPD), pneumonia, and congestive heart failure also may cause an organic mental syndrome and either confuse or complicate the picture. Digitalis delirium is often a harbinger of the more serious and potentially lethal side effects of digitalis.

DISULFIRAM TOXICITY

Disulfiram (Antabuse) is used in the management of well-motivated patients with alcohol dependence to prevent sporadic unconsidered drinking. The disulfiram alcohol reaction consists of the rapid onset of diaphoresis, facial flushing, hypotension and tachycardia after an individual who is on disulfiram drinks or is otherwise exposed to alcohol. Disulfirum alone, however, has a toxicity that is felt to be due to the biochemical and histopathologic effects of disulfiram and its three major metabolites: diethyldithiocarbamate, diethylamine, and carbon disulfide (Rainey, 1977). Clinicians should be aware of these symptoms and signs so that they are not confused with other clinical syndromes such as schizophrenia.

Symptoms

1) Delirium
2) Lethargy

3) Loss of libido
4) Psychosis
5) Depression

Signs

1) Unilateral weakness
2) Meningeal signs
3) Peripheral neuropathy
4) Optic neuritis

Differential Diagnosis

1) Disulfiram toxicity
2) Manic-depressive illness
3) Schizophrenia
4) Other neurological and psychiatric illness

Management

1) Reduction of the dose of or complete cessation of the disulfiram will usually bring about amelioration of the symptoms.

DISULFIRAM AND ALCOHOL

1) Disulfiram (Antabuse) interferes with the metabolism of alcohol in the body. As a result of its interaction, the level of blood acetaldehyde begins to rise. Symptoms appear within 15 minutes to 1½ hours after ingestion.

2) Individual response to alcohol varies among people taking disulfiram. Some show very little response to the ingestion of a considerable amount of alcohol, while others respond dramatically to very little.

3) The typical response after a small amount of alcohol is unpleasant and includes:
    a) a sensation of heat over the face
    b) sweating
    c) facial flushing
    d) bloodshot eyes
    e) throbbing headache
    f) tachycardia
    g) nausea
    h) vomiting

   i) dyspnea
   j) apprehension
   k) hyperventilation
   l) hypotension
   m) sleepiness
High doses of alcohol may lead to coma and death.

4) Some individuals on disulfiram are so sensitive that exposure to fumes of substances containing alcohol (e.g. rubbing alcohol) may set off a reaction.

5) The treatment of a disulfiram reaction involves:
   a) antihistamines
   b) having the patient lie down if hypotensive
   c) if shock is present, the usual means of treating circulatory collapse such as intravenous fluids, and levarterenol (Levophed).

6) The usual maintenance dose of disulfiram is 0.25–0.50 gm daily.

7) Its use is contraindicated in patients with psychoses, cardiac disease, diabetes, cirrhosis, epilepsy, organic brain syndromes, nephritis, psychosis and in pregnancy.

8) Those who advocate the use of disulfiram feel that the unpleasant symptoms that follow alcohol ingestion will reduce the amount of impulsive drinking.

GILLES DE LA TOURETTE'S SYNDROME

Gilles de la Tourette's syndrome is described as a triad of explosive vocal utterances, tics, and imitative phenomena.

History

1) Patients with this rare disease give a history of explosive involuntary utterances, either in the form of obscenities (coprolalia) or inarticulate noises such as yelps, grunts, coughs and barks. These may be accompanied by sudden involuntary movements including vulgar gestures (copropraxia) and both verbal and behavioral imitative phenomena (echolalia and echopraxia).

2) Diagnosis is based on the presence of coprolalia or the more rarely occurring copropraxia.

3) The disorder occurs more frequently in males than in females.

4) Onset usually occurs before age 7 with an age range of 2 to 18 years.

5) The course is usually progressive with waxing and waning of symptoms, but arrest may take place at any stage.

6) The disease is not believed to result in psychoses or any mental or neurological deterioration.

Symptoms

1) The first symptoms are usually uncontrolled, often explosive, in the area of the head, neck, and shoulder girdle.

2) These may progress to include movements of the upper extremities, shoulder and chest. Lastly, if at all, the lower extremities may be affected.

3) The movements tend to be brief and explosive.

4) After several months or even years, the vocal tics become apparent and consist of obscenities or inarticulate sounds.

5) Sometimes the coprolalia or verbal tics may be the presenting symptom.

6) Imitative phenomena are often seen such as echolalia and/or echopraxia.

7) Stress, anger, excitement and fatigue may increase the intensity of symptoms while fever, relaxation, sleep and drowsiness bring about improvement.

Signs

1) Sudden involuntary movements.

2) Explosive involuntary utterances and imitative phenomena.

3) The pathognomonic feature is the uncontrolled repetitive utterances of obscenities. The abnormal movements are *not* associated with a paroxysmal dysrhythmia on the electroencephalogram.

Differential Diagnosis

1) Gilles de la Tourette's disease
2) Syndenham's chorea
3) Schizophrenia
4) Encephalitides such as encephalitis lethargica
5) Wilson's disease
6) L-Dopa toxicity

Management

1) The treatment of choice is haloperidol given in a dosage of 2

mg–10 mg per day. Dosage is regulated by disappearance of symptoms or the occurrence of severe side effects of the drug and therefore much higher doses than 10 mg may be tried.

2) Antiparkinsonian medication should be given to counter the extrapyramidal side effects of haloperidol.

The symptoms and signs of Gilles de la Tourette's syndrome resemble the movement disorders seen as a side effect of L-dopa therapy. Interestingly, while its etiology still remains veiled in mystery, the disorder is treated by haloperidol, the most potent dopamine blocking agent currently available.

GRIEF

It is normal and expected following a loss, expected or unexpected, that an individual mourns. Erich Lindemann, in his landmark paper on the history of crisis intervention, described in 1944 the course of bereavement in relatives of those who died in the catastrophic Coconut Grove nightclub fire in Boston. His findings indicated that those individuals who were most stoic in their adjustment to death are eventually most affected by it. Mourning is a necessary and important part of psychological adjustment to the loss of a loved one. Encouragement of mourning and support for grief during the first three months following loss has been demonstrated empirically to lower post-bereavement morbidity (Raphael, 1977). It is only when mourning becomes melancholia that grief becomes pathological and psychopharmacological, somatic (e.g. electroshock) and/or more specific psychotherapeutic approaches become necessary.

History

1) The first step in evaluation of individuals whose response to tragedy is interfering with their functioning is a determination of the nature of the loss as well as the circumstances surrounding it. If a friend or relative died, what was the cause of death (e.g. a car accident, suicide, cancer, homicide)? Who was present when the patient died (e.g. spouse, children, lover as opposed to spouse)? What was the relationship of the patient to the deceased? How frequently did they see each other? Was there any sexual involvement? Did the patient argue with the deceased before his or her death?

2) The way an individual has managed loss in the past is a good

predictor of how it will be handled in the present. If there is a past history of loss, how did the patient deal with it?

3) Information should be obtained as to the degree to which the loss will alter an individual's life. Will their income decrease? Are there outstanding business obligations? Debts? Medical bills? Funeral costs? Is there a Will or will there be a delay in settlement of an estate because of the absence of a Will? Is it going to be necessary for an individual to sell his home or a family business? Is there tension among family members over the inheritance?

4) The absence of grieving at the time of a loss does not invariably mean that an individual will subsequently develop a pathological grief reaction, but many who do not express grief at the time of a death, do later develop symptoms of pathological grief.

5) Normal grief should be differentiated by history and symptoms from depressive reactions of psychotic proportions and abnormal grief. Normal grieving does not usually extend much beyond 4 to 6 weeks.

Symptoms of Normal Grief

1) Restlessness
2) Guilt with feelings of not having done enough for the deceased
3) Preoccupation with the image of the deceased
4) Self-blame
5) Inability to organize daily activities
6) Hostility toward the doctors and other medical professionals who attended the deceased
7) Insomnia
8) Irritability
9) Appetite loss
10) Somatic symptoms such as headache and diarrhea

Symptoms of Abnormal Grief

1) Panic attacks
2) Taking on the symptoms of the last illness of the person who died
3) Imprudent business transactions
4) Apathy
5) Personally destructive behavior
6) Agitated or retarded depression
7) Overactivity without a sense of loss
8) Increased use of alcohol or drugs

Management

1) Allow the patient to ventilate his or her feeling of loss in a supportive atmosphere.

2) Help to identify and to complete necessary tasks at the time of a death such as preparation for the funeral, burial, and settling of the estate.

3) Relatives and friends should be encouraged to stay with the bereaved during the first few days after a loss. If it seems indicated, suggest that a relative or friend move in with the bereaved or that the bereaved stay at a relative's or friend's house for a few days.

4) Sleep medication may be required for the first few nights following a loss. A small dose of a benzodiazepine such as flurazepam hydrochloride (Dalmane), oxazepam (Serax), diazepam (Valium) or chlordiazepoxide (Librium) is usually sufficient.

5) Assess suicide risk. If this is significant and the patient is without social supports to reduce risk, he or she may have to be hospitalized.

6) Evaluate the use of alcohol and other drugs. Some individuals first develop alcoholism or drug abuse in an attempt to self-medicate the pain of a loss and the anxiety of living alone and redirecting the course of their life.

7) If grieving extends beyond the usual course (i.e. 4 to 6 weeks), the need for antidepressant medication should be assessed.

8) Common sense is the best guide for care of individuals during the immediate few days following a loss. Friends, relatives and familiar clergy should be encouraged to help take care of the patient and help to "people" the empty space created by the loss. The patient should be provided with good and tasty food and helped out with mundane household tasks.

GROUP HYSTERIA

Sometimes after a personal or collective tragedy such as a death, rape or fire, a number of individuals may present bereaved to a psychiatrist or other health professional in an emergency room. It soon becomes apparent what has happened, but unlike the evaluation of an individual alone in crisis, evaluation and treatment of a group of stressed individuals is more difficult. There may be much crying, anger, hostility and hopelessness. At times some may give evidence of psychophysiologic responses such as fainting. The group may be composed of all members of one family, all tenants of one building that burned, or some other combination like two families—one of a murdered girl, the other the family of her murderer (who was also her husband). As the members of the group continue to interact there is sometimes a spiraling increase in symptoms.

Symptoms and Signs

1) The symptoms predominating in the group are often those of one or two key persons. When the key person screams, others scream in a way in which one might assume there is competition to see who will be the most vocal. When a key person cries, others may follow suit. If one faints, others comparably may faint.

2) The overt display of emotion seems to vary from one subculture to another. Some ethnic groups such as the Puerto Ricans allow a much greater display of grief than others such as Anglo-Saxons who may be cautioned by a relative to keep a "stiff upper lip."

Management

1) The key figure or figures should be separated out from the rest of the group, evaluated, and treated, using the crisis intervention approach to therapy.

2) Calmer supportive family members, friends and community leaders, such as the family's clergy person (minister, priest or rabbi), should be called upon both to help in the management of the acute crisis as well as to make them aware of the family or group's need for support during the critical period.

3) If an individual has died in the emergency room friends and family members should be allowed to see the body before it is taken to the morgue. This is best done by having an aide take a few people at a time to view the body, then have them go on home, and another few brought in until all have seen the body.

4) Offering coffee or another beverage sometimes calms a family faced with a crisis.

5) In some cases oral antianxiety agents may be necessary such as 10–25 mg of chlordiazepoxide (Librium) p.o. or diazepam (Valium) 2–10 mg p.o. to take the edge off the anxiety.

6) Sleep and good food are simple considerations often neglected in the management of bereaved patients. Those less directly involved with the deceased, but supportive and interested as friends of a bereaved person should be encouraged to either stay with him if he

lives alone, or invite him over to their own home, and/or prepare some food for him. It may be necessary to prescribe a sleep medication such as flurazepam (Dalmane) 15–30 mg or benadyne 50 mg q hr p.o. for 1 to 5 days.

HALLUCINOGEN HALLUCINOSIS, DELUSIONAL SYNDROME AND AFFECTIVE SYNDROME

Hallucinogenic drugs include lysergic acid diethylamide (LSD), mescaline, 2,5 dimethoxy-4 ethyl-amphetamine (STP), diethylhyptamine (DET), psilocybin, and dimethyltryptamine (DMT). Phencyclidine (PCP), marijuana and its active ingredient tetrahydrocannabinol (THC), hashish, nutmeg and atropine-like substances such as Angel's Trumpet are also sometimes referred to as hallucinogens, but differ structurally from those discussed in this section and are, therefore, considered separately. Most hallucinogens are structurally related to catecholamines (e.g. mescaline) or to serotonim (e.g. lysergic acid diethylamide).

History

1) Frequently, but not always, individuals presenting with a hallucinogen hallucinosis will give a history of having taken a hallucinogen by name (e.g. mescaline, DMT) of "dropping acid," of "taking dope" or of having eaten morning glory seeds, nutmeg, cactus buttons or other substances with hallucinogen properties.

2) The effects of many hallucinogens are difficult to distinguish clinically. Stimulants such as cocaine and methedrine may be added to provide a kick. Strychnine is also sometimes added and may result in serious medical consequences including death.

3) Morning glory seeds and nutmeg (myristica) are readily available in food stores and garden shops and produce symptoms of psychosis if ingested in sufficient quantities.

4) The symptoms of a hallicinogen hallucinosis generally occurs in a state of full alertness.

5) The symptom picture represents an interaction of:
    a) a given drug
    b) the dosage taken
    c) the duration of action
    d) the effects of other drugs the individual has taken concurrently or which adulterate the hallucinogen
    e) the rate of onset of the drug

    f) the user's premorbid personality and physical health

    g) the expectations of the user

    h) the setting in which the drugs are taken

6) Hallucinogen users unlike most schiozphrenics or individuals toxic with sympathomimetic substances or atropine-like drugs are frequently aware that what is happening to them is the effects of a drug.

7) Low doses of hallucinogens will create a clinical picture resembling cannabis intoxication and may be mistaken for it.

8) Prolonged psychosis following hallucinogen use may relate to a genetic vulnerability to schizophrenic or affective illness. The fact that several hallucinogens are indole derivatives (e.g. LSD, DMT, DET and psilocybin) or catecholamine derivates (e.g. mescaline) raises the possibility that the psychosis may reflect a particular vulnerability of central serotonergic or catechol neuronal symptoms to the biochemical stressor (Bowers, 1977).

9) Onset of symptoms generally begins within one hour of ingestion. The typical hallucinogen hallucinosis resolves in 4 to 16 hours untreated, but may last as long as two to three days.

10) Organic delusional syndromes or affective syndromes that persist beyond the period of direct effect of the hallucinogen used are referred to as hallucinogen delusional syndromes and hallucinogenic affective syndromes.

Symptoms

1) Distortions of body image
2) Kaleidoscopic and other visual hallucinations
3) Synesthesia (e.g. a sound produces a sensation of color)
4) Increased vividness of both real and fantasized sensory perceptions
5) Confusion
6) Visual illusions
7) Alteration of mood, often in the direction of euphoria, but depression may also occur
8) Pseudohallucinations (appearance of geometric figures and forms which the patient knows are not real)
9) Increased distractability
10) Impaired judgement
11) Paranoia
12) Anxiety sometimes of panic proportions
13) Fear of going crazy
14) Lability of mood
15) Feeling of having special insights or religious experiences

16) Blurring of vision
17) Depersonalization
18) Derealization
19) Difficulty expressing thoughts
20) Hyperacusis
21) Distortion of time such that everything appears to be happening more slowly
22) Over-attention to detail
23) Auditory hallucinations (rare)
24) Tactile hallucinations (rare)
25) Palpitations
26) Violence to self or others (rare)

Physical Signs

1) Dilated reactive pupils
2) Sweating
3) "Gooseflesh"
4) Slight increase in body temperature
5) Tremors
6) Slight increase in blood pressure
7) Tachycardia
8) Incoordination

Differential Diagnosis

1) Hallucinogen hallucinosis, delusional syndrome or affective syndrome
2) Atropine-like drug intoxication
3) Sympathomimetic intoxication
4) Other toxic organic states
5) Acute schizophrenic episode
6) Exacerbation in chronic schizophrenia
7) Micropsychotic episode in a patient with borderline personality
8) Mania

Management

1) The level of some hallucinogens may be detected in the serum if the appropriate assay equipment is available.

2) The patient should be placed in a well-lighted, quiet, nondistracting room away from disturbing noises and intrusive people.

3) Reassure the patient that he is not becoming insane, but that the alterations in his perception is due to the drug he took.

4) Help orient patients by mentioning where they are, the day and the time. This process may have to be repeated several times and is referred to as "talking down" the patient.

5) Have a close friend or relative, if available, stay with patient to support, to avert and to keep them from harming themselves or others.

6) If sedation is necessary, diazepam 20–40 mg, may be given followed by 10 mg q hour until calm. Alternately, an equivalent dose of another benzodiazepine may be utilized.

7) If a patient is particularly disturbed, haloperidol may be given. There have been reports that administration of chlorpromazine is not safe with STP and as the exact nature of the offending drug may not be known, a benzodiazepine is preferred and any antipsychotic given only with caution.

8) If psychosis persists, the possibility that the patient was psychotic prior to hallucinogen use should be considered and the psychosis treated appropriately. Contaminant drugs, and underlying predisposition to psychosis or hysterical character features may contribute to prolongation of psychotic symptoms. It is, of course, also possible, although not proven, that an hallucinogen may cause biological changes in the brain that result in a more enduring psychosis.

9) Lack of response to medication or to "talking down" within 6 to 16 hours may necessitate hospitalization.

10) It should be understood if a patient is medicated that the symptoms may return after the effect of the medication wears off and the patient presents a risk to himself or others. Therefore, if a patient is not hospitalized following a bad trip, care should be taken to assure that the patient is with another person such as a family member, lover, or friend. This person should be charged with the task of staying with the patient for 24 hours and to provide the prescribed medication if symptoms reemerge and to return the patient to the emergency room if needed.

HALLUCINOGEN FLASHBACKS

Flashbacks are recurrences of symptoms experienced by the hallucinogen drug user long after the original experience or experiences.

History

1) Flashbacks are usually brief, lasting only minutes and signifi-

cantly attenuated in intensity. When they do last longer or are more intense they can be quite frightening and confused with the micropsychotic episodes experienced by some individuals of borderline personality makeup

2) Flashbacks may occur after one or several episodes of hallucinogen use.

Symptoms

1) Intense panic
2) Intensification of colors
3) Visual illusions
4) Synesthesias
5) Pseudohallucinations
6) Paresthesis
7) Depersonalization
8) Derealization
9) Intense loneliness
10) Depression sometimes to near or actual suicide proportions
11) Paranoia

Physical Signs

None.

Management

1) Flashbacks are usually self-limited and do not require any treatment other than reassurance.

2) Ten–20 mg of diazepam or the equivalent dosage of another benzodiazepine can be given if there is an excess of anxiety at the time of recurrence.

3) If there is considerable depersonalization or derealization or psychotic symptoms, such as paranoia, an antipsychotic such as 5–10 mg of thiothixene or 50–100 mg of chlorpromazine should be given.

4) The patient should be instructed to avoid all further hallucinogen use including marijuana.

5) Persistance of flashback or intensification of symptoms may require extended neuropsychiatric evaluation to rule out an insidious organic process or more severe psychopathology.

HOMICIDAL AND ASSAULTIVE BEHAVIOR

The term "violence" denotes a spectrum of self- and other-destructive behavior. Self-destructive behavior ranges from suicide to more subtle forms of damage to one's personal integrity, such as tendency to repeated accidents ("accident proneness"), drug abuse and alcohol addiction. Other directed violent behavior spans from careless automobile driving to robbery, assault, rape, manslaughter and homicide. On the whole, such behavior is extremely difficult to predict although there are some factors which have been identified that characterize those who behave violently. In this section, homicidal and assaultive behavior will be discussed.

History

1) Ex-mental patients have not been demonstrated to be responsible for any more crime than those without a history of psychiatric treatment. In fact, Cohen and Freeman (1945) reported that the incidence of violent crimes or of any crime is much lower among former psychiatric patients than among the general population. Previous psychiatric hospitalizations and diagnoses are therefore not necessarily indicants of violence.

2) The majority of murders are committed by a relative of the victim or by a person acquainted with the victim. Comparably, the majority of aggravated assaults occur within a family, among neighbors or among acquaintances.

3) Age is related to violence with almost 80% of violent acts performed by those under fifty years, in one study.

4) Those who are most likely to be violent tend to have histories of previous criminal activity. More explicitly, violent behavior is most frequently found to occur by people who have a number of previous arrests, have a juvenile police record, or have a history of a conviction for a violent crime. The more severe the original offense, the greater the likelihood of future violence.

5) Those who are violent as adults have a higher incidence of self-mutilation and other self-destructive behavior. While in psychiatric practice, wrist cutters tend to be women, two-thirds of wrist cutters with police records are men (Bach-Y-Rita, 1974).

6) As children, adults who go on to commit violent acts tend to be impulsive and stimulus seeking. History taking may reveal that they set fires. In addition, their home life is often characterized by violence or deprivation.

7) Individuals who live in subcultures characterized by excessive violence tend to be more inclined to violent acting out at times of stress.

Signs

1) Shouting
2) Display of weapons (There should be a weapon control policy)
3) Threatening talk
4) Pacing
5) Shaking fist
6) Shooting
7) Knifing
8) Chair swinging
9) Acid throwing
10) Pounding fist
11) Slamming door

Diagnosis

The first task of a psychiatrist evaluating a potentially violent person is to attempt to get some indication of its cause. Etiology directs treatment. If a patient has a thought disorder characterized by common hallucinations telling him to kill his mother, he requires psychiatric hospitalization and antipsychotic medication. If he does not accept this plan, medical commitment would be necessary both to protect the relatives *as well as* the patient. Those who take extreme civil libertarian views often fail to recognize that medical commitment not only has evolved legally to protect society from the violent patient, but also to protect the patient from the consequences of his own uncontrollable behavior. Patients who, while psychotic, destroy their family's and friend's property, as well as threaten them with, or actually commit, violent assault, destroy the social supports which may be needed to help them function after their aberrant mood swings or delusional ideation is corrected with appropriate antipsychotic agents.

Differential Diagnosis

1) Temporal lobe epilepsy
2) Explosive personality
3) Acute organic mental syndrome secondary to drug intoxication such as PCP and amphetamine-induced psychoses

4) Paranoid states
5) Schizophrenia, especially paranoid schizophrenia
6) Catatonic excitement
7) Alcoholic intoxication
8) Antisocial personality
9) Uncontrollable violence secondary to interpersonal stress (e.g. domestic quarreling)
10) Other organic states (e.g. cerebral neoplasia and other space-occupying lesions, infections, or chemical lesions involving primitive centers in the brain)
11) Decompensating obsessive compulsive neurosis
12) Dissociative states
13) Homosexual panic
14) Side effect of barbiturate, tricyclic or benzodiazepine therapy (Rampling, 1978)
15) Social maladjustment without manifest psychiatric disorder

Management

The approach to treatment of all patients with other destructive behavior is analogous to that of suicidal behavior after initial diagnosis.

1) Does the patient need to be hospitalized? If he needs to be hospitalized, will he go voluntarily, or does he require medical certification? What type of milieu will be necessary to contain his behavior? Will he need a locked ward or individual 24 hour surveillance? The answer to all these questions rests on a clinical judgement as to what the evaluating psychiatrist feels patients are likely to do, given their past medical and psychiatric history, what patients say they will do, what patients have done recently, patients' moods and quality of thought and perceptions, and the patients' social situations.

2) If the decision is not to hospitalize, appropriate family members and/or friends should be made aware of the risk to their lives. Those at whom violent behavior might be directed, or who know a violent patient well, should be made aware of what behavior changes will necessitate immediate hospitalization. For example, a mother plagued by obsessive homicidal thoughts toward her child that cause her anxiety may be managed outside the hospital as long as she has good impulse control. But if the anxiety begins to diminish and her control begins to disintegrate, she will have to be hospitalized.

3) Medication should be given when indicated. If patients have

clear-cut thought disorders with command hallucinations telling them to kill their own brother, they should be given antipsychotic medication just as should any patient with paranoid ideation. If they are in catatonic excitement, tranquillization will be needed. Episodic outbursts of violence may respond to a trial of lithium carbonate. If the history is more suggestive of seizure disorder, an evaluation should be performed on an inpatient or outpatient basis dependent upon the nature of the violence. If studies prove positive, anticonvulsants should be commenced. Treatment of other organic states may involve other medications or, as in the case of PCP and amphetamine-induced psychoses, simple conservative measures may lead to resolution of behavior aberrations. Typical medications used as chemical restraints are sodium amytal (125–375 mg IM), Valium (15–45 mg p.o. or 5–15 mg IV), Paraldehyde (10 cc IM or 8–12 cc p.o.), Haldol (5–10 mg IM or 5–20 mg p.o.), Navane (10–20 mg IM or 15–60 mg p.o.), and Thorazine (50 mg IM or 100–200 mg p.o.).

4) Patients' social supports should be assessed as well as the nature of their home environment. An individual who becomes violent with his spouse may only require a change in living arrangement to a friend or relative. A person who is paranoid and suspicious may be more inclined to act out in a neighborhood characterized by violence and muggings than in one where most individuals are quite law abiding and keep to themselves.

5) Finally, it must be stressed that the great majority of patients who perpetrate violent acts, especially homicide, do not have a psychiatric or medical condition, strictly defined, as the basis for these acts. Some of the individuals have personalities which may be characterized as sociopathic or antisocial. This means that they appear unsocialized and repeatedly come in conflict with the values of society. They are callous, grossly selfish, impassive and unable to feel guilt or to learn from experience and punishment. Their frustration tolerance is low, and they are incapable of significant loyalty to groups, individuals, or to social values. It is unclear at this time whether psychiatry has anything to offer these people which will significantly alter their behavior. In fact, it can be seriously argued that while, as with all human behavior, genetic or early environmental factors play significant roles in the genesis of this behavior, as in *all* behavior, this is not an illness but a style of life or pattern of personality. It may be necessary to protect society as well as these individuals themselves from abuse and fatal consequences by protective confinement. Social factors that contribute to this behavior cannot be dealt with by a psychiatrist engaged in treating psychiatric

emergencies any more than it can be by psychiatry as a profession. It is a challenge facing all contemporary society and one that will not readily yield a simple solution.

6) Unipolar and bipolar illness is felt to be especially high among criminal and unprosecuted offender populations. In one study (Good, 1978), ten percent of the offender population studied was found to have primary affective illness.

7) Violent outbursts should be prevented whenever possible. Staff should be aware of issues and problems and work to minimize the need for chemical or physical restraints. Written policies and procedures should be understood and have been practiced by the staff. Patients should be seen in areas that have adequate space, appropriate lighting, an alarm system, and ready availability to security officers. Self-defense courses may be in order for clinicians working in areas of high crime and predictable violence. The interviewing room should have multiple exits and a minimum of dangerous materials and furnishings that could be used as weapons.

8) If the violence has occurred, the clinician should document any personal or bystander injuries as well as damage to furnishings and equipment. The waiting room attendants and other patients should be approached as to what happened. Staff should meet to review the events in order to see what steps may be taken to avoid future occurrences.

HOMOSEXUAL PANIC

Included in the differential diagnosis of violent behavior is homosexual panic. Contrary to popular belief, homosexual panic does not usually involve individuals who are same-sex oriented but rather individuals who are ostensibly heterosexual who have difficulty integrating their homosexual feelings or activity.

History

1) Homosexual panic usually occurs when an individual with strong latent homosexual drives is placed in a situation such as dormitory or barracks where there is much visual stimulation of homoerotic fantasies or by the physical encounters common to these situations such as playful wrestling. It also may occur when a predominantly heterosexual man is "seduced" or "raped" or finds himself impotent in a heterosexual encounter and feels a desperate

need to prove himself to be heterosexual or bisexual.

2) Individuals in homosexual panic, most often men, feel extremely anxious, agitated, fearful and paranoid. They are intensely fearful of members of the same sex. They may panic and attack if touched and threaten any same-sex person's life who dares to take advantage of them.

3) They may appear to be decompensating and disintegrate into a paranoid psychosis.

4) The psychodynamic basis of the fear and panic is thought to be the emergence of repressed homosexual feelings that are intolerable consciously to the individual. They, therefore, are projected onto other same-sex people. Ideas of reference may develop and the individuals feel that others, rather than themselves, are accusing them of "being homosexual." The individual defends against acting out their feelings by avoiding same-sex people or actually being hostile to them.

Treatment

1) Patients in homosexual panic should preferably be (although this is not always possible) interviewed by someone of the opposite sex in the acute phase. The clinician should be particularly attuned to the intensity of patients' fear and the threat of violence (either self or other) created by the emergence of strong latent homosexual drives.

2) The patient should not be touched other than for routine procedures such as vital signs or a physical examination which should be performed in the presence of another person if done by a same-sex physician. A gentle slap on the thigh can give genesis to a physical attack. Examination of the genitals or rectum should be deferred until a patient has become more integrated.

3) Patients should be reassured and allowed to ventilate about their experience and fears.

4) Exceptionally anxious patients should be given a minor tranquilizer such as 5–10 mg of diazepam orally. Intramuscular injection may be seen as a further attack by a male patient, but if required, should be given.

5) Particularly paranoid or psychotic patients (e.g. those with delusional thinking or hallucinations) should be given an antipsychotic such as 100 mg of chlorpromazine or 5–10 mg of haloperidol or thiothixene orally.

6) Crisis-oriented therapy and medication may not be sufficient for particularly violent patients who may try to defend themselves

from a fantasized sexual assault. These patients may need to be hospitalized for a brief period until their potential for violence is diminished and their paranoia and ideas of reference subside.

HYPERSOMNIA

Feeling excessively tired or sleepy is a common complaint. The cause is usually readily apparent. Individuals with active lives such as college students and those working two jobs or shifts will be more tired and require more sleep. Individuals who are depressed (especially if the depression is part of manic-depressive illness) may be hypersomnic and sleep 12 to 16 hours a day rather than be insomnic. Finally, there are a number of physical illnesses in which increased sleep may be a part. These include narcolepsy, sleep apnea, hypothyroidism, encephalitis, and the Pickwickian syndrome.

History

1) Individuals complain of some form of increased sleep or sleepiness. For some these are isolated episodes. An individual is overcome with an intense irresistable desire to sleep. For others, there is an increased number of total hours of sleep at night. For instance, a patient will report sleeping 14 hours, whereas, 5 months ago he or she only slept 7 to 8 hours. Still others will complain of a constant feeling of exhaustion with a need for napping. The character of the need for increased sleep provides a clue to diagnosis.

2) The setting of the onset of the increased desire to sleep is important. Narcoleptics can fall asleep during activity while typically Pickwickians do not. A person who is depressed or has functional hypersomnia, is generally tired and "washed-out" all of the time.

3) Associate symptoms and changes in behavior should be ascertained. A narcoleptic classically complains of sleep paralysis (episodes either just before falling asleep or on awakening at which time the individual feels awake but unable to move), hypnogogic or hypnopompic hallucinations (vivid visual or auditory hallucinations just before falling asleep or on awakening that seem so real the individual may act on them) and cataplexy (attacks at which time an individual becomes akinetic and falls down while remaining fully awake) in addition to sleep paralysis. Patients with sleep apnea characteristically do not feel rested at night because of airway obstruction and recurrent awakening. Their snoring and sonorous breathing

may be commented upon by those who live with the patient. Attacks of sleep with sleep apnea occur at times when a patient is inactive which differs from those of narcoleptic. Pickwickian's are usually quite large (in excess of 300 lbs. in weight) and have compliance problems with resultant hypercapnia.

4) In the Kleine-Levin syndrome, personality changes are coupled with hyperphagia and hypersomnia. In all instances of hypersomnia, organic causes for increased sleep should be considered. Only in the absence of some intercurrent physical illness or obvious major psychopathology such as manic-depressive illness should a diagnosis of functional hypersomnia be made.

Differential Diagnosis

1) Narcolepsy
2) Sleep apnea
3) Cerebral neoplasia
4) Functional hypersomnia
5) Pickwickian syndrome
6) Seizure disorder
7) Encephalitis
8) Side effects of medication or illicit drug use (e.g. tranquillizers, barbiturates)
9) Hypoglycemia
10) Hypothyroidism
11) Kleine-Levin syndrome
12) Sequelum to cerebral trauma
13) Depression

Management

1) The first step in management of an individual presenting with hypersomnia is taking a careful history and performing a physical examination.

2) In some instances electroencephalograms will be helpful. A patient with a seizure disorder may show a dysrhythmic pattern or even an epileptogenic focus. The sleep EEG of a narcoleptic shows REM sleep as a patient falls asleep and increased REM activity throughout natural sleep.

3) After a diagnosis is made, disposition should be made to the appropriate specialty for treatment. Obviously, an individual found

to have a cerebral tumor should be referred to neurosurgery. Most other sleep disorders are treated by neurologists except when increased sleep is seen as part of an identifiable psychotic disturbance. An exception is the treatment of narcolepsy for which both psychiatrists and neurologists are qualified to manage. Methylphenidate dextroamphetamine, impramine and protriptyline have all been used to manage patients with the narcoleptic tetrad.

4) Individuals with functional hypersomnia usually have histories of rapid sleep onset, prolonged deep sleep (more than 9 or 10 hours), irritability, daytime sleepiness and postdormital confusion. A tendency to worry and depression are also part of this syndrome. Excess stress may lead to the disorder. Methylphenidate or d-amphetamine administered about one-half hour before awakening is usually significant to manage well motivated patients or patients with conscientious family members or roommates who will monitor medication intake. Alternately, imipramine may be used for functional hypersomnia and given at the usual times.

5) CNS stimulants and imipramine have been found to have REM suppressing properties and, therefore, are useful in the management of a number of other sleep disorders such as pavor nocturnus (night terrors), somnambulism (sleep walking) and enuresis (bed wetting).

HYSTERICAL PSYCHOSES

Hysterical psychoses is distinguished from an acute schizophrenic episode by the suddenness of onset and by the dramatic array of hallucinations, derealizations, delusions and bizarre behavior. Hallucinations tend to be visual rather than auditory as seen with schizophrenia. Affect tends to be expansive and effervescent rather than flat or blunted. If there appears to be a disturbance of thought processes, it does not resemble the loosening of associations seen with schizophrenics. The delusions and hallucinations when present are less like that of a schizophrenic adult than like the disturbance of a fearful angry child.

Hysterical psychosis tends to be a response in an individual with the appropriate psychodynamics to an affect laden situation. As anxiety mounts, the patient becomes overwhelmed, distraught and unable to mobilize himself in an integrated manner. After the psychosis runs its course, no chronic disability remains. Hysterical psychosis most frequently occurs in people described as having an hysterical personality with traits such as suggestibility, seductiveness, emotional lability, self-centeredness and vanity. Hysterical personalities tend to be excitable, attention-seeking and dramatic. They are often quite dependent, shallow and superficial. Their thinking pattern tends to be dominated and controlled by their prevailing mood (Cavenar et al. 1979).

Management

A hysterical psychosis is usually ameliorated by judicious use of benzodiazepines, ventilation and crisis oriented therapy. A sodium amytal interview may be helpful if the psychosis is precipitated by a traumatic event which the individual has difficulty discussing.

L-DOPA INTOXICATION, DELUSIONAL STATES, AND DELIRIUM

L-DOPA, a precursor of dopamine, is used in the treatment of patients with idiopathic Parkinson's disease. The amelioration of the symptoms of Parkinson's disease is thought to be mediated by an increase in dopamine synthesis in the central nervous system. It would be expected and in fact is borne out by clinical experience that alterations in mood, thought and behavior would result from use of this drug that resemble a number of clinical states. Mania, depression and schizophreniform psychoses have all been reported. In one series of 88 patients with Parkinson's disease without prior psychiatric symptoms or dementia, nearly half reported psychological changes within a year of treatment (Moskovitz, et al. 1978). These changes included hallucinations vivid dreams, illusions and nonconfusional as well as confusional psychoses. Cessation of the drug or lowering its dosage where possible will generally bring about remission of symptoms. If the dosage cannot be reasonably altered without considerable detriment to the patient, a trial of lithium carbonate has been found in at least one instance to be of benefit (Braden, 1977).

MARITAL CRISES

Crisis within marriages and around the dissolution of a marriage are one of the most common situations confronting psychiatric clinicians in emergency psychiatric services.

History

There are a number of questions that should be asked when one or both members of a couple appear because of a domestic crisis.

1) Is it the first emergency room visit of the couple?

2) What are the events that led up to the presentation at the emergency room?

3) Does either have a past psychiatric history?

4) Is there a personal or family history of divorce?

5) Are there any children? If so, what are their ages? When did they, or are any planning to, leave home? Marry?

6) Is either individual contemplating divorce?

7) Is a third party involved? Has, or is, either partner having an extramarital—heterosexual or homosexual—affair? (Questions regarding affairs should be asked each spouse privately as some who protest vehemently that they would never "wander" or experiment with homosexuality outside of a marriage will be found on tactful questioning to be involved in extramarital liaisons of some duration.)

8) Does either use drugs or alcohol?

9) Has eigher attempted or threatened suicide? Are there fantasies of such? And, if so, how strongly are they defended against?

10) Is the spouse who appears the sicker of the two a symptom "cover" for the other? (e.g. A wife may take an overdose acting out the suicidal preoccupations of her husband or his covert or overt homicidal messages).

11) Does it seem that the latent issue is that one spouse desires hospitalization or commitment for the other? If so, are there clinical indications for this or is it a maneuver to get rid of the spouse temporarily or permanently?

12) Be alert to the usual conflict areas in every marriage. Are and where are the in-laws living? How many children do they want and when? Are there arguments over religious, ethnic, or socioeconomic class differences? How are finances regulated and are they balanced to each other's satisfaction? Has there been a recent loss or attainment of financial security or wealth? Has or is either about to retire? How is discipline of the children handled? Is there child abuse? Have there been any recent entrances or exits from the family system? Are they sexually satisfied with each other?

13) Inquire about physical health and attitude toward age. Has either just turned 50? Is the wife menopausal? Is either seriously ill? Has either had any recent operations? Mastectomy? Prostatectomy? Hysterectomy? Vasectomy? Is the husband impotent? Has either lost interest in sex?

14) Is help being sought for a crisis when one member of union has already independently decided to divorce the other? Have lawyers already been contacted and alternate living arrangements made?

Management

1) After obtaining a good history observe the couple interact. If possible, interview them together as well as independently.

2) Obtain additional information from children, the family physician, or clergy as needed.

3) Consider hospitalization for one if he is homicidal, suicidal, or overtly psychotic. In rare instances it may be necessary or advisable to hospitalize both, either on the same treatment unit or on different units.

4) Attempt to clarify the key issue, but be alert to deceptions, half truths and family secrets when assessing the couple and planning disposition. More than one interview may be necessary to determine the appropriateness of a disposition. Trust may have to be firmly established before the real issues emerge.

5) Gauge the therapeutic intervention to the flexibility of the family system. In some cases ventilation at the time of crisis may be all that is needed. Other situations may require a variety of other approaches including medication, referral to family agencies, referral to AA, and separation, at least during the crisis. One party may be advised to return home while the other stays with a friend or relative. If there has been a heated row and the couple has been brought in by the police but now seem to have calmed down enough to return home, the police may be willing to check on them in a couple of hours to see if the truce has continued.

6) Medication may be needed for sleep or anxiety.

7) If either has been drinking, risk of homicide or suicide increases. If they are truly hostile to each other, help arrange alternate living arrangements.

8) Long-term disposition depends on motivation, diagnosis, and

resources. Private psychotherapy, family services, private marital counselors, legal aid and community mental health center services are all possibilities.

9) If one is depressed and divorce is being contemplated, crisis clinicians should be firm in the recommendation that lawyers be involved early so that one party is not exploited by the other. This is particularly important if children are involved and decisions are being made regarding both their living arrangements and support.

The comments made in the preceding section are not limited to conventional marriages but are also applicable to crisis work with individuals living together in a variety of alternate life styles such as a man and woman who do not wish to marry but live together with/without children or homosexual lovers living together with or without children from a previous marriage, an affair or from adoption.

MEPERIDINE TOXICITY

Meperidine (Demerol) causes both agitation and confusion if its renal clearance is decreased as suggested by elevated serum creatinine levels. Disorientation, hallucinations, visual disturbances, and dysphoria have been reported. Management consists of switching the patient to methadone or some other analgesic of equal potency with fewer side effects.

MINIMAL BRAIN DAMAGE (MBD)

Children as well as increasing numbers of adults are being found to have minimal brain damage. The etiology often remains unclear. Cerebral trauma perinatally, in utero or occult cerebral infections in early childhood, the fetal alcohol syndrome, and transient episodes of anorexia while the brain was developing are a few of the causes posited. The children and adults with MBD are found to be easily distractable. They have a limited attention span and great need for activity (hyperactivity). These individuals are rarely seen first in the emergency room. When they are, however, it is usually because of some delinquent behavior and the clinician finds that rather than a sociopathic or depressed child or adolescent, he or she has discovered an undiagnosed case of minimal brain damage. Hyperactive children are also seen when they develop a sympathomimetic psychosis on the drugs they are taking for their MBD. The usual treatment consists of the use of one of several agents found to have a paradoxically calming effect on these children. These include methylphenidate hydrochloride, dextroamphetamine sulfate and caffeine (Arnold, et al. 1978; Barkley and Cunningham, 1979; Reichard and Elder, 1977; Weiss, et al. 1979). Side effects of methylphenidate have not been found to correlate with dosage in at least one study (Satterfield, et al. 1979). The lack of a simple dose relationship of side effects to the amount of amphetamine-like substances taken has also been observed in adults who take the drug either therapeutically or recreationally.

NITROUS OXIDE

Nitrous oxide or laughing gas is used by teenagers and health professionals such as dentists who have ready access to it to develop a mild euphoria high and light headedness. Younger adolescents may obtain it by using the gas from aerosol cans of whipped cream. Holding the can upright without shaking and pressing the release may allow them as many as 5 to 6 hits. (Block, 1978).

NUTMEG INTOXICATION

Nutmeg, derived from the seeds of the aromatic evergreen, *myristica fragrans*, native to the Spice Islands, is one of the oldest spices in use. The psychoactive substance myristicine is found both in the seed coat and in the oil of the seeds. Individuals seeking an inexpensive hallucinogenic experience may purchase the drug at the spice counter of a grocery store and take it directly or mix it with food. Hallucinations and agitation have been reported when inadvertently a naive person has used inappropriate proportions of nutmeg in preparation of a pie.

Severe headaches, restlessness, visual hallucinations, muscular excitement, numbness in the extremities, palpitations, flushing and changes in time and space perceptions have been reported. Death due to fatty degeneration of the liver has been reported in severe cases of poisoning (Faquet and Rowland, 1978).

OPIATE DEPENDENCE

The distribution of methadone is carefully governed by federal regulations. The practicing physician should be aware of what these are as he is bound to obey them or suffer the penalties. Generally speaking, it is not legal to provide methadone on an outpatient basis, without a license, to maintain and addict. In an emergency situation, *at the time of hospitalization,* it may be necessary to provide a dose to avoid the painful withdrawal symptoms, but the patient must be already hospitalized. The law is *very strict.* The usual mistake made by the novice is providing a sociopathic addict, well aware of the federal laws, a dose on an outpatient basis. In so doing the physicians break the law, opening themselves up to penalties. It is therefore incumbent upon physicians to learn what outpatient, inpatient and other live-in drug treatment programs are available in their community so that when they are confronted with an addict who expresses interest in ending his habit, they may outline what is available, and direct them to the appropriate agency. When patients in early withdrawal present themselves it is usually best to explain the law and the fact that physicians themselves do not make it but are bound to obey it. The physician should then explain what is available, and if the patient wishes to be admitted for withdrawal, arrange hospitalization. If the patient desires an outpatient program, it is good practice to phone the agency and make the contact for the patient by providing his name and some identifying data (with the patient's permission). If it is possible that patients may be seen the same day, they should be sent to the agency immediately to maximize the probability that they will follow through on the referral.

Opiate abuse generally follows or is part of a general pattern of poly-drug abuse which includes use of alcohol, marijuana, hypnotic-sedatives, cigarettes, amphetamine-like substances, hallucinogens and prescription or nonprescription cough syrups. Untreated, most opiate dependent individuals either die before age 40 as a result of their life style, or "mature out" and cease opiate abuse.

OPIATE INTOXICATION

History

1) The signs and symptoms of opiate intoxication as the result of recent overuse of opiates include a number of psychological and neurological signs and symptoms.

2) In the extreme, opiate intoxication can lead to coma and death.

3) The signs and symptoms of opiate intoxication can be reversed by intravenous administration of a narcotic antagonist if irreversible cerebral anorexia has not occurred. Narcot antagonists include nalophine, naloxine and levallorphan.

4) The effect of a single dose of intravenous or subcutaneous morphine peaks at about 20 minutes or one hour respectively and nearly entirely diminishes in 4 to 6 hours. There is usually a "down" feeling after the effect wears off.

Symptoms

1) Euphoria or dysphoria
2) Apathy
3) Drowsiness
4) Reduced visual activity
5) Constipation
6) Analgesia
7) Nausea

Signs

1) Flushing
2) Hypertension
3) Decreased heart rate
4) Decreased body temperature
5) Pupillary constriction (Pupillary dilation may result from severe overdose)
6) Psychomotor retardation
7) Slurred speech
8) Dysattention
9) Memory defect
10) Impairment of judgement
11) Doses of meperidine (Demerol) exceeding 1,200 mg/day can cause psychosis, muscle twitching and seizures.

Differential Diagnosis

1) Opiate intoxication
2) Barbiturate intoxication
3) Alcohol intoxication
4) Hallucinogen hallucinosis

OPIATE WITHDRAWAL

1) The prognosis for successful permanent cessation of opiate abuse in young people is guarded. Many young addicts who present for withdrawal either have been coerced by legal authorities, relatives or friends, or wish to reduce the amount needed to give them a high by withdrawing and recommence their drug use at lower doses.

2) Physicians who are used to working with addicted populations should be aware that many users of heroin are quite sociopathic and will lie about their symptoms and the extent of their habit in an attempt to obtain drugs.

3) In taking a history the physician should ascertain the type of drugs used, the amount used, the time of the last dose, and the duration of use. Additional information should be obtained about the frequency of use, the routes used, the source and the cost. Symptoms and signs of opiate withdrawal may be seen in withdrawal from codeine, morphine, dilaudid, Demerol, Darvon, Methadone and Talwin.

4) Individuals addicted to drugs are prone to certain medical problems that may become apparent during history or physical exam. These include psychiatric illnesses such as schizophrenia or affective illness, hepatitis, tuberculosis and other infections.

5) When a patient has been admitted to an inpatient facility, physical examination should include a pelvic and rectal exam for the presence of hidden drugs. Arms should be carefully examined for evidence of needle marks, tracks (i.e. scarring along the veins of the arms), tattooing over veins, ulcers and abscesses. The nasal mucosa should be checked for erosion and the presence of perforations of the nasal septum. Examination of the needle marks may give a clue to the time of the last injection.

6) Opiate withdrawal may be precipitated by either abrupt cessation of opiad administration after a one- or two-week period of continuous use or by administration of an opiate antagonist such as naloxone or nalorphine after therapeutic doses for as little as 3 or 4 days.

7) It is uncommon for opiate craving to occur after opiate administration for pain associated with physical disorders.

8) Usual withdrawal symptoms from morphine or heroin commence within 6 to 8 hours following previous dose and peak in 2 or 3 days. In 7 or 10 days they have run their course. Withdrawal from meperidine commences within hours after the last dose, peaks within 8 to 12 hours and is over in 4 or 5 days, while withdrawal symptoms

from methadone may not begin for 1 to 3 days and continue as long as 10 to 14 days.

9) Death rarely occurs from opiate withdrawal unless there are attendant medical problems such as coronary heart disease.

10) History and blood and urine analysis should be used to distinguish opiate withdrawal from other substance withdrawal.

Symptoms

1) Anxiety and panic
2) Craving for opiates
3) Myalgia and joint pains
4) Decreased appetite
5) Hot and cold flashes
6) Nausea
7) Irritability
8) Depression
9) Weakness
10) Aggressiveness

Signs

1) Yawning
2) Perspiration
3) Lacrimation
4) Rhinorrhea
5) Pupillary dilation
6) Decreased pupillary reaction to light
7) Pilomotor erection ("gooseflesh," "cold turkey," "kicking the habit")
8) Muscle twitches
9) Fever
10) Increased blood pressure
11) Vomiting
12) Weight loss
13) Insomnia
14) Orgasm
15) Diarrhea
16) Restlessness
17) Tachycardia
18) Increased respiratory rate and depth
19) Tremor

Differential Diagnosis

1) Opiate withdrawal
2) Influenza
3) Barbiturate and other hypnotic withdrawal

Treatment

1) Because of its cross tolerance with a number of opiates, methadone, a long acting oral synthetic narcotic is substituted for the opiate. The patient is then slowly withdrawn from methadone over a week or two.

2) The general basis of this approach is to provide a sufficient amount of methadone in the beginning to control the symptoms of abstinence. Sufficient time is then allowed for detoxification so that there is a gradual reduction in the patient's physical dependence.

3) The minimum time to allow for detoxification of a heroin addict is about one week. If detoxification is attempted more rapidly, signs of abstinence such as muscle and joint pains, insomnia, malaise, gastrointestinal disturbance, and sweating occur.

4) Typically, in the absence of any serious medical problems, the physician usually should wait for signs of withdrawal and then give methadone. Usually 10 mg either b.i.d. or q.i.d. will suffice. Then after giving the same dose for 2 days, the physician begins to cut the dose by 5–10 mg daily. For instance, 30 mg may be given for the first two days, 25 mg on the third, 15 mg on the fourth, 10 mg on the fifth and 5 mg on the sixth and last day.

5) Acute inflammatory or febrile illnesses increase opiate tolerance and the severity of withdrawal symptoms, thus requiring higher initial doses, a longer period of withdrawal, and a greater number of doses (e.g., q.i.d.)

6) Because of the general discomfort occasioned by medical or surgical problems, withdrawal may be of longer duration to minimize any additional stress for the patient.

7) The nurse and physician should check daily for signs and symptoms of toxicity or withdrawal and adjust the doses properly. In no instance should the rate of withdrawal be greater than 20% of the daily dose above 20 mg of methadone per day.

8) Seizures are not usual with opiate withdrawal, unless the patient is addicted to meperidine (Demerol). If they do occur, the physician should suspect that the patient either has a mixed addic-

tion and the withdrawal seizures are due to cessation of another drug such as barbiturates or alcohol, that the patient is epileptic, or that the seizures are hysterical or feigned. The barbiturate tolerance test may be used to corroborate the diagnosis. If there is no evidence of mixed addiction, seizures should be worked up to ascertain their etiology and then appropriately treated.

9) Patients who are intoxicated should not be allowed to smoke in bed unless attended and if they are able to get about, they should have a staff member assigned to accompany them to protect them from injuring themselves.

10) Antipsychotic agents are usually not required to control the patient unless he is psychotic in addition to his addiction.

11) Vomiting is a symptom of withdrawal. However, some patients adequately covered with opiates for withdrawal experience nausea and vomiting coupled with fantasies of getting the "poison" out of the system. Intramuscular trimethobenzamide (Tigan) or hydroxzine (Vistaril) can be used to manage this.

PERIODIC CATATONIA

Periodic catatonia is characterized by the rapid onset and subsequent disappearance of catatonic excitement or stupor. The sudden onset of catatonic symptoms in an individual who is otherwise without manifest psychopathology is felt to be due to a shift from a predominantly cholinergic state to an adrenergic state characterized by salivation, pallor, mydriasis, inhibited peristalsis, tachycardia, increased blood pressure and sleep disturbance. Urinary steroids and catecholamines and their metabolites are often increased.

Management

Lithium carbonate has been proposed to have a specific therapeutic effect (Wald and Lerner, 1978).

PHENCYCLIDINE INTOXICATION, DELUSIONAL STATE AND DELIRIUM

Phencyclidine is a potent hallucinogen. It was originally marketed as Sernylan, a veterinary anesthetic with sympathomimetic properties. In 1978, all legal manufacture was discontined as it was classified as a class II drug under the criteria of the Comprehensive Drug Abuse Prevention and Control Act of 1970.

History

1) Phencyclidine is sold and taken under a number of names including PCP, Angel Dust, Kay Jay, Hog, Pill, Peace, Crystal and Rocket Fall.

2) Ketamine, a structurally comparable anesthetic is still sold. Some individuals have reported adverse reactions to this drug comparable to that reported with phencyclidine.

3) Phencyclidine is a white crystalline solid that may be taken by mouth, snorted, smoked or taken intravenously. Chronic users prefer to smoke it. Oral ingestion is rare among sophisticated users save as a suicide attempt.

4) It is quite easily manufactured in a kitchen laboratory.

5) Phencyclidine may be misrepresented as cocaine, tetrahydrocannabinol (THC), psilocybin, mescaline and LSD or may contaminate any of the above.

6) Phencyclidine's presence in the body can be documented by serum assay.

7) The onset of symptoms is rapid with a bizarre clinical picture that is sometimes confused with schizophrenia. Symptoms can be quite incapacitating and the patients may be at risk of injury to themselves or others.

8) The clinical picture following phencyclidine use seems less dependent on the users personality structure than do the clinical presentations of other hallucinogenic drugs.

Symptoms

1) Thought disorders
2) Hostility and combativeness
3) Tangentiality
4) Ideas of reference
5) Agitation
6) Grandiosity
7) Disorientation
8) Euphoria
9) Depression
10) Body image distortion
11) Paranoia
12) Irritability
13) Suspiciousness
14) Tactile, auditory and visual hallucinations
15) Suicide ideation

16) Negativism
17) Anxiety
18) Paresthesias or analgesias
19) Circumstantiality
20) Disassociation of somatic sensation

Signs

1) Clouded sensorium
2) Constricted or normal sized pupils
3) Elevated blood pressure
4) Hypersalivation
5) Diaphoresis
6) Hyperpyrexia
7) Tachycardia
8) Increased deep tendon reflexes
9) Ataxia
10) Rigidity
11) Myoclonus
12) Psychomotor excitement
13) Mutism
14) Decreased peripheral sensation to pain and touch
15) Decreased position sense
16) Stereotypies
17) Loss of motor control
18) Vomiting
19) Loss of consciousness
20) Nystagmus (at first horizontal than vertical)
21) Hiccoughs
22) Muscle spasticity
23) Hyperacusis
24) Tachypnea

Differential Diagnosis

1) Phencyclidine intoxication
2) Other hallucinogenic intoxications
3) Amphetamine and other sympathomimetic intoxications
4) Schizophrenia
5) Mania
6) Encephalitis

Management

1) Phencyclidine intoxication is always considered serious until proven otherwise. Medical consultation should be sought if there is any question of a medical complication or a change in status for the worse.

2) The measurement of phencyclidine in the urine, serum or gastric contents, requires chromatographic essay and, therefore, is not practical for emergency diagnosis.

3) Individuals with mild intoxication can be expected to clear in a short while. In these instances, diazepam and minimal stimulation may be all that is required for treatment.

4) In some instances, the psychosis may persist for weeks or be attended by severe medical complications. In these instances, life support measures may be necessary with transferral to an intensive care unit and protection of patients from harming themselves or others. Haloperidol, 5 mg I.M. q one hour as indicated is usually sufficient to handle these patients.

5) Patients who have intentionally or unintentionally taken large doses of the drug may develop status epilepticus and adrenergic crises. Respiratory failure is a late sequelum.

6) Some authors (Rappolt et al. 1979) divide PCP intoxication into three stages for treatment. In Stage I, the patients are conscious but disoriented. They may harm themselves or others. In Stage II, patients are unconscious but without other serious medical complications. In Stage III, patients are in adrenergic crisis. Status epilepticus may occur and the patients die of respiratory failure.

a) Stage I Management: External Stimuli are reduced and vital signs monitored. Voice contact is established and some attempt made to talk down the patient. Instrumentation is avoided where possible. Muscles are massaged and diazepam 10–30 mg are given. Cranberry juice and 0.5–1.5 of ascorbic acid are given to acidify the urine and enhance excretion of PCP. If adequate facilities are not available for prolonged observation, the patient will need to be hospitalized. Serum half life in overdoses is 1 to 3 days. Samples of blood, urine and gastric contents are sent for analysis. Patients must be protected from harming themselves or others. Oropharyngeal and bronchial secretions are markedly increased but because laryngeal and pharyngeal reflexes are accentuated, a patient, if necessary, should be suctioned carefully from the corners of the mouth. Propranolol 40–80 mg orally three times a day may be given to protect patients from adrenergic crises. It is said to have both adrenolytic cardiac effects as well as a central calming effect since it crosses the blood brain barrier. Ipecac is contraindicated in all stages because of the risk of convulsions in PCP intoxicated patients.

b) Stage II Management: Patients in this stage are comatose but responsive to noxious stimuli. In addition to the measures taken in Stage I, a patient is sponged and other measures taken to dissipate heat and obviate hyperthermic crisis. Intubation and deep suctioning should be avoided save where absolutely necessary. Intramuscular diazepam, 10-30 mg, relieves muscle spasm and may restore consciousness. Intravenous infusion should be instituted using a large bore cannula and ascorbic acid given in solution by drip. Propranolol is given to minimize or avoid hypertension and tachycardia. Bladder catheterization may be needed as PCP and other sympathomimetic intoxications may be accompanied by retention. Administration of furosemide enhances PCP excretion. As the patient regains consciousness, voice contact is instituted as in Stage I Management and an attempt made to orient the patient and restore functioning.

c) Stage III Management: In Stage III, the intoxicated patient is comatose and unresponsive to deep pain: The overdose may represent a suicide attempt and the possibility of death quite real. The patient is hospitalized, medicated, airway established and every effort made to maintain vital life processes. Fluid is given intravenously and furosemide and ascorbic acid administered in an attempt to hasten excretion of the drug. Anticonvulsants are used as indicated to control seizures. A large bore nasogastric tube is used to flush gastric contents. Temperature is kept down by sponging and propanolol used to titrate hypertensive spikes. Cholinergics should be avoided because bronchial secretions are already in excess.

PHENELZINE-INDUCED PSYCHOSIS

Monoamine oxidase inhibitors are increasingly being used for clearly defined affective illness as well as for heterogeneous groups of disorders of which depression does not appear with neurovegetative signs as part of the clinical picture. This latter group includes "hysteroid" dysphoria, the phobic-anxiety-depersonalization syndrome and atypical depression. Phenelzine has been reported to induce a psychosis in some patients with these disorders treated with the monoamine oxidase inhibitor (Sheehy and Maxmen, 1978). The mechanism may be similar to the psychoses precipitated in borderline patients treated with tricyclic antidepressants and lie at a central catecholamine level.

PHOBIAS

Phobias are characterized by the persistant avoidance of a specific object, activity or situation based on an irrational fear. Individuals with phobias are more commonly seen in outpatient psychiatric clinics or in private consultation than emergency psychiatric services. When seen on crisis units, they are often flooded with anxiety or panic following an encounter or near encounter with the phobic object. Management of the crisis entails ventilation, support and use of a benzodiazepine such as Serax or Tranxene. Longer-term management involves use of one or more of a number of therapeutic modalities including behavioral techniques, tricyclic antidepressants, monoamine oxidase inhibitors and supportive psychodynamic psychotherapy (Jobson, et al. 1978; Zitrin, et al. 1978).

POSTCARDIOTOMY DELIRIUM

Delirium may follow cardiac surgery. The usual sequence is a lucid interval followed by a period of illusions and/or disorientation and at times progression to hallucinations and/or delusions (Heller, et al. 1979). A number of factors have been posited for these changes including:
1) A reaction to the impact of the open heart surgery recovery room in patients made vulnerable by cardiac disease and surgery.
2) Change in the postoperative cardiac index (cardiac output/surface area)
3) Postoperative infection
4) Atelectasis
5) Blood loss
6) Pain
7) Effect of anesthetic agents used
8) Electrolyte imbalance
9) Effect of other medication the patient is on
10) Prehistory psychopathology exacerbated by the surgical trauma

POSTCATARACTECTOMY SYNDROME

The postcataractectomy syndrome refers to the acute changes in mental status seen following cataract surgery. Anticholinergic intoxication is posited as one explanation for the changes (Summers and Reich, 1979). Mydriatic agents have access to the vitreous because of the disruption in the usual ocular physiology. The anticholinergic drug, therefore, can be taken up by the neurons and transported by anterograde axonal transport into the central nervous system and give rise to a central nervous system anticholinergic psychosis.

Signs and Symptoms

1) Disorientation
2) Disturbance of recent and remote memory
3) Delusions
4) Hallucinations
5) Illusions
6) Depersonalization
7) Anxiety
8) Fear
9) Depression
10) Euphoria
11) Increased psychomotor activity

RAPE

History

1) While women will come to the emergency room and state that they were raped, this is not always the case.

2) Some women who have been raped may present with complaints of appetite loss or sleep disturbance. They may be suffering from what is referred to as the "silent rape reaction." Many of these women have been raped or molested in the past, especially in adolescence or childhood, and the current trauma has reactivated early feelings that have never really been talked about and worked through. When given the opportunity, they may talk as much about the earlier incident as about the recent rape.

3) A high index of suspicion that a woman has experienced a previous rape should be entertained when she begins to show signs of increasing anxiety, such as minor stuttering, blocking of associations,

physical distress, and long periods of silence during the evaluation.

4) It is always important to find out what a woman means when she states she has been raped. A histrionic housewife may label a sexual advance by her husband, at a time she prefers not to have intercourse, a "rape." In other instances, a "rape" may be the label attached to an aggressive sexual advance by a husband after a trial separation or a boyfriend after heavy petting and mutual drinking. In other cases, "rape" is clear physical assault in which sexual gratification is not a primary end, but rather a violent act in which sex is a weapon.

5) Men, as well as women, may have been raped and be embarrassed to talk about it. Both men and women can be homosexually raped. Rapists spare no age group. Young children and women in their eighties have been raped.

Symptoms and Signs

Burgess and Holmstrom (1974) describe a two phase reaction to rape: an initial phase of disorganization followed by a phase of reorganization. During the former phase the rape victim's predominant feeling is fear, with notable physical symptoms. There is a reevaluation of her life style during this stage. The second phase, reorganization, usually commences two to three weeks after the attack. During this stage the victim reorganizes her life style, often switching living residence and phone number. Phobias, nightmares and increased motor activity are found during this stage.

In a study of a number of rape victims, Burgess and Holmstrom found in the initial stage either an open expression of emotions such as fear, anger, anxiety through crying, tenseness, smiling, and restlessness, or a more controlled emotional countenance in which feelings appear submerged behind a calm subdued style. Signs and symptoms seen over the course of the first several weeks included:

1) Symptoms resulting from physical trauma such as soreness and bruising of the legs, arms, breasts, thighs and neck. (In women forced to have oral sex, trauma to and irritation of the throat were also noted)
2) Tension headaches
3) Sleep disturbance, including delayed onset and sleep interruption
4) Irritability and startle reactions
5) Stomach pains and appetite loss
6) Vaginal discharge, itching and dysuria
7) Rectal bleeding and pain (in women reporting forced anal sex)

8) Psychological feelings such as fear, anger, revenge, self-blame, humiliation and embarrassment
9) Upsetting dreams and nightmares
10) Increased motor activity
11) Traumatophobia, including fear of outdoors, fear of indoors, fear of being alone, fear of crowds, fear of people being behind them, and sexual fears

Management

1) The immediate psychotherapeutic approach to the rape victim is modeled on the crisis intervention techniques of allowing ventilation and encouraging return to the previous level of functioning as soon as possible. Previous problems are not as important as the current difficulties.

2) If there appears to be a more fundamental psychiatric problem, such as schizophrenia, or alcoholism, which may have led the patient to take the risks that led to her rape, she should be referred for long term therapy for appropriate psychopharmacotherapy, psychotherapy or sociotherapy.

3) Not all patients will want more than the initial opportunity to ventilate their feelings and to receive legal counsel and medical care at the time of their rape. Others, however, may want to return for a few follow-up sessions to talk more about what happened and perhaps also talk about earlier comparable experiences that have been reactivated.

4) To prevent pregnancy, the patient should be offered one of several methods available presently. Methoxyprogesterone or diethylstilbestrol orally for 5 days has been recommended. If menstruation does not commence within one week after cessation of the estrogen, all alternatives, including abortion, should be made available to the patient. If the patient has been using either an oral contraceptive or an intrauterine device, no further treatment should be necessary to prevent pregnancy.

5) The rapist may have had a venereal disease, so the physician should, with written consent, provide appropriate antibiotic therapy. If the patient is not allergic to penicillin, benzathine penicillin G should be given. Alternately, probenecid could be given orally followed in 30 to 60 minutes by intramuscular procaine penicillin or oral ampicillin may be given simultaneously with probenecid. If the patient is allergic to penicillin or to penicillin-like drugs, treatment recommendations are:
    a) oral tetracycline HCl

b) streptomycin I.M.

6) A swab should be taken from the vaginal pool to be saved for the police laboratory to inspect for acid phosphatase, and blood antigen of the semen. In addition, both cervical and rectal cultures should be obtained for gonorrhea and a serology sent off for syphilis. Six weeks later, these tests should be repeated and compared to baseline. Of all the above recommended treatments, only penicillin is effective for the treatment of simultaneously incubating syphilis and gonorrhea, so when an alternate treatment regime is used, there must be a follow-up serology for syphilis.

7) Witnessed written permission should be obtained to protect the physician for examination, for photographs, for collection of specimens, and for the release of information to the proper authorities.

8) The question as to whether or not rape has actually occurred is a legal decision and not a medical diagnosis. Physicians may be subpoenaed to justify their statements. Therefore, for protection of the patient and themselves, they should obtain consent, record the history in the patient's *own* words, obtain the required laboratory tests, record the results of their examination, save all clothing, make no diagnosis, and provide protection against disease, psychic trauma and pregnancy.

9) When constucting rape teams, both men and women should be represented. This serves several purposes. Men, as well as women, are raped and may feel more comfortable discussing the rape with a man. Rape is a violent act and many women have a disinterest or aversion to sexual intercourse following rape. A warm supportive relationship with a man in crisis intervention following a rape allows a woman to separate out the male cum sexual component from the violent physical assault. This helps to immediately desensitize women from seeing men or sex as bad and place the rape in its proper perspective as a brutal violent assault on person and not a male sexual involvement as such. Finally, male members of rape teams are valuable in talking to spouses and fathers concerning their feelings about having had their wife or daughter raped. Husbands and fathers may unjustly see their spouse or daughter as having colluded in the act (e.g. "asked for it").

REFILL REQUESTER

Patients who are unfamiliar to the emergency psychiatric clinician may appear in the emergency room seeking a renewal of a prescription written by someone else. All patients requesting refills for psychotropic medication ordinarily received elsewhere should be seen so that the immediate situation can be assessed. Some patients who have discontinued therapy seek a refill at the time of crisis. The hidden agenda is the need for help, not medication or at least not primarily medication. These individuals should be encouraged to return to the original clinic or clinician who knows their complete psychiatric and treatment history. An attempt should be made to contact the clinic or clinician at the time of the request for renewal of medication to alert them to the patient's problem. The emergency psychiatric clinician should resist any desire to take over the patient's care as this undermines the patient's treatment and reinforces sporadic use of emergency services rather than supporting the continuity of care and commitment to therapy that is needed to provide more long-lasting resolutions of psychological problems. If medication is given, it should be only a sufficient amount to cover the days until the patient's next clinic visit or visit to his clinician.

RESERPINE INTOXICATION

The rauwolfia alkaloids are used clinically for a variety of reasons and, in particular, the treatment of hypertension. Psychiatric uses include the treatment of acute and chronic schizophrenia, mania, delirium tremens and senile agitated states. Reserpine is used experimentally in animals by researchers interested in studying the effect of depletion of catecholamines on behavior.

History

1) In therapeutic doses, resperpine can produce sedation, tranquilization and antihypertensive effects.

2) Small doses of reserpine can produce nightmares and a depression accompanied by serious suicidal ideation. The depression may be insidious in onset.

3) Elderly patients are particularly prone to depression with this drug.

Symptoms

1) Depression
2) Nightmares
3) Suicidal ideation and attempts

4) Decreased libido
5) Lassitude
5) Increased appetite
7) Weight gain
8) Nasal stuffiness
9) Abdominal cramps
10) Symptoms of peptic ulcers
11) Diarrhea
12) Fluid retention
13) Lactation
14) Drowsiness
15) Dizziness

Signs

1) Cutaneous flushing
2) Drooling
3) Extrapyramidal symptoms
4) Hypotension

Differential Diagnosis

The differential diagnosis includes all causes of the depressive syndrome of both neurotic and psychotic proportions.

Management

1) Carefully reduce the dose of reserpine and, if possible, discontinue its use and begin the patient on a suitable alternate drug.
2) These patients can really be quite suicidal and the usual precautions may be necessary to prevent the patient from harming himself.
3) Antidepressant medication or electroshock may be required if the depression is profound and persistent following cessation of reserpine use.

SCHIZOPHRENIA

Early recognition and treatment of a patient undergoing a schizophrenic break can reduce the emotional pain to both the patient and his family as well as reduce or actually obviate the need for inpatient psychiatric care.

History

1) Gradual withdrawal from interpersonal relationships is an ominous sign and especially suggestive of an insidious schizophrenic deterioration in adolescence or in the twenties. A patient may give a history of increasing difficulty at school (which can be objectively quantified by progressively poorer grades) after promise of a sterling academic career.

2) In many instances interest in sex diminishes; in others there may be evidence of increased libido with more time committed to autoerotic behavior (i.e. masturbation) and promiscuous hetero- and homosexual activity.

3) Interests may turn from sports and the mundane to a preoccupation with unanswerable philosophical and religious questions. A previously politically or religiously indifferent individual may become heavily involved in extreme religious or political groups which, in some cases, dynamically appear to represent an attempt to organize the external world while the internal one is in chaos.

4) Decreasing functioning at work manifests itself by an inability to hold jobs or by a gradual constriction of the patient's responsibilities by superiors.

5) Symptoms seen with psychoses of a variety of etiologies may be seen. Ideas of reference, paranoid ideation and hallucinations may be separated historically and the advent of these symptoms may serve to document the time course of the illness.

6) Classically, hallucinations, when reported in schizophrenia, are of the auditory variety although all types can occur and often do.

7) The age of onset of the illness is early, with a peak for admissions to hospitals, of schizophrenics in the age range 25 to 34 years.

8) Family history is always important in providing clues. This is especially true when there exists confusion as to whether a patient is schizophrenic or suffering from an affective disorder. A family history of schizophrenia would incline the diagnostician to think of a thought disorder. Conversely, one should be cautious about diagnosing schizophrenia in a person with a family history of affective disorder.

9) A "schizophrenic" break often appears in retrospect to have been a manic or mixed manic-depressive psychosis.

10) Obtaining a good history from a schizophrenic or his/her family is not always an easy task. The ability to critically evaluate a patient's history is the hallmark of the skilled interviewer. Many patients, when asked the number of close friends they have, will reply "many", "several", or even quantify them (e.g. "10 to 15").

Diagnosticians should then ask the patient to name them even though they themselves will not usually recognize the names. They will be impressed with the hesitation, or even in some instances, the inability to name any at all! In other cases, a person may be named who, when the patient is asked "When is the last time you saw him?" will reply, "Last year," "Several years ago," etc. In other instances, another patient who is incapable of any supportive or close relationship will be named. Sometimes a famous actor or actress or psychiatric aide or a member of a janitorial staff may be mentioned. This again reflects that the patient has few close friends of his own.

11) In the family history, it is important to ask about any member of the family who was "institutionalized," committed suicide, spent long times in a hospital for "nervous reasons" or behaved strangely. When the last mentioned is answered in the affirmative, the patient should be asked what was strange. A mother may have left a family when the patient was 8 and become a prostitute by picking up men or women at bars. The abandonment of the family and rapid change from the previous pattern of behavior would suggest that the patient may have had an undiagnosed schizophrenic parent.

12) Schizophrenics, especially chronic schizophrenics, have significantly more anhedonia than nonschizophrenics (Harrow, et al. 1977).

13) History bears on diagnosis. An insidious onset, impoverished or absent affective component, inability to hold a job, no friends or intimate relationships, no clear precipitant, and a family history of schizophrenia are all associated with a poor prognosis. Good prognosticators include marriage, strong affective component, acute onset, ability to make and maintain close friends, ability to hold a job, a family history of affective disorders and a clear precipitating event. In a study by Carpenter, et al. (1978) constricted affect was the only symptom found in a group of schizophrenics capable of predicting poor outcome. Anxiety, depression and nuclear symptoms of schizophrenia were not.

Symptoms

1) The symptoms originally described by Eugene Bleuler in 1911 in his monumental work *Dementia Praecox oder die Gruppe der Schizopheniem* are still held to be cardinal symptoms of schizophrenia although other symptoms such as those referred to as Schnieder's first-rank symptoms have proven more useful

diagnostically, and more replicable for investigators studying schizophrenics.

2) Bleuler's symptoms included a change in affect. The patients' affects are inappropriate or constricted. They are more concerned with what is going on inside them rather than in the reality of the world about them (they are autistic). Their associations may be loose; that is, their thoughts do not seem to follow logically one upon another; and they are unusually ambivalent. We are all obviously ambivalent about people we are close to, or about what we do; but we weigh pros and cons about a person or choice and arrive at a conclusion, almost in an algebraic manner. For instance, we may dislike somewhat the fact that a friend smokes, but are considerably more impressed by his kindness and consideration toward others and therefore, like him and choose to be his friend. A schizophrenic in his ambivalence is unable to make such a decision and may say "I love you, I hate you, I don't know how I feel about you."

3) More practical for use in the mental status are Schnieder's first-rank symptoms. If a number of these are present, the diagnosis is probably schizophrenia. These symptoms include:

a) Hearing voices arguing
b) Hearing voices commentating
c) Audible thoughts
d) Thought broadcast
e) Thought withdrawal
f) Thought insertion
g) Forced feelings, impulses and volitons

4) Obviously, there are clinical signs such as extreme passivity of schizophrenic patients and their lack of personal rapport with the examining physician which may also serve as guides to diagnosis in some cases, but are not as easy to objectify. The presence or absence of Schneider's first rank symptoms may be determined by the following questions:

a) Do you sometimes hear voices arguing about you among themselves without directly talking to you?
b) Do you hear voices commenting on what you do, think or say?
c) Do you hear thoughts as if others in a room nearby could also hear them?
d) Do you ever feel your own thoughts are being broadcast about you as from a radio so that everyone is aware of what you are thinking?

e) Do you ever feel that your thoughts are being taken from your head, leaving your mind empty?

f) Do you ever feel thoughts are being inserted into your mind which are not your own?

g) Are you ever made to have feelings which you do not believe are your own?

h) Do you ever feel you are forced to want things that you would otherwise not want yourself?

i) Do forces outside yourself make you do or say things that you yourself feel you do not otherwise want to do or to say?

Signs

1) There are, unfortunately, no pathognomonic signs of schizophrenia.

2) As in all cases of an acute psychosis, there are certain non-specific psychophysiological changes which may be observed.

3) Physical examination is most useful in helping to identify one of the symptomatic schizophrenics, i.e. clinical pictures which look like schizophrenia but have a potentially identifiable organic base such as hyperthroidism and frontal lobe tumors. In the former instance, patients may appear acutely excited, anxious, and feel they are going crazy, but also have an elevated resting pulse and other stigmata of an excess of thyroid activity. In the latter instance, there may be a gradual social withdrawal and deterioration of personal habits coupled with an emotional distance or inability to develop rapport often used as a clinical indicant of schizophrenia.

4) Frontal lobe signs such as the grasp reflex, the snout reflex and the palmo mental reflex would suggest frontal lobe disease such as one of the dementias (e.g. Pick's or Alzheimer's disease) or a frontal lobe neoplasm.

Differential Diagnosis

1) Schizophrenic
2) Manic
3) Psychotic depression
4) Alcoholic hallucinosis
5) Pick's disease
6) Frontal lobe neoplasm
7) Idiosyncratic alcohol intoxication
8) Symptomatic schizophrenia

9) Adolescent turmoil
10) Hysterical psychosis
11) Alcoholic paranoia
12) Drug-induced (e.g. PCP, amphetamine) psychoses
13) Steroid psychoses
14) Syphilis
15) Endocrine disease
16) Pernicious anemia
17) Huntington's chorea
18) Alzheimer's disease
19) Temporal lobe epilepsy
20) Schilder's disease
21) Arteriosclerotic brain disease
22) Senile degeneration of the brain

The symptomatic schizophrenias, as mentioned earlier, include those illnesses of organic nature which may present a clinical picture of schizophrenia. Of the toxic states, amphetamine and phencyclidine psychosis are remarkable in their resemblance to schizophrenia. Amphetamine psychosis may arise after as little as a single dose of amphetamine. There is no impairment of orientation, or memory, nor any alteration in the level of consciousness. Visual hallucinations may be absent and a marked delusional system may be manifest. Auditory hallucinations and feelings of thought control or audible thoughts may be part of the picture of chronic intoxication. The presence of amphetamine in the serum urine supports the suspicion of an amphetamine psychosis although a patient undergoing an acute schizophrenic break may have also taken amphetamines. Recovery generally occurs rapidly following withdrawal from the drug. Chronic alcoholic hallucinosis resembles chronic amphetamine psychosis. The character of hallucinations in alcoholic paranoia are often auditory.

A variety of cerebral lesions may present like schizophrenia. Temporal lobe tumors, like temporal lobe epilepsy, may be accompanied by symptoms suggestive of schizophrenia such as feelings of impending doom, déjà vu, derealization, depersonalization and aural phenomena. Cerebral syphilis may present as a number of schizophrenic syndromes, including acute paranoid episodes and catatonia. Tumors of the frontal lobes as well as of other areas such as the brain stem and diencephalon resemble schizophrenia. Endocrine dysfunction can cause behavioral alterations and for this reason routine thyroid function studies and electrolyte studies should ideally be obtained. Cerebral trauma should also be ruled out and evidence of head injury should be sought. Degenerative diseases that resemble schizophrenia include Huntington's chorea and Schilder's disease. In the early stages of Huntington's chorea, paranoid features may predominate the clinical picture. Deficiency states such as pernicious anemia may also mimic schizophrenia when central nervous system involvement is present. Schizophrenia with a late onset (called paraphrenia by some) may be confused with a senile or arteriosclerotic psychoses. If an individual has been anxious and is taking phenothiazines, there may occur an intensification of the anxiety to apparent psychotic proportions with or without a need to pace. Oral or intramuscular benztropine mesylate (Cogentin) should reduce this feeling if it is caused by a phenothiazine. One should be careful in making the diagnosis of schizophrenia when there is a strong family history of affective psychoses. An affective disorder may present with schizophrenic-like symptoms in adolescence, and like adolescent turmoil is often difficult to distinguish from schizophrenia. A history of affective disorder in first degree relatives lends support to the diagnosis of a manic-depressive psychosis. A severe weltschmerz should make one suspicious of schizophrenia, especially if it has lasted for several months without remission.

Management

1) There are a number of treatment approaches to the management of an acutely psychotic patient which are nonspecific in nature which can be generalized to the management of all acutely psychotic patients (Anderson and Kuehnle, 1974). The principle tasks that should be achieved in an emergency situation are:
    a) Ascertain whether there are signs of delirium
    b) Determine whether a patient is homicidal, suicidal, or severely depressed
    c) Determine the amount of social support present
    d) Determine whether a psychosis will clear substantially with medication in 4 to 6 hours
    e) Ascertain whether the remission of symptoms continues over several days
2) Admission to an inpatient unit for evaluation and treatment is indicated if there are signs of a delirium. In addition, if a patient is seriously suicidal or homicidal, if no viable social supports are present, if the psychosis does not clear with the use of high-potency antipsychotic chemotherapy, or if a remission obtained does not persist longer than a few days then the patient should be hospitalized.

3) The clinician should always aim to manage a patient outside the hospital. This reduces the stigmatization of hospitalization and counters the regressive tendency so often encountered in patients undergoing a psychotic break. In addition, it reduces the cost of treatment to the patient and the pessimism often felt by the patient's family. The ability to choose the proper antipsychotic medication and use it in the dose and for the duration needed obviates many hospitalizations. In addition, it allows the clinician to work with the patient and his family or other social supports in the community in which the patient ultimately must function to survive.

4) History and physical examination supplemented by data from friends and relatives should help exclude delirium.

5) Special care should be given to clues to endocrinopathies, seizure disorders, head injuries, cardiopulmonary disease, nutritional disorders, renal and hepatic disease, electrolyte imbalances, and to a history of alcohol, drug or poison ingestions.

6) Physical examination is usually possible although at times sedation may be needed.

7) High potency antipsychotic drugs which produce little sedation and is less likely to confuse the picture than the more sedating drugs such as barbiturates and chlorpromazine. Five–10 mg of intramuscular haloperidol is recommended. Vital signs should be routinely obtained on all psychiatric patients seen in emergencies and force the clinician to explain abnormalities such as an elevated pulse rate, or temperature. The diagnosis of hyperthyroidism would be much less frequently missed if the diagnosis was included in the differential of all patients with elevated pulse rates. Evidence of trauma should be sought and the fundi observed for evidence of increased intracranial pressure. Signs of meningeal irritation and of focal neurological dysfunction must be sought.

8) A psychiatrist should be able to evaluate the cranial nerves, motor, cerebellar and sensory function and reflexes. Certain signs have localizing value such as the Babinski, grasp, sucking, glabellar, snout and palomental reflex. If there is evidence of Wernicke's disease with oculomotor palsies, ataxia and the amnesic-confabulatory syndrome (Korsakov's psychosis), it would be necessary to give thiamine hydrochloride and large doses of other B vitamins immediately. Evidence of a tremor, asterixis, or aphasia should also be recorded.

9) Identification of an acute or chronic organic mental syndrome is usually obtained by careful mental status examination. Disorientation to time and place are often intact in considerably disturbed manic or schizophrenic patients, while those with organic mental syn-

dromes show deficits. In the latter, recent memory is usually impaired. The character of hallucinations is also helpful. Olfactory and visual hallucinations are more suggestive of organic disease, while auditory hallucinations are more frequent with schizophrenia.

10) The last step in the evaluation of an acutely psychotic patient is the assessment of suicide and homicide potential and the nature of the social supports. Moderately suicidal patients may be managed in outpatient therapy if they have a very supportive family or circle of friends. A mildly suicidal patient without any supports may have to be hospitalized even if outpatient follow-up is available. Command hallucinations in schizophrenics and depressives are ominous even if the patient does not report feeling destructive to himself or others. It should be remembered that persecutory delusions always increase risk. Paranoid patients becoming fearful may either attempt to "defend" themselves from the "persecutors" or to escape from them by a potentially self-destructive route, e.g. jumping out of a window.

11) The presence of a family alone does not mean that a patient has a viable social matrix. Families must be willing to recognize the seriousness of patients' illness, be truly interested in their welfare, and be willing to take some responsibility in them. If medication is needed, they must be able to guarantee that they will take it; if they become unmanageable or more depressed and less communicative of their intents, they must be willing and able to bring them back to the hospital. Even with the best intentions, families may have an unconscious need to deny the seriousness of a patient's condition and the extent of his potential for violence. In other instances, there may be an unconscious desire to have the patient commit suicide and they may neglect to observe him or ensure that he takes the medication. They may, in their ambivalence, fail to insist that he follow through on a recommendation for outpatient care. This neglect may unconsciously represent a desire that he either end his life or become so psychotic that he has to be hospitalized.

Initital Management Of Acute Schizophrenic Patients

1) Anderson and Kuehnle (1974) feel that good initial treatment is based on an awareness of:
    a) the constant risk of self-destructive, or other destructive behavior in the acutely psychotic patient, regardless of the immediate physical or social constraints.

b) the fact that acute psychosis is a painful state to the individual, and delay in treatment is not a humane alternative.

c) that delayed treatment may lead to chronic changes in behavior (although this has not been proven as yet).

2) The high potency antipsychotic agents such as trifluoperazine (Stelazine), haloperidol (Haldol), fluphenazine (Prolixin), and perphenazine (Trilafon) are preferred in emergency situations. The dosage of perphenazine when given intramuscularly is 5–10 mg and of haloperidol 5–10 mg. This may be repeated in one-half an hour if agitation persists. Fifty mg of chlorpromazine may also be given intramuscularly, but it is more sedating than the higher potency antipsychotics and tends to cause more hypotension.

3) Sedation itself is often not as important as the antipsychotic effect and sedation may confuse the picture in some cases. Hypotension is less frequently seen with the piperazine phenothiazines and haloperidol. If a patient is able to take medication orally, it is the preferred route.

4) The initial oral dosage for a mild to moderate schizophrenic psychosis of commonly used antipsychotics is:

100 mg chlorpromazine (Thorazine) q.i.d., or
100 mg thioridazine (Mellaril) q.i.d., or
8 mg perphenazine (Trilafon) q.i.d., or
5 mg trifluoperazine (Stelazine) q.i.d., or
5 mg fluphenazine (Prolixin) q.i.d., or
5 mg thiothixene (Navane) q.i.d., or
2 mg haloperidol (Haldol) q.i.d.

5) The choice of antipsychotic agent should be based on how much sedation is desired (chlorpromazine is much more sedating than the piperazine), how a patient responded to a drug in the past (Was he allergic? Did he respond better to butyrophenone [Haldol] than he did to a phenothiazine?) and the extrapyramidal and other side effects. If the patient is moderately or severely schizophrenic, much higher dosages may be needed, especially in the acute stages and for sleep:

e.g. Perphenazine (Trilafon) 16 mg p.o.q.i.d. and 8–16 mg q one hour until sleep

e.g. Chlorpromazine 200 mg p.o.q.i.d. and 100–200 mg p.o.q. one hour until sleep

6) Side effects such as hypotension and extrapyramidal dysfunction should always be monitored. In addition to severity of illness and the presence of side effects, age and weight consideration should determine the dosage used.

7) If there is some question that the medication is not being swallowed, the liquid form may be given.

8) In the acute stage, it may be necessary to repeat the dosage every hour until improvement occurs. For example, 5–10 mg of haloperidol may be given every hour until a patient's symptoms decrease, or they fall asleep (up to about a total of 60 mg). If fluphenazine is given intramuscularly, the hydrochloride should be used rather than the enanthate or decanoate which is long acting (10 to 14 days) and cannot as easily be titrated in an emergency situation.

9) In all instances of use of the major antipsychotic agents—the phenothiazines, the thioxanthenes, and the butyrophenones—extrapyramidal changes may occur. The question, therefore, is whether or not to give an antiparkinson agent prophylactically.

10) If using the piperazine phenothiazines, the thioxanthenes, and butyrophenones in doses sufficient to keep down a psychotic process, we recommend giving an agent such as benztropine mesylate (Cogentin), 0.5–1 mg t.i.d. or q.i.d.

11) Even though in many instances the use of an antiparkinson agent may not be necessary, when extrapyramidal effects do occur, they are quite frightening to someone already terrified of the chaos within. After a few weeks, the antiparkinsonian agent could be withdrawn to see if it is really needed.

12) The antiparkinson agents, like the phenothiazines, have anticholinergic properties; therefore, they increase blurriness of vision, constipation, dry mouth, etc.

13) If a dystonic reaction occurs, 50–100 mg of diphenhydramine (Benadryl) or 1–2 mg of benztropine mesylate can be given intramuscularly.

14) There is no significant increase in onset of action when benztropine mesylate (Cogentin) is given intravenously.

15) If there is little or no improvement in major schizophrenic symptomatology after six hours of the above plan of treatment, the patient should be hospitalized.

16) A number of new antipsychotic agents have been introduced and are reported to have specific advantages to recommend them. Clozapine, belonging to the dibenzazepine group, is said to be low on extrapyramidal side effects and have strong anxiolytic and hypnotic properties. Hypotension, hypersalivation and sedation are its more common side effects (Shopsin, et al. 1979). Molindone has a central anorexigenic effect with a weight reducing property (Gardos and Cole, 1977). Penfluridal is said to show an overall low incidence of side effects (Lapierre, 1978).

CATATONIC SCHIZOPHRENIA

The critical feature of catatonic schizophrenia is a marked psychomotor disturbance coupled with other features of schizophrenia. The disturbance in motor activity may take the form of rigidity, stupor, posturing or excitement. In some instances, stupor may alternate excitement.

History

1) Catatonic schizophrenia, like schizoaffective schizophrenia, has a relatively good prognosis. This is especially true if the onset is acute, if there exists a clear precipitating factor, and the patient has functioned well socially and at work prior to the onset.

2) The usual age of onset is between fifteen and twenty-five years of age.

3) Catatonic schizophrenia is now relatively uncommon.

4) If a patient has had several catatonic episodes, either of excitement or stupor, the course of the illness may take on the characteristics of other forms of schizophrenia with a more permanent alteration in psychosocial functioning. Sometimes one sees a spontaneous remission without any treatment. Remission, in fact, may occur overnight.

5) Before the introduction of electroshock therapy and the widespread use of phenothiazines, catatonic stupor often lasted as long as several months. Without psychiatric intervention, catatonic excitement can result in death.

Signs

1) Waxy flexibility (flexibilitas cerea): This term refers to the tendency of mute catatonic schizophrenics to allow their bodies to be molded into position, sometimes positions that are extremely uncomfortable. For instance, one such patient in a crowded big-city emergency room was thought to be in a coma. After an extensive medical evaluation including vital signs, medical and neurological examination, chest and skull films, CBC, blood glucose, BUN, creatinine, electrolytes, calcium, phosphorus, liver function studies, blood alcohol, toxicology screen and EKG, all of which were negative, it was discovered that she had a previous psychiatric history, and in fact, had previously presented mute. The patient's arm and legs were maintained in positions which looked most uncomfortable. Each finger could be placed in a position which was still main-

tained 10 minutes later. It is important to remember that such patients retain awareness during this state despite their ostensible "coma." Later they may recount all that was said by examining medical and psychiatric staff.

2) Catatonic excitement: Catatonic excitement may occur with or without alternating episodes of stuporous behavior. Excited behavior in catatonic schizophrenics is differentiated from manic episodes in manic-depressive illness by its more bizarre and regressed character. Self-destructive and assaultive behavior may be part of the clinical picture.

3) Stupor: Very difficult to distinguish from coma in the absence of a psychiatric history, catatonic stupor is characterized by the nearly total absence of any movement. Saliva may flow from the patient's mouth, and they are often incontinent and unresponsive to most stimuli. It may be necessary in extreme cases to feed, dress and take over the toilet and bathing care of such patients.

4) Mutism: Loss of speech may occur for days or months in catatonic schizophrenia. In some cases the mutism may be episodic. Some of these patients will respond only monosyllabically.

5) Characteristic schizophrenic thinking may also be observed especially in patients who have had several episodes or who have family histories of schizophrenia.

6) Stereotypes.

7) Negativism.

8) Mannerisms.

Differential Diagnosis

Physical examination as with the other forms of schizophrenia serves the primary function of ruling out organic causes for the stupor or excited behavior. The differential diagnosis is that of other forms of schizophrenia. In particular, catatonic stupor may be confused with the numerous other causes of coma, all of which could occur in addition to schizophrenia. Catatonic excitement resembles toxic states. Both stupor and excitement can be part of an hysterical psychosis. Catatonic-like symptoms have been reported as a side effect of high potency neuroleptics (Gelenberg and Mandel, 1977; Brenner and Rheubon, 1978).

In this latter instance, cessation of the neuroleptic medication and use of amantadine have been reputed to alleviate the symptoms. Periodic catatonia, thought to be due to a rapid switch from a predominantly cholinergic state to an adrenergic state, is discussed elsewhere in this book.

Management

1) Catatonic schizophrenics need careful supervision because of the risk of exhaustion, starvation, and self or other injury.

2) The treatment approach is identical to that discussed under acute schizophrenic episode, with a heavy emphasis on a careful differential diagnosis being elaborated and followed through. In an emergency situation treatment intervention such as electroshock, tube feeding, and personal care are not immediately relevant. In addition to appropriate doses of antipsychotic medication, these are part of a long term treatment program. Some catatonic patients, both excited and mute, respond quite rapidly to intramuscular antipsychotic medication. If excited, chlorpromazine 50 mg every ½ to one hour may be required, but blood pressure and pulse rate should be carefully followed. Alternatively 5–10 mg of haloperidol can be given at hourly intervals. Even though the risk of hypotension is significantly less, blood pressure and pulse should still be monitored. Response to treatment is sometimes dramatic.

PARANOID SCHIZOPHRENIA

Paranoid schizophrenia tends to have a later age of onset than other subtypes and has greater stability over time. Paranoid schizophrenics tend to be less disorganized and less acutely psychotic than catatonic or hebephrenic schizophrenics.

History

1) Paranoid schizophrenics may have a history of being in treatment, although if their delusions are well compartmentalized, they have often remained outside psychiatric care for months or even years. If they have been in treatment, history often reveals that they have stopped their medication and become psychotic.

2) Frequently, the delusion of paranoid patients revolves around the idea that someone is trying to control them. Insistence that they continue to take medication obviously corroborates this delusion.

3) The onset of the illness is usually in the fourth decade.

4) Paranoid patients often seem more intelligent than patients with other sub-types of schizophrenia. The complexity of their delusional systems frequently reveals how they brought their intelligence to bear on the problem of organizing their world as the chaos in their mind increases.

5) Deterioration may occur over time although it is usually not

as severe as in forms such as hebephrenic.

6) While such patients have a poor prognosis as to complete permanent remission of symptoms, they often can maintain some level of functioning in the community and more contact with reality than in the dementia praecox type.

7) Premorbid personality is often one of coldness, suspiciousness, aloofness, resentfulness and distrust.

Symptoms

1) A marked delusional system usually more persecutory in nature and more organized than in other schizophrenic conditions. The content of the delusions may be persecutory, grandiose or jealous.

2) Ideas of reference.

3) Feelings that others are trying to control their thoughts, wills or bodies.

4) Feelings they or others are giving off electric or other sources of energy to control others or themselves, (e.g. a patient may feel his sex is being changed by magical powers).

5) Delusions of grandeur may exist alone or in combination with persecutory delusions.

6) Auditory hallucinations, (e.g. Voices may be calling the patient a "faggot").

7) The patient's suspiciousness and ideas of reference may lead to violent behavior. This may be other-directed and take the form of antagonistic, aggressive and even homicidal behavior if the patient feels others are after him to bring him physical harm or to sexually abuse him.

8) If there has been deterioration over time, the delusions may be less systemized and other signs of schizophrenia may dominate the clinical picture such as apathy, mannerisms, preocccupation or incoherence.

9) Nihilistic and other depressive and somatic delusions are not infrequent.

Obviously, not all of the above symptoms are always present, nor are those present of the same degree. Personal history and cultural factors appear to influence the character of the predominant symptoms as with all schizophrenic syndromes. Individuals from strongly guilt-inducing religions may have predominating religious delusions of personal destruction. An individual from a highly technical subculture may present with the belief that electric or cosmic beams from outer space are being used to control his behavior, or a machine located elsewhere in the city is being used to control his thoughts.

Signs

As with the other schizophrenic syndromes, physical examination is helpful in ruling out the symptomatic schizophrenias such as syphilis and amphetamine or PCP toxicity. In the former, there may be a variety of other diffuse and localizing neurological signs including the classic pupillary changes (i.e. a pupil which accommodates but does not respond to light). In the latter, one may observe tachycardia and pupillary dilation. In a study by Freedman and Schwab (1978) only one half of those who were admitted to a general hospital psychiatric ward with paranoid delusions were found to have paranoid schizophrenia. A significant number had affective illness or organic mental syndromes. A clinical sign of paranoid schizophrenia frequently mentioned by seasoned clinicians is the patient's tendency to wear dark glasses. This supposedly seems to mask his own identification and allows him to watch others who may be "talking about" him or "plotting" to seduce or otherwise harm them. It is unwise to perform a rectal examination or to examine the genitals of a paranoid schizophrenic without proper precautions because of the frequent homosexual fears. Such action may be misconstrued as a homosexual assault and the patient might then take violent action to counter the "attack."

Differential Diagnosis

The differential diagnosis of schizophrenia in general is presented in an earlier section. Obviously, a change in mental status could be due to physiological dysfunctioning. Both psychiatrists and internists may forget that schizophrenics are more prone to physical injury as well as to drug or alcohol abuse. Therefore, a change in a chronic paranoid schizophrenic's clinical status could be due to a physical injury such as subdural hematoma. Paranoia can also result from a transient decrease in blood flow to the brain secondary to a cardiac arrhythmia. Alcoholic paranoia and hallucinosis may be mistaken for paranoid schizophrenia. Some authors, in fact, feel that those with a genetic or psychological predisposition to schizophrenia are more prone to develop these states with chronic alcohol abuse. Amphetamine and PCP-induced psychosis is especially worthy of mention here to remind the reader that these syndromes can perfectly simulate paranoid schizophrenia. It may occur after as little as one large dose. The physiological signs of sympathetic hyperactivity (e.g. tachycardia, pupillary dilation) are not always present. Cocaine toxicity is very comparable in its presentation to amphetamine psychoses. Nasal perforations may be present from "snorting" cocaine.

Management

1) The treatment is as outlined in an earlier section. The first consideration again is whether or not the patient need be hospitalized. If he is suicidal or homicidal, has an acute toxic psychosis superimposed, or lacks sufficient social supports, they should be hospitalized. A toxic psychosis can in some circumstances be treated in an emergency room. In addition, an emergency room setting allows a 4–6 hour trial of aggressive medication. If a patient responds to medication, it may be possible to follow him on an outpatient basis, at first by brief daily contacts, and then by the initiation or resumption of a weekly treatment appointment. If response to medication is equivocal, the clinician may wish to give the patient a 3–5 day trial on an outpatient basis. If symptoms do not remit, hospitalization then would be necessary for medication stabilization.

2) Paranoid schizophrenics are extremely difficult to manage on medication expecially when they are acutely psychotic. Taking medication may be seen as an attempt to control or of trying to poison them. In reality, of course, the medication does represent an attempt to control the patient's symptoms. However, if this is mentioned by the patient, it may be explained that we are trying to help the patient control the symptoms so he has the freedom to act without his psychotic thoughts dominating his existence. If medication is refused, intramuscular medication may need to be given to prevent violent assaultive behavior. In addition, paranoid patients, if left unmedicated, may also kill themselves in an attempt to escape their persecutors. If they feel trapped in a room, and fearful of assault, they may jump out of a window. Long term psychotropic management in a reliable patient may necessitate use of long acting fluphenazine (e.g. Prolixin Decanoate or Enanthate).

3) In dealing with such patients, it is necessary to be as flexible as possible. However, a psychiatrist should be prepared for a show of force. Once the diagnosis becomes apparent patients' families and/or security guards, or other available hospital or clinical staff should be alerted if there is a need. The door of the clinician's office should be kept open. If patients appear particularly fearful, it may be better to interview them in the lobby or waiting room.

4) External stimulation should be minimized. Beepers and other

paging systems may be seen as modes of control, and the voices or other electronic stimuli misconstrued. The clinician should talk calmly. If a clinician is given due cause to be angry he should attempt to control it as any direct expression of it may provoke patients to assault.

5) Patients should not be touched. Be genuine and real. Long silences should be avoided as well as questions about sex, and, in particular, homosexual experiences and thoughts.

6) Medication should first be offered orally, preferably in a liquid form so patients can't "cheek" it and absorption is quicker. If patients refuse oral medication, then the intramuscular route should be used. Sufficient help should be summoned if there is any hesitation on the part of patients to accept medication.

7) If patients have command hallucinations, (i.e. voices telling them what to do), or if very fearful of harm coming to them by an external agency they should be hospitalized because of the high homicidal and suicidal risk in such cases.

CHRONIC SCHIZOPHRENIA IN EXACERBATION

History

1) Generally speaking, recognition of chronic schizophrenia in exacerbation is somewhat easier than that of an acute schizophrenic break by the fact that patients usually have a history of psychiatric treatment and often repeated hospitalizations. Their relatives may, in fact, know the diagnosis, and a family history often reveals relatives who are schizophrenic, have been hospitalized, have committed suicide, or were known for their "unusual ways." When asked what is meant by "unusual" the psychiatrist may be told, "Oh, he dropped out of college and went off to study mysticism in India and never returned." If there is a question of what a patient's previous diagnoses may have been, they should be asked, as should their relatives, as to what treatment was given. If the patient previously received the high doses of phenothiazines, thioxanthenes, or butyrophenones, schizophrenia is suggested, although, if they have functioned extremely well between episodes and have a family history of affective disorder, they may have been given the drugs for mania. Lithium carbonate suggests a cyclic mood disturbance which may have been part of the picture of manic-depressive disease. Lithium, however, is also given for schizoaffective schizophrenia or other disorders with a phasic pattern.

2) Sometimes a clear precipitant will be identified such as a recent death, divorce, sexual encounter, drug experience, job loss or change in social supports. Other times, the patients may have simply stopped their medication. This may have represented an unconscious need to be hospitalized or become psychotic at a time of stress. There is little evidence to support any notion that verbalization of this interpretation, however, will lead to acceptance of it by the patient and alteration of medication-taking behavior in the future.

3) Early signs of a psychotic decompensation include:

    a) Increasing sleep disturbance

    b) Increasing social withdrawal

    c) Increasing difficulty at work or school

    d) A need for more medication such that patients begin to take one or more extra pills

    e) Increasing paranoia with ideas of reference

    f) Increasing concern with religious and philosophical problems

    g) Increasing grandiosity

4) When a patient decompensates, the pattern of breakdown frequently follows that of previous breaks. This is true of both recurrent schizophrenic episodes and recurrent depression or mania. If a patient began to spend more time in empty churches while missing work with his first break, he may, as he relapses, begin to spend more time in empty churches or be absent from work again.

5) In other instances, patients who are obviously schizophrenic by history may have survived for years in a well structured and minimally stressful environment. The intensity of their psychotic symptomatology may be due to an accumulation of a series of undesirable life events and losses in the face of minimal coping ability. This is frequently seen in patients from compromised socioeconomic circumstances who lack both the internal adaptive ability ("ego strength") and external economic or political or social power to cope with the stresses of their environment. These patients may have long histories of an inability to make or maintain friends, hold jobs over sustained periods of time, or even care for themselves in habits of personal hygiene. Their affect often appears blunted or flat. They appear to be without drive and incapable of investing emotionally in anything. They may be laborers or prostitutes or members of other marginal groups. Sexual life is impoverished for many and their hetero- or homosexual acts represent a futile attempt to make contact with the world rather than represent any real closeness. Decision making is difficult, and, if married, they seem to float in a role fairly well-defined by society.

Symptoms

Chronic schizophrenics in exacerbation may present with any of the range of symptoms seen with a schizophrenic break. If their history, however, is more consistent with simple schizophrenia, a clinician may be less impressed with florid symptomatology than with the presentation of an extremely passive and disorganized individual who is unable to make decisions or care for him-/herself even at the most rudimentary level. The spectrum of symptoms and signs seen in, but not necessarily restricted to, schizophrenia include:

1) Disturbance of thought, perception, and speech
   a) Hallucinations
   b) Disturbance of body image
   c) Neologisms
   d) Delusions
   e) Concrete thinking
   f) Paralogical thinking
   g) Ideas of reference
   h) Vagueness in thinking
   i) Withdrawal
   j) Fusion and loss of ego boundaries
   k) Magical thinking
   l) Preoccupation with mysticism and philosophy
   m) Incoherence
   n) Symbolism
   o) Blocking
   p) Overinclusive thinking
   q) Word salad
   r) Verbigeration
   s) Mutism
   t) Echopraxia and echolalia
   u) Suggestibility
   v) Fragmented speech
   w) Hypochondriasis
   x) Ambivalence
   y) Depersonalization and derealization
   z) Thought broadcasting
   aa) Thought withdrawal
   bb) Thought insertion
   cc) Delusions of being controlled
2) Disturbances of affect
   a) Paucity of affect
   b) Inappropriate affect

3) Disturbances of behavior
   a) Negativism
   b) Stupor
   c) Waxy flexibility
   d) Mannerisms
   e) Catatonic excitement
   f) Stereotypies
   g) Deterioration of activity
   h) Conative disturbance
   i) Impulse disturbance (e.g. homicidal and suicidal behavior)

Signs

1) The signs of an exacerbation of a chronic schizophrenic process are like those of an acute one and include much of what is listed above. Whether these are signs or symptoms which a patient or family complain about, is semantic. Strictly speaking, mannerisms, excitement, waxy flexibility, mutism, and the like are "signs" in that a patient does not complain of "mutism" or "waxy flexibility." None of these are, however, pathognomonic and physical examination is more important for the identification of signs suggestive of a symptomatic schizophrenia superimposed upon a patient with a documented thought disorder.

2) It is always important to remember that an original diagnosis may have been incorrect, and the patient may have a degenerative disease such as Huntington's Chorea or Schilder's disease. In addition, another process may be active in addition to schizophrenia. A patient may have contracted syphilis which has gone untreated. Schizophrenics in past times were more likely to contract tuberculosis in crowded state mental hospitals, and the alteration in behavior may be due to a tuberculous meningitis or tuberculoma. Alcoholic or epileptic schizophrenics are more inclined to trauma and may have a subdural hematoma causing what appears to be an exacerbation of their schizophrenia. Finally symptoms reported by schizophrenics are more likely to written off as hypochondriacal. Thus a neoplastic process, either primary in the brain or metastatic, may be overlooked.

Differential Diagnosis

The differential diagnosis of schizophrenia is discussed in a previous section.

Management

1) The first step in treatment is the same as for an acute psychotic break of any nature. An organic process presenting as schizophrenia must be ruled out. The quality of a patient's social supports should be assessed, and the risk of homicide or suicide evaluated. Initial response to medication should be observed to see if a patient can be managed outside the hospital.

2) If patients are in treatment, their therapists should be called. Calling therapists serve several purposes.

a) Therapists can provide information as to what was transpiring in therapy (e.g. Was termination being discussed?).

b) Therapists may be able to provide other information such as which and how much medication might be needed to manage the patient.

c) Therapists may be able to identify the precipitant from their knowledge of patients and their histories.

d) Therapists may be aware of social manipulations which may allow patients to be handled outside the hospital.

e) Therapists may have names and addresses of relatives or friends who may provide an alternate disposition if it is felt that a patient should not go home, but still is not sick enough for hospitalization.

f) Therapists may come in or speak to the patient on the phone, which may be sufficient to calm the patient down.

g) Therapists should be alerted to any contemplated change in medication, and given an opportunity to participate in a decision to hospitalize.

h) Therapists and their patients should set an appointment to meet together soon after the emergency room visit (if the patient is not hospitalized).

i) Assessment of the *real* suicidal or homicidal potential may only be possible if a therapist who knows the patient well is given the opportunity to place a current threat in the context of the patient's history and what is known about previous attempts, gestures, and threats.

3) An evaluation should be made of why the patient is psychotic at this time. Is there an intolerable situation at home, work, or school that he wants to get out of? Was there a recent loss, move, job change or other change in social matrix which has compromised his ability to cope? Is it an anniversary of a parent's death or other significant date such as the time a woman would have given birth if she had not been aborted? Is the exacerbation simply due to a reduction

or discontinuation of medication by him or his therapist? Has he just changed therapists or terminated therapy? Even something as ostensibly simple as discontinuation of medication may have been motivated by an unconscious need to be rehospitalized by an intolerable situation such as completion of college and facing the job market, or a marriage.

4) Critical to the outpatient management of chronic schizophrenics be it during a crisis or at other points during the trajectory of their illness, is a knowledge of the efficacy of all the major groups of antipsychotic medications, the antidepressants, and the antianxiety agents. Schizophrenics in exacerbation usually need more medication during crisis as well as an increase in their daily dosage for some time after. This is not to belittle the importance of sociotherapeutic interventions at times of crisis such as family or couples therapy. However, it is difficult to engage a grossly (or even moderately) psychotic patient in any meaningful therapy until their psychosis is under control. An acutely psychotic chronic schizophrenic may be given liquid medication orally on an emergency basis such as 16 mg of perphenazine, 100–200 mg of chlorpromazine, 100–200 mg of thioridazine, 5–10 mg of haloperidol or 5 mg of fluphenazine. If they are unwilling to take the medication, 5–10 mg of haloperidol can be given every hour intramuscularly up to about 60 mg without the fear of the hypotensive risk associated with chlorpromazine use. Chlorpromazine 50 mg intramuscularly may be given if sedation is desired, but blood pressure and pulse rate should be monitored very carefully, i.e. recorded before it is given and at regular intervals after. This should be done with all intramuscular medications, but one should anticipate problems associated with chlorpromazine. In addition, perpherazine (5–10 mg) or fluphenazine (5 mg) may also be given intramuscularly. Additional medication should be given for sleep during the acute episode as with the first acute schizophrenic episode. For example:

    a) chlorpromazine 100 mg p.o. qlh until asleep

    b) perphenazine 8 mg p.o. qlh until asleep

5) Medication should be continually reevaluated during the acute phase until the appropriate amount is arrived at which then may be given in divided doses during the day and at bedtime. Alternately, the clinician may give all the medication at bedtime. Antidepressants may be added if there exists a strong depressive character to the illness, but this should be done by the patient's therapist, and not in an emergency situation. Chlordiazepoxide may be given in divided doses for anticipatory anxiety. Whether or not an antiparkinsonian agent should be given concurrently with an antipsychotic agent depends on the amount and the particular agent

given, as well as a patient's current and past history of need for these agents.

6) Psychiatric clinicians should discuss with patients and, when indicated, their families, the importance of continued medication and involvement in therapy. If there exists particular signs which foreshadow a decompensation or give warning of increased risk of suicide or homicide, these should be identified, and articulated, and the route to hospitalization outlined. Namely, who should be called? Where could he go? A patient's insurance and eligibility for a veteran's hospital should be known. If violent or suicidal, and the patient protests hospitalization, how can he be hospitalized? Ambulance crews cannot legally bring patients to the hospital by force when they have not been committed or are not under arrest. If a patient's family finds it impossible to bring a patient into the hospital themselves and he is grossly psychotic, suicidal or homicidal, it will either be necessary for a physician to go to the patient's house with the permission of his spouse or parents to evaluate him, or the patient's relatives may need to have him arrested for destroying property or threatening to kill them. If either of these have happened, one can give the police information about his psychiatric history so that he might be brought to the emergency room rather than to jail.

7) A patient's relatives and friends should be instructed as to the continuing need for medication. If a patient has had one psychotic episode, it is not usually good to discontinue medication for one year, although it may be possible to taper the dosage significantly. After two psychotic episodes, it is generally best to wait at least two years, and if there have been three episodes, medication may have to be continued indefinitely.

8) Always use the rule of thumb of *minimal dose for maximal functioning*. Patients and their relatives must be made aware of both the need to keep down the undercurrent psychotic process to avoid regressive rehospitalization as well as the possibility of tardive dyskinesias from long-term antipsychotic therapy. Drug holidays with weekends off or one week a month off may help this. In addition, it may be necessary to switch to another agent if a patient becomes psychotic off medication, but also has developed a tardive dyskinesia with a particular drug.

9) If a patient is unreliable, and cessation of medication quickly results in rehospitalization, a regimen of long acting fluphenazine in the form of Prolixin Decanoate or Prolixin Enanthate may be needed. The dosage to be given every 2 weeks is determined by calculating the total amount of Prolixin that would be given orally over 14 days and then take one-fourth to one-sixth that dose and give it in the enanthate or decanoate form by deep intramuscular or sub-

cutaneous injection. If a patient has not had the medication before, a test dose of 1/10 cc should be given subcutaneously while monitoring blood pressure and general reaction. This is to test both for allergy to the fluphenazine (i.e. Prolixin) as well as to the vehicle (i.e. decanoate or enanthate). If there is no indication of sensitivity after one-half hour, the calculated dose, usually between 25–75 mg, can be given intramuscularly or subcutaneously.

10) The long term treatment approach to any patient with chronic schizophrenia involves an integration of psychotherapy, sociotherapy and psychopharmacotherapy. This includes structuring patients' environment, such as making sure they keep their job, pay their rent and take care of other mundane activities such as eating and bathing. If they are not working and have discontinued medication, this alone may indicate a need for inpatient hospitalization. Such might allow the patient to obtain a job and recommence his medication. If he has had several exacerbations due to a failure to take medication, long acting fluphenazine would be started and the patient's response monitored.

11) Family therapy should also be undertaken in an attempt to help the family become aware of the chronicity of the patient's illness and how they may respond in a way that will promote optimal functioning. Obviously, it is not infrequent to find a sibling or a parent with schizophrenia. This complicates matters for both parents and therapist. All the therapist can do is work with the reality of the family situation if no other disposition is possible, or if other dispositions have been tried, but are nonviable. If other members of the family are healthy it may be possible to explain that despite the fact that the patient appears well on medication, a chronic psychotic process is bubbling along underneath. It may be explained that as little as 20 years ago patients with even one schizophrenic episode often spent months to years in a state or private psychiatric hospital, acting bizarrely, with great pain within them, and at great emotional and financial expense to their family. Only through the advent of the antipsychotic agents has it been possible to manage such patients outside a hospital. This is, however, only symptomatic relief. If medication is stopped, the psychotic symptoms return and sometimes become more florid than before. At these times, neither psychotherapeutic nor sociotherapeutic interventions are successful. Only after a psychosis has run its course or is in remission, is it possible to reduce or discontinue medication. The potency of our antipsychotic agents is attested to by the extent to which psychotic thinking and behavior returns when they are discontinued.

12) It takes a long time for some families to face the reality that one among them is recurrently or chronically psychotic. A few families may never feel this reality. Most families, however, first re-

spond with denial; a patient is seen as "eccentric" or "going through a stage." Later, when denial is no longer possible, there is anger. This may be directed at a spouse, parents, or siblings. Each may blame the other; or a family may turn its anger toward the patient and extrude him from the family circle. Only in later stages when a family is willing to acknowledge that a patient is ill and that they may have played some part in the genesis of the illness, or may be able to play some part in the healing process, is it possible to form a working relationship in which therapist, patient, and family work together to achieve the best milieu for a patient's continued functioning. Raymond et al. (1975) have called this a "healing alliance." The therapist's awareness that the family (like the therapist) may at times feel frustration, anger, guilt and hopelessness and want to deny the seriousness of a patient's illness, allows him to work better with the reality of the family's dynamics. It is obviously impossible to make any realistic plans for the family to participate in the effort to keep the patient in therapy and take medication while they still must deny the illness. At the stage of guilt, there may be such overwhelming self-flagellation that the family may need to be helped to look forward, rather than backward, as to what must now, and in the future, be done. It neither helps the family nor patient to recount a litany of psychological indiscretions from the past. To know the past will help a therapist to make realistically viable plans for the future and reduce a repetition of past mistakes by a knowledge of what has failed or made a patient worse or better. Unfortunately, there is little controlled evidence that intellectual insight in patients themselves necessarily leads to modification of maladaptive behavior.

SEIZURE DISORDERS

Long-term management of patients with seizure disorders usually falls within the domain of neurology. Psychiatrists may, within the routine of daily practice or in emergency consultation, be called upon to determine whether aberrations of mood, thought and behavior are due to a seizure disorder or a process more strictly psychiatric. In some cases, the diagnosis may be apparent, as with most instances of grand mal epilepsy. At other times, the diagnosis may be extremely difficult, particularly if the seizures are temporal lobe in origin. In addition, a patient may have a psychiatric disorder such as schizophrenia as well as seizures. According to Hill (1958), 50% of patients with temporal lobe epilepsy have abnormal personalities, and 25% have episodes of psychosis. It is, therefore, important for a psychiatrist to know the manifestations of the various forms of epilepsy.

Grand Mal Seizures

Grand mal seizures typically last 5 to 30 minutes. They may or may not be preceded by an aura. When an aura occurs, it may be experienced as a feeling that a seizure is about to occur, or as weakness, numbness, paresthesias, auditory hallucinations, scintillating scotomata, fear, or pain in the abdomen. A shrill cry often heralds the onset of a seizure, and the patient loses consciousness. The body then stiffens tonically, with rigid extension of all four extremities, simultaneous clonic movements of the extremities, trismus and opisthotonus. This may be followed by bilateral simultaneous clonic movements of the extremities, head and jaw. During the seizure, the patients may bite their tongue, ejaculate, or have fecal or urinary incontinence. If they fall, there may be evidence of trauma. Because of the temporary paralysis of the respiratory musculature, they may appear cyanotic. Afterward there is coma followed by sleep. When they awake, there is often headache, muscle aches and vomiting. Clinicians observing a grand mal seizure, should record the side to which the head and eye turns. If consistent, it suggests a lesion of the opposite cerebral hemisphere. Post ictal motor weakness (Todd's paralysis), sensory, speech or visual changes also suggest localization. Grand mal seizures may occur as frequently as one or more a day or as far apart as years.

Petit Mal Seizures

Petit mal seizures, while usually considered a disorder of childhood, may continue into adulthood. They do not have any aura or warning and usually are quite brief, frequently less than a minute in duration. They may occur several times daily. They can be broadly subclassified into three types: myoclonic jerks, absence (staring episodes) and akinetic. The last mentioned consists of either falling to the floor suddenly, or dropping objects. Electroencephalograms recorded at the time of a seizure will show a characteristic bilaterally synchronous three per second spike and wave over the entire brain. In fact, the eyelids may flutter at a rate of three per second at the time of a seizure. Patients may be aware that they had a petit mal attack.

Jacksonian Seizures

Jacksonian seizures are a result of discharge in the motor or sensory areas of the cerebral cortex. When motor in nature, convulsive twitchings or clonic movements typically begin at the angle of the mouth, great toe or thumb. They then often progress to involve part of the face or extremity, or go on to include an entire side. In some cases, they may become generalized with a resultant grand mal seizure. Jacksonian sensory seizures follow the same pattern as the motor, with or without an accompanying clonic component. The march of movement follows the train of discharges across the contralateral cerebral cortex.

Temporal Seizures

Psychomotor or temporal lobe seizures typically last 3 to 5 minutes and consist of involuntary, purposeful, but irrelevant movements for which the patient has no recall. Any attempt to assist the patient in what he seems to be doing during an attack is resisted. These seizures are often confused with psychiatric states such as fugues and psychogenic amnesia. Their aura may resemble symptoms of an anxiety neurosis. The patient may appear to be chewing or having other abnormal mouth movements, tug at his clothes, walk, drive a car or perform a variety of complex tasks. A sleep EEG may reveal spikes or other dysrhythmias over the temporal lobes. A variety of emotional changes have been reported with these seizures including rage attacks, anxiety, and euphoria. The mental cloudiness that sometimes occurs resembles that of a psychosis.

Other Seizure Disorders

Uncinate seizures present by momentary episodes of strange odors or tastes—usually of an unpleasant nature. Gelastic epilepsy is a convulsive disorder with laughter as a manifestation of an attack. Auditory hallucinatory seizures may consist of vague noises or complex scores of music. Both hyperacusis and hypoacusis can occur with the latter. Well formed images or flashes of light may be seen with visual hallucinatory seizures. These unusual variants of epilepsy can occur alone or as an aura of one of the major convulsive disorders.

Status Epilepticus

The term status epilepticus is used to refer to persistent recurrence of seizures without episodes of consciousness between. They are usually grand mal in nature, but may be also petit mal or psycho-motor. Status epilepticus is a medical emergency requiring immediate medical intervention.

Differential Diagnosis

1) Idiopathic epilepsy
2) Alcohol withdrawal
3) Barbiturate withdrawal
4) Cerebral neoplasia
5) Cardiac arrhythmias
6) Uremia
7) Asphyxia
8) Granuloma
9) Hypocalcemia
10) Carotid sinus sensitivity
11) Hypoglycemia
12) Hepatic coma
13) Meningitis
14) Cerebral abscesses
15) Encephalitis
16) Recent and old infarcts
17) Cerebral vascular insufficiency
18) Atrophic lesions
19) Traumatic scarring
20) Degenerative brain diseases
21) Conversion symptoms
22) Meperidine intoxication
23) Other organic causes

Pseudoseizures

Psychogenic seizures (pseudoseizures) like bonified epilepsy may occur in rapid succession simulating status epilepticus. Clinicians should be aware of this so as to avoid administration of large and unnecessary doses of medication to patients with pseudoseizures. Patients with pseudoseizures tend to show the absence of any post-convulsive stupor or sleep (Gross, 1979). In some instances, in fact, they may recall the seizure and describe how they behaved. Postictal confusion and mental cloudiness is common after grand mal seizures and a period of brief coma may follow an episode of status epilepticus. During a pseudoseizure the electroencephalogram is normal. Babinski's sign is absent and the patient is not cyanotic. This is just the opposite of the clinical picture with grand mal seizures (Paulose and Shaw, 1977). Patients with pseudoseizures often appear bizarre and respond the same to placebo and active medication. Patients' eyes may go up when someone is present (i.e. secondary gain). Psychogenic seizures should be suspected when there is no tongue biting or fecal or urinary incontinence. Bodily injury is rare with pseudoepilepsy (Gross, 1979).

Management

1) Pharmacological, surgical and behavioral (as in the instance of some of the sensory epilepsies) management of seizures and the side effects of anticonvulsant medication is discussed in neurological textbooks.

2) Patients may have both pseudoseizures and real seizures. In such instances, patients must be treated with anticonvulsants in addition to psychotherapy.

3) Patients with ictal seizure disorders may also have nonictal seizure disorders with such symptoms as well circumscribed episodes of fear, derealization, depersonalization, déjà vu or rage attacks. These are most commonly seen in patients with temporal lobe epilepsy. Sphenoidal electrodes with simultaneous audiovisual monitoring is sometimes helpful in diagnosing these patients.

SOCIOECONOMIC EMERGENCIES: RESOURCELESS PATIENTS

A difficult problem that all psychiatrists and perhaps all physicians sooner or later face is confrontation with a patient who asks nothing more than food and shelter. The answer is not always as simple as it may seem at first. Many of these individuals have no serious psychiatric or medical problems which require inpatient care. At times, these individuals are inappropriately admitted to a psychiatric unit because the psychiatric clinician could either think of no alternative or did not wish to take the time to explore what possibilities existed.

Management

1) It is important at all times to protect the patient's self-esteem. Despite the fact that these individuals may appear as the disinherited of the earth, and some of them to collude in maintaining dependent posture, the clinician should not express anger at them out of frustration in being confronted with what seems an impossible

task to perform. Treat the patient with respect and try to empha-
thize and understand what it means to be in such a situation for
either psychological reasons or because of extremely limited
economic opportunities to better oneself because of social circumstances, age, illness, etc.

2) Clearly identify exactly what the patient wants. While at first
glance it may appear that the patient wants a place to stay, he may
only want someone to talk to for a while to relate how badly life has
treated him.

3) If there is a need for a particular service, then the psychiatric
clinician should review in his mind the possible alternatives and
present the most realistic and readily available. Long enumeration of
multiple agencies available in emergencies to one's colleagues may
be impressive, but to people in such circumstances it may just be
another reminder of how limited they are in their resourcefulness
compared to the clinician. It is good to develop a written list of agencies which provide emergency services. Increasingly, mental health
professionals are finding that they must rely on themselves to
develop alternatives in such circumstances. As social workers have
begun to move away from this area in many centers to spend their
time in the practice of psychotherapy and other tasks common to a
number of professions, no group has clearly emerged to take over the
responsibility of becoming expert in knowledge of community
resources and how to use them ("case work").

4) The first choice should be to assess which relatives and friends
are available to provide the service the patient requests. Sometimes a
simple call to an aunt or friend may provide a room and the
companionship the patient wants for the night.

5) If friends and relatives are not available, there are a number
of other agencies which may provide financial aid, food or shelter to
a patient for a time. There is Traveler's Aid, Fish, The Salvation
Army, and Christian Community Action, to name but a few. Some
church groups maintain hostels to provide shelter for an evening, and
knowledge of these sometimes only comes from experience. Grass-
root drug drop-in centers exist in some cities and provide a special
resource for the distraught adolescent; and there generally are a
number of less expensive hotels or branches of the YMCA with
available resources for those with compromised means. For those
who require nursing care (e.g. geriatric patients), nursing homes
vary, and some receive referrals at unexpected hours for reasonable
rates.

6) If patients are able themselves to contact the agency and follow through, it is best to allow them to take the needed step. If, however, it seems doubtful that the patient can manage for himself, the

clinician should phone to see what is available and provide referring information with the patient's permission.

7) If legal or accounting advice is required, the clinician should provide the name of either free services (e.g. Public Defender Service) or of those individuals in town who will provide services on a sliding scale or for a nominal fee.

8) Explorative psychotherapy may be helpful in some instances in aiding patients in obtaining an understanding of how they got themselves in such situations and to determine what psychological blocks may exist in preventing the patient from resolving socio-economic crises himself. Obviously, in some instances, the reality of the patient's life is so overwhelming that if any form of therapy is indicated, it may only be of the crisis intervention supportive variety. Sometimes, however, counselling in how to handle money is more important than any psychological maneuvers.

9) Avoid pushing. If what seems to be a minor intervention appears to relieve patients, do not force them into more than they want at the time. An aggressive approach may appear to the patient paternalistic or overwhelm the patient who never wanted more than support and a possible suggestion.

10) Finally, hospitalization may be a needed step to begin the patient in a program of social and economic rehabilitation. Use of hospitalization is always a delicate issue. The patient may regress and it may make it difficult for him to be discharged to a world he feels by contrast cold and unfriendly. If it is concluded that there appears to be no alternative to hospitalization, it should be on a crisis type unit that works with a philosophy to help the patient maximize his own internal resources, is antiregressive, and moves toward a speedy discharge with good follow-up care.

SOMATOFORM AND DISSOCIATIVE DISORDERS

The somatoform disorders are discussed together with the conversion and dissociative disorders because of the tendency of clinicians to confuse these terms and the occurrence, frequently, of patients presenting with two or more of these disorders at various times in their lives.

History

The essential feature of somatoform disorders is the occurrence of physical symptoms and signs for which no demonstrable organic pathology may be found to explain the clinical findings. These symptoms, unlike those of malignancy or factitious illness are not under voluntary control. The individual does not consciously feign illness. Symptom formation is unconscious and the primary management is psychological. No physical basis can be found by exact laboratory procedures and physical examination.

1) Briquet's Syndrome (Somatization disorder) is characterized by recurrent and multiple somatic complaints for which no physical basis can be found. The disorder is said to begin prior to age 25 and menstrual difficulties may be one of the earliest signs. Complaints are often vague or presented in a dramatic way. Patients with Briquet's syndrome have complaints referrable to many systems and have seen many physicians. According to Guze (1975) these patients often have a clinical history of nervousness, marital and sexual maladjustment, menstrual difficulties, anxiety symptoms, various pains, gastrointestinal disturbances, urinary symptoms, disorders of mood and conversion symptoms. They tend to use a great number of medications, seek medical consultation frequently and get hospitalized. Sometimes they are found to have had excessive surgery. The natural history of Briquet's Syndrome is decades, with fluctuations in intensity. Interpersonal difficulty is common, marital problems, depression, anxiety and suicide threats or attempts may bring these patients to the attention of a psychiatrist. This disorder is most frequently diagnosed among women. Seldom a year goes by without patients with Briquet's Syndrome seeking help from a physician.

2) Patients with conversion disorders present with a loss or alteration of physical functioning suggesting physical pathology as a direct expression of a psychological conflict or need. A conversion disorder is most likely to involve a single site during a given episode but may vary in site or nature if there is more than one episode.

3) The predominant feature of psychalgia is the complaint of pain in the absence of any physical findings to explain the symptoms and in the absence of any other mental disorders. Psychological factors are usually present to suggest a psychological etiology.

4) Dissociative disorders are characterized by sudden, temporary alteration in the normally integrated functions of consciousness, identity, or motor behavior so that one or more parts of these functions are lost. An individual may be amnesic for a certain period of time (psychogenic amnesia) or another personality or personalities may be taken on at various times which are distinct and separate (multiple personalities). The sudden onset of unexpected travel away from one's usual place of living or working with the assumption of a new identity and inability to recall the former one without evidence of an underlying organic mental disorder is a dis-

sociative disorder referred to as a psychogenic fugue. Depersonalization disorder is a dissociative state in which there is an alteration in the perception or experience of self that the feeling of one's own reality is temporarily lost.

5) Conversion disorders are not restricted to patients with Briquet's Syndrome. Histrionic personality disorders and antisocial personality disorders are two of the most common personality disorders seen with conversion disorders.

6) Antisocial men tend to marry histrionic women and histrionic character disorders are often coupled with sociopathic traits in hysterical women. Women later diagnosed to have Briquet's Syndrome may have an earlier history of antisocial and delinquent behavior.

7) Malingering must be distinguished from conversion symptoms and dissociative disorders. Secondary gain is less apparent with conversion and dissociative disorders. Lawsuits may be found to be pending with malingerers.

8) Just because a patient may have some histrionic characteristics or has a past documented history of conversion symptoms does not mean that his present symptoms are not organic. Real physical illness can occur in patients with Briquet's Syndrome and in patients with a past history of conversion disorders.

9) Some studies have demonstrated a significant number of individuals diagnosed to have conversion disorders turn out to have documented physical illness that can well explain the original symptoms. In Slater's (1965) well known study, it was found that after a follow-up averaging nine years on a group of 85 patients diagnosed as having conversions, as defined by the British, 28 were found to have no organic basis that could be identified on admission for the symptoms, but were later discovered to have organic illnesses that could account for them.

10) A symptom to be labeled "conversion" should be one without any readily identifiable physical basis. There are certain features of a patient's personality that suggest conversion or Briquet's Syndrome. The patient often shows a lack of concern for the seriousness of the symptom ("la belle indifference"). Patients with Briquet's Syndrome usually have a multitude of symptoms. Sometimes a plausible psychological explanation seems readily apparent (e.g. a fugue state as a flight from an impending marriage about which the patient is strongly ambivalent).

11) Conversion symptoms first appearing late in life are often associated with an organic disorder or a psychotic depression.

12) Somatoform disorders and conversion disorders should be

distinguished from factitious disorders. The latter includes physical and psychological symptoms that are produced by the individual and under his voluntary control. These include Ganser's Syndrome and Munchausen's Syndrome. The former is sometimes referred to as pseudostupidity. Patients with a Ganser's Syndrome seem to understand a question, but give ridiculous answers (e.g. How many legs does a three-legged stool have? Four. How many eyes does a man have? Seven). Munchausen's Syndrome is a label given to those individuals who seem addicted to surgery and medical care. They sustain numerous operations without much pathology ever being found.

Symptoms and Signs of Briquet's Syndrome

The diagnosis of Briquet's Syndrome entails the manifestation of at least one symptom in five of the following six groups for women. For men, a symptom need only occur in four of the groups.

Group 1

The individual believes he/she has been sickly for most or a good part of his/her life.

Group 2

1) Dissociative reaction (e.g. amnesia)
2) Conversion symptom (e.g. deafness, aphonia, loss of sensation)

Group 3

1) Vomiting spells
2) Abdominal pain

Group 4

More severe or frequent than in most women
1) Dysmenorrhea
2) Menstrual irregularity (e.g. amenorrhea or more severe bleeding)

Group 5

For the major part of an individual's life following opportunities

for sexual activity
1) Lack of interest in having sex
2) Sexual indifference
3) Lack of pleasure during intercourse
4) Pain during intercourse

Group 6

1) More headaches than most people
2) Back pain
3) Joint pain
4) Pain in extremities

Symptoms and Signs of Conversion Disorders

Symptoms and signs suggesting neurological disease such as:
1) Paralysis
2) Aphonia
3) Seizures
4) Dyskinesia
5) Akinesia
6) Coordination disturbance
7) Blindness
8) Paresthesia
9) Anosmia
10) Vomiting
11) Sensory loss—especially in a stocking or glove distribution with a sharp border or total analgesia
12) Urinary retention
13) Hysterical psychosis
14) Choreiform and athetoid movements
15) Tics
16) Tremors
17) Dysphonia
18) Hallucinations
19) Hoover's Sign—used to distinguish a psychogenic lower limb paralysis from an organic paralysis, this consists of the examiner placing his hand under the ostensibly paralyzed leg and feeling its downward movement when the patient is asked to raise his normal leg.
20) When a patient who is not too intelligent presents with a suspect psychogenic anesthesia, he may be asked to say blindfolded, "Yes" when he feels a pinprick, and "No" when he doesn't.

21) There is often an inconsistency in the border of a psychogenic sensory loss, or the loss may not follow the anatomical distribution of a dermatome or peripheral nerve. Sometimes the border is sharper than it normally would be.
22) Visual fields may show a tubular constriction.
23) The reflexes are usually symmetrical with conversion symptoms.
24) There are inconsistencies in examination of muscle strength and the sphincters are not affected in psychogenic paraplegia.
25) La belle indifference
26) Psuedocyesis (false pregnancy)
27) Astasia—abasia (inability to walk or stand even though all leg movements are normal)
28) Globus hystericus (difficulty swallowing on an hysterical basis)

Signs and Symptoms of Psychalgia

1) Complaint of pain in the absence of adequate physical findings.

Signs and Symptoms of Dissociative Disorders

1) Amnesia
2) Fugue
3) Multiple Personality
4) Depersonalization

Differential Diagnosis

1) Briquet's Syndrome
2) Conversion disorder
3) Multiple sclerosis
4) Schizophrenia
5) Vitamin deficiencies
6) Toxic nerve damage
7) Temporal lobe epilepsy
8) Anxiety states
9) Other forms of epilepsy
10) Tabes dorsalis
11) General paresis
12) Basal ganglia disease
13) Cerebral neoplasia
14) Psychalgia
15) Dissociative disorder

16) Collagen diseases (e.g. lupus erythematosus, polyarteritis nodosa)

17) Other organic disorders

Management

1) Carefully take a medical history; do a general physical and neurological examination and order appropriate diagnostic tests to rule out any organic disease.

2) Find out any recent life events which may have stressed the patient. What is his personal past history? His family history?

3) Do not focus on the symptoms. When interviewing the patient, remove him from friends and relatives who may be a source of secondary gain.

4) Allow the patient to ventilate in a supportive psychotherapeutic relationship.

5) If a crisis intervention mode of psychotherapy does not work with patients with conversion symptoms, dissociative disorders or psychalgia, try suggestion, hypnotherapy or an Amytal interview using the proper precautions.

6) If a patient appears excessively anxious, it may be necessary to use an antianxiety agent such as 2–10 mg of diazepam (Valium) p.o.

7) If none of the above succeed in removing the symptom, it may be necessary to hospitalize the patient, but both neurologist and psychiatrist should work together in the evaluation.

8) Long-term supportive limit-setting psychotherapy may be needed with various degrees of health education and explorative psychotherapy to get at the underlying psychogenetic roots. For instance, if a patient repeatedly becomes psychogenically paralyzed when dating married men, she should be advised not to do so and to explore the reasons why she is attracted to them rather than to unmarried men who offer a more stable relationship.

STEROID PSYCHOSIS

Steroids such as prednisone may be prescribed for a number of illnesses. These include the management of collagen disease, Addison's disease, and a number of allergic and neoplastic diseases. Nonspecific psychoses, mania, delirium, dementia, depression and schizophreniform psychosis may be seen if the patient becomes toxic. It is not necessary to reduce or discontinue the steroid being given if the primary clinician feels that it must be continued. Antipsychotic medication may be prescribed in doses sufficient to control symptoms. Haloperidol, 2 mg p.o. t.i.d. is usually sufficient to manage a steroid psychosis.

It should be remembered that a psychosis may be developed while a patient's dose is being increased, while it is being decreased, or while at a steady state. If psychosis develops during reduction of dosage, it is possible to return to the original dose and decrease dosage more slowly. If it develops while increasing a patient's dose, decrease the dose and increase more slowly. If psychosis develops while at a steady dose, either reduction of dose or the addition of antipsychotic medication may be used to manage the patient.

SUDDEN DEATH ASSOCIATED WITH ANTIPSYCHOTIC MEDICATION USE

Sudden death has been reported with patients on neuroleptic medication and attributed to seizures and asphyxiation, cardiovascular causes, postural hypotension and laryngeal-pharyngeal dystonia. Chlorpromazine acts directly on autonomic centers in the midbrain producing a blocking effect on sympathetic ganglia resulting in hypotension (Flaherty and Lahmeyer, 1978). In elderly people and others with compromised cerebral or cardiac vascular status this may result in strokes or myocardial infarctions. In patients treated with phenothiazines there is a diminution of the gag reflex that may result in aspiration asphyxia secondary to regurgitation due to loss of control of the esophageal sphincters and impairment of swallowing (Weiner, 1979). Solomon (1977) reported a case of drug-induced bulbar-palsy-like syndrome in a man receiving fluphenazine enanthate. He postulated that phenothiazine-induced bulbar-palsy may cause laryngeal and/or pharyngeal dysfunction that are responsible for aspiration in patients with aspiration asphyxia.

SUDDEN DEATH OF PSYCHOGENIC ORIGIN

Emotional factors are sufficient to bring about death in individuals not otherwise predisposed by immediate physical factors. An individual may die of a heart attack after he learns that his entire family has been killed in an airplane crash on the way to meeting him. Some people die of "fright" and others "give up" and die. Powerlessness, hopelessness or other intense emotions usually precede these deaths. The cardiovascular system responds to stress under such conditions to make sudden death more likely from cerebrovascular accidents or arrhythmias. People with coronary heart disease would be particularly at risk (Dimsdale, 1977).

Voodoo deaths a particular subtype of sudden death. "Root doctors," "conjure doctors," and "two headed doctors" exist in both isolated rural communities in the deep South as well as in the large urban areas of the West and Northeast and are believed able to cause insanity, sickness and death. They are also felt able to cure those who have been hexed using a mixture of herbs, stones, powders, insects, charms, roots and incantations (Golden, 1977). These items are sometimes purchased at folk medicine stores for use by interested lay people. In order for a hex to work it is felt that victims must believe in the power of the person who places the curse and must have some knowledge that they have been hexed.

Management

1) Management of patients who believe they are hexed is often quite difficult without the involvement or support of lay or community healers.

SUICIDAL BEHAVIOR

The evaluation of suicidal and homicidal potential is one of the most stressful aspects of emergency room psychiatry. Obviously if there is significant suicidal or homicidal potential, a patient must be hospitalized. Most states have laws which allow a physician to medically certify those individuals whose behavior presents a significant risk to themselves or others when under such circumstances they or their families resist hospitalization. In rare instances, a family may be able to provide round-the-clock surveillance of a suicidal person under the supervision and responsibility of a physician but this is a relatively unusual circumstance, and a patient who truly desires to take his life should not be considered adequately protected unless he is hospitalized. In addition, a family may be ambivalent and while overtly displaying concern and support may harbor covert death wishes which patients may pick up and act out. Obviously not everyone who states they wish to end their life really intends to. The question then arises: who are the individuals who, if not hospitalized, will be likely to take their lives and what are the gestures of the people who seek some secondary gain and convey a message by an abortive self-destructive act. Fortunately, a body of data has been accrued that enable the clinician to arrive at a probabilistic statement on suicide risk based on epidemiological and sociological studies of self-destructive behavior.

Incidence

The United States ranks about average on an international scale of rates of successful suicides. The annual incidence is about 10 to 12 per 100,000 population. In 1976, there were 27,000 recorded suicides. It is the fifth major cause of death in the United States. Chile, Ireland and New Zealand have rates below 6/100,000. Rates above 20/100,000 have been reported in Austria, Denmark, Hungary, Japan, Sweden and West Germany. Data presented by Mintz (1964) indicate that in Los Angeles, 3-4% of adults will attempt suicide at sometime during their life. In the United States, it is believed that ten times as many people attempt suicide as succeed. Weissman (1974) has reviewed incidence rates of suicide attempts over the past decade. She found an alarming rise, which underscores the need for psychiatric clinicians to sharpen their skills in distinguishing between those who are intent on killing themselves and those who use self-destructive behavior as a cry for help or to convey other messages. The incidence rates for attempts in 1960 in Philadelphia was 59/100,000 compared to 183/100,000 in 1970-1971 in New Haven, Connecticut. This trend has been observed elsewhere. Western Australia had a rate for attempts in 1961 of 90/100,000 and the city of Melbourne had a rate of 160/100,000 in 1970. A dramatic increase was observed in Great Britain over the decade when data taken from Sheffield, England in 1960-1961 is contrasted to rates in Glasgow, Scotland in 1970. The rate in the former city was 82/100,000 in the early sixties whereas the latter had a rate of 300/100,000 one decade later!

Questions to be Asked in an Evaluation of Suicide Risk

The following questions may serve as a practical guide to assessing suicidal potential in people who have either threatened to take their lives, are entertaining self-destructive thoughts, or who present to an emergency facility after a suicide attempt. If several of the factors that increase risk are present, the clinician should be most hesitant to consider management on an outpatient basis. Hospitalization may be the only medically sound and ethically acceptable choice to protect patients from their own self-destructive aims.

Considerations in the Evaluation of Suicidal Risk

1) *Marital status*—The suicide rate for single persons is twice that of the married. Divorced and widowed individuals have rates four to five times those of married persons. In the widowed population, risks are greatest during the first year of widowhood. Rates are lowest among married persons, especially if they have children. One exception is the married female adolescent who is a greater risk than the single teenage girl (NAMH Reporter, Winter 1972/3).

2) *Sex*—Women attempt suicide more but men succeed more. In Farberow and Schneidman's (1965) study, the percentage of successful suicides was 70% for men and 30% for women. Women tend to overdose while men use more lethal means such as firearms. Ratios of male and female suicide range 2:1 to 7:1. This is changing. Women, especially professional women, are having increased rates of suicide, alcoholism and coronary heart disease. In a study at the Massachusetts General Hospital in 1972 (O'Brien, 1977) it was found that as many males as females were attempting suicide by overdose.

3) *Age*—Suicide risk and age are positively correlated. In 1976, in the United States the annual rate in the 15- to 24-year-old range was 11.7/100,000 and in the 25-34 year range, 16.5/100,000. In the age group 55 to 64, it was 20.0/100,000. Suicide is the fourth leading cause of death in the age group 15 to 44 years. There has been a 250% increase in suicide rates for males, age 15 to 24 over 20 years from 6.8/100,000 to 17.4/100,000/year. After adolescence, there is a decline in rates until age 40 at which time they again begin to rise. The rate of the 20- to 24-year-range, however, is not equaled again until age 55. Rates continue to rise then to a peak of 42.5/100,000/year at age 75 to 79, the highest in any age group (Frederick, 1978). There has actually been a decrease in suicide rate in past years for the elderly considering the increase in population in this age group suggesting that the attention given in recent years to the need for social supports in the older age groups is helping.

4) *Religion*—Suicide rates are lowest among Jews and Catholics. Protestants have significantly high rates. Active membership in a religious organization seem to be the important factor (Breed, 1966).

5) *Socioeconomic status*—In the United States, the incidence of

suicide is greatest in the lower social classes. Unskilled laborers and agricultural workers have rates significantly higher than the national average. Professional groups and highly skilled workers have suicide rates below the average. In Europe, one sees high rates at both socioeconomic extremes. The peak for suicide in this country was 17.4/100,000 after the Great Depression (Frederick, 1978).

6) *Race*—Suicide rates of nonwhites which have characteristically been lower than whites have increased in recent years to rates equal to or greater than white rates. In Schneidman's and Farberow's group (1965), 95% of successful suicides were white and at that time the rate among blacks was generally felt to be about 1/3 that of white rates save in urban centers where it approximated white rates. In 1960, the rates for nonwhites in the age groups 20 to 24 were 4.9/100,000/year. In 1973, it was 14.1/100,000/year—nearly that of whites. Suicide is a special problem among Native Americans who have rates 64% higher than whites. Some tribes, in fact, have rates five times the national average (Frederick, 1978; Frederick and Lague, 1972).

7) *Depression*—Suicide risk increases with depressed mood, especially if vegetative signs are present such as loss of appetite and weight, decreased libido, difficulty falling asleep, awakening during the night, and early morning wakening. It is also increased in the presence of psychomotor retardation and feelings of worthlessness and hopelessness. Suicide risk may increase early during treatment with antidepressants as the return of energy brings about an increased ability to act out self-destructive wishes. Self-inflicted death is 500 times more common in those who are seriously depressed (Frederick and Lague, 1972).

8) *Severe insomnia*—Even in the absence of depression, severe insomnia is associated with increased suicide risk.

9) *Alcohol and drug abuse*—Suicide risk is difficult to predict in alcoholics and many "accidental" deaths on the highway may represent suicides. Alcohol may trigger self- and other-directed violence. Barbiturates and alcohol represent a particularly lethal combination. Use of alcohol and drugs may be an attempt to self medicate a depression or schizophrenic psychosis.

10) *Schizophrenia*—Suicide risk is difficult to evaluate in schizophrenics and borderline schizophrenics. The combination of a thought disorder, depressed mood, and suicidal ideation in male schizophrenics is particularly ominous (Tsuang, 1978).

11) *Command hallucinations*—Hallucinations telling a person to kill him-/herself or calling them to join those in the world beyond remarkably increases risk.

12) *Sexual orientation*—Individuals with a predominantly homosexual orientation have a higher risk, especially if depressed, aging, or if alcoholic.

13) *Physical illness*—There is an increase in risk if patients have a physical illness, especially if they have previously been independent and robust and are afflicted with a painful and/or disabling illness such as cancer. In one study (Neuringer and Lettier, 1971) a third of those who attempted suicide were found to have a serious physical complaint and another third reported that a family member was sick or had been hospitalized just before the attempt.

14) *Family history*—Risk is increased if there is a family history of suicide, especially in a same-sexed parent. In Schneidman and Farberow's series, 25% of those individuals who attempted suicide had a history of suicide in the immediate family. A family history of suicide particularly increases risk if the suicide occurred before pubescence of a survivor and his relationship to the victim was close (Frederick, 1973).

15) *Giving away personal property*—If an individual has begun to dispose of his property, especially of his cherished personal possessions, risk is increased. This in essence represents making out a Will and executing it.

16) *Previous attempts*—Fifty to 80% of those who ultimately commit suicide have a history of a previous attempt. The ratio of attempted suicide to completed suicide has been given as between 5.5:1 to 7.2:1 (Pederson, et al., 1973).

17) *Lack of future plans*—No plans for the future increases risk. This is especially so if patients talk of how they will be viewed at their own funeral and what friends and relatives will do after they are gone.

18) *Lethality of attempt*—If individuals have made an attempt on their life that would have resulted in death if they had not been found and brought for treatment, their risk is much greater for another attempt than if they had employed a method which was more benign (e.g. 10 aspirins). Hanging, jumping from high places, and gunshot wounds are associated usually with quick deaths and represent, therefore, lethal attempts. Wrist cuttings and minor ingestions are significantly less lethal. The more violent and painful the attempt, the greater the risk. Overdose of tricyclic antidepressants, thioridazine (Mellaril) and mesoridazine (Lidaner and Serentil) are particularly lethal because of the potential of cardiac arrhythmias and death (Donlon and Tupin, 1977). In 1975, 60% of deaths by substances were by women while 82% of deaths from firearms and 62% of deaths by jumping were by males (Frederick, 1978). People tend

to use the methods available to them. In New York City where there are many tall buildings, 33% of those who commit suicide do so by this means whereas, only 3% of all suicides in the United States are by jumping (Frederick and Lague, 1972). Suicide risk correlates highly with lethality *when* the attempter has sufficient knowledge to assess the lethality of the attempt (Beck, et al. 1971).

19) *Living alone*—There is an increased risk if a person lives alone.

20) *Recent loss*—Risk is increased if a person recently experienced a loss of a loved one through death or separation.

21) *Hypochondriasis*—Hypochondriacal prooccupation increases risk.

22) *Recent surgery and childbirth*—Both these events are associated with increased risk. Self-inflicted death during pregnancy is unusual (Resnick and Wittlin, 1971). Refusal to grant an abortion at the time when medical permission was necessary did not appear to influence suicide rates.

23) *Unemployment or financial difficulty*—Economic problems due to lack of employment or increased financial burden increase risk.

24) *No secondary gain*—The absence of any apparent secondary gain for a self-destructive act such as "message value" increases risk.

25) *Accident proneness*—An increase in accidents may be due to underlying unconscious suicidal wishes.

26) *Ethnic origin*—Within the United States, rates among the foreign born tend to be higher than among the native born and the rates tend to be those of the country of origin.

27) *Education*—Suicide rates among college students are higher, especially at the more prestigious schools. Lyman reported the annual suicide rates per 100,000 population in the age group 20 to 24 years in England as follows:

Oxford University	26.4/100,000
Cambridge University	21.3/100,000
University of London	16.3/100,000
Seven unnamed British Universities	5.9/100,000

The rates at that time for England and Wales was 4.1/100,000 for this age group. In the United States where the usual rate for this age group was 7-10/100,000, the rate at Yale was 14/100,000 (Parrish, 1957) and at Harvard 15/100,000 (Temby, 1961).

28) *Urban versus Rural existence*—In Europe, suicide rates in urban areas have been strikingly higher than in rural areas. While this was also the case in the United States until 45 years ago, presently the difference between rural and urban areas has become negli-

gible. Suicide rates vary with the vicissitudes of the country's economy, with the rates of whites more sensitive to business fluctuations than nonwhites. A study in Chicago, reported by Henry and Short (1954), found that those of upper socioeconomic status reacted more violently to fluctuations than those of the lower social classes and that suicide rates for men were more sensitive to economic shifts than those for women. An exception was the black woman, who is more sensitive to economic shifts than the black man. In addition, those in the age group 15-65 were more sensitive than those above age 65. While the suicide rate in higher rent districts of Chicago fell sharply from 1930-32 to 1939-41, the rate in low rent areas was found to remain relatively constant. Suicide rates (as well as admissions to mental hospitals) decrease at time of war.

29) *Degree of tension*—In deciding on a disposition following a suicide attempt, the degree of tension that remains at the end of the clinical interview should be assessed. If a patient is able to consider alternatives to the self-destructive act, such as a commitment to a program of therapy, this becomes a positive factor in favor of outpatient care.

30) *Occupation*—Rates differ remarkably among professions with physicians, business executives and other professionals ranking quite high. Rates are lowest among farm workers and artisans. Male health professionals on the whole show an excess of 2.3:1. Female health professionals have an excess of 1.7 to 1. Physicians over 65 show the highest rate. Half of suicides by physicians occur during the most productive decades of 35 to 54. Excess ratio after retirement for physicians is 12:1 compared to 3:1 for the general population. Divorced physicians are 13 times more likely to kill themselves than their married colleagues. Psychiatrists, ophthalmologists, and otolaryngologists have the highest rates with pediatricians and pathologists, the lowest. Other groups with equally high rates are chemists, pharmacists, nonmedical technicians, dentists, lawyers and engineers.

31) *Location*—Rates of suicide vary by state. Nevada has the highest with Wyoming, California, Maine and Vermont close behind. New Jersey and New York have low rates (Frederick, 1978).

32) *Time*—In the 1950's and 1960's, April and May were the months with the highest incidence of suicide but since then there has been a bimodal distribution with high rates in both spring and fall. December has low rates, save for during the Christmas holidays when both depression and suicide increase.

Other questions which should be asked in an evaluation include:
What setting did an attempt occur in?
Was there a likelihood of immediate discovery?
Did the patient inform anyone that he was going to take his life?

Individuals who do not give off any signals that they intend to take their life represent a greater risk, especially if they seek out a place for the attempt where there is little likelihood of discovery except by accident.

Management

1) Primary care clinicians should be taught to identify potentially suicidal patients and means of reducing risk. Approximately 75% of individuals who kill themselves see a family physician within three months of killing themselves. Eighty percent of those who kill themselves have given a warning.

2) If an individual has attempted suicide, the risk for a future attempt should be considered. If significant, the patient should be hospitalized. If risk is low and there are sufficient supports in the community, the individual may be treated as an outpatient.

3) The decision as to whether or not to hospitalize is based on a combination of assessment of risk from history, the patient's current living situation, the degree of depression, the availability of social supports and the effect of evaluation and initiation of treatment. A moderately suicidal individual may be managed outside of the hospital if there are supportive family members and friends while a mildly suicidal person who is a loner may not be.

4) If suicide ideation and depression is secondary to an organic process that is treatable, consultation should be sought and appropriate therapy initiated. For instance, if depression is a side effect of an antihypertensive medication, the medication should be, after consultation with the patient's internist, discontinued, reduced, or substituted for by another drug with less likelihood of depression.

5) If the patient is to be managed as an outpatient:
a) social support should be rallied
b) appropriate psychopharmacotherapy, psychotherapy, or sociotherapy should be initiated.
c) the patient and his family and friends should be given the psychiatric clinician's telephone number as well as that of a backup clinician or emergency room where they can go if the clinician is unavailable.

d) reduction of patients' and families' anxiety during the acute phase to see how the patient is doing.

e) a return visit (even the next day if it is felt the decision to not hospitalize may need to be reconsidered) should be scheduled.

f) friends and families should be alerted to ominous signs such as increasing withdrawal, preoccupation, silence and moroseness.

g) careful records should be kept in all instances documenting why a patient was or was not hospitalized.

6) The thrust of crisis work with a suicidal patient is opening lines of communication, identifying and exploring resources and options, establishing social supports and initiating therapeutic interventions. Frequency of visits, if the patient is treated as an outpatient depends on how much the psychiatric clinician can depend on others in the community such as friends, family, lovers, and clergy to provide social support, an opportunity for ventilation, and exploring options, and to call the clinician if the patient's condition worsens.

TARDIVE DYSKINESIA

The widespread use of antipsychotic medication has lead to rising awareness of their potential for adverse side effects. One such side effect is the bucco-lingual-masticatory dyskinesia referred to as tardive dyskinesia.

History

1) Patients presenting with tardive dyskinesia have a history of prolonged use of antipsychotic medications. All subgroups—phenothiazines, butyrophenones thioxanthenes—are reported to play a role in the genesis of this disorder in predisposed individuals although risk is said to be greater when the high potency lower dosage neuroleptics are used.

2) Symptoms first appear after prolonged use of a drug or when drug dosage is lowered or is discontinued. Increasing the dose of a drug may make the dyskinesia disappear but contributes further to the problem.

3) A higher incidence of the disorder is reported for older people, women, those with brain damage, those with long records of hospitalization, those where neuroleptic medication had little effect and those treated with fluphenazine (Chournard, et al. 1979).

4) The longer patients are on an antipsychotic drug, the more likely they are to develop the disorder.

5) Youth is not a protection against development of a tardive dyskinesia. Children and adolescents are at risk. A case has been reported in a 15-year-old boy that responded to use of deanol (McLean and Casey, 1978).

6) Prompt detection of early signs of the disorder and neuroleptic withdrawal may result in amelioration of symptoms.

7) Duration of symptoms prior to drug withdrawal appears to be a more important factor than age of onset in determining reversibility of symptoms (Quitkin, et al. 1977). In one study, persistence of tardive dyskinesia, after cessation of neuroleptic and antidepressant drugs, was related to significantly longer neuroleptic treatment and a greater number of drug interruptions of at least two months (Jeste, et al. 1979). This latter finding is surprising as periods of drug interruption is usually deemed a preventive measure and suggests when drugs are given for a significant duration to patients predisposed to development of a dyskinesia, risk is high regardless of drug holidays.

8) Dopamine receptor supersensitivity is purportedly responsible for the abnormal movements. (Tamminga, et al. 1977; 1979).

Signs and Symptoms

1) Lip smacking
2) Chewing movements
3) Choreoathetoid movements of the tongue
4) Puckering of the lips
5) Choreoathetoid movements of the limbs and trunk (less frequent) (Wegner, et al. 1979).

In addition to the above, potentially life-threatening ventilatory and gastrointestinal disturbances may develop that require rapid reinstitution of neuroleptic therapy (Casey and Robins, 1978).

Treatment

1) Cessation of neuroleptic drugs at the first sign of the development of a tardive dyskinesia is recommended if the patient's condition allows. Early cessation may lead to total disappearance of symptoms.

2) If a patient's condition is such that psychotic symptoms which prevent functioning of the individual in his environment will reemerge on cessation of medication, another antipsychotic, prefer-

ably from a different class, should be substituted at equivalent doses. For instance, if the patient develops a tardive dyskinesia on 24 mg a day of perphenazine (Trilafon) substitute 6 mg a day of Navane.

3) Deanol in doses of 1600–2000 mg/day has been considered helpful in some cases. The success of its use in well established cases, however, is frequently not beneficial (Davis, et al. 1977).

Prevention

1) The best approach to tardive dyskinesia is to minimize its occurrence by judicious use of neuroleptic medication. Only use antipsychotic medication when absolutely necessary and then only at the minimum doses required. Risk is minimized by systematically monitoring side effects and reducing drug doses as soon as a patient's condition permits (Crane, 1977).

2) Patient and family should be apprised of the risk and the ethical necessity to always balance continuation of patient functioning in the community and alleviation of psychic pain against the development of what is sometimes permanent neurological dysfunction and which makes both the patient and those around him feel uncomfortable.

3) Drug holidays should be given. Neuroleptic medication can usually be discontinued during weekends with a well managed chronically psychotic patient without return of psychotic or aggressive symptoms. Sometimes it is possible to take patients off medication one week a month without difficulty.

4) Switching from drugs in one class to another (e.g. a butyrophenone to a thioxanthene) or from one subgroup of a class of drugs to another subgroup (e.g. aliphatic phenothiazine to a piperazine phenothiazine) is felt to decrease risk if done at relatively frequent intervals (e.g. six months to one year) in patients who are chronically psychotic.

5) There is some evidence to suggest that use of higher-dosage lower-potency neuroleptics is associated with less risk than use of the higher-potency low-dosage drugs.

THYROID STORM

Stress and infection can give rise to thyroid storm characterized by marked tachycardia, gastrointestinal dysfunction, hyperthermia, and a variety of neurological and psychiatric symptoms such as overwhelming anxiety and psychomotor agitation. It is an exaggeration of thyrotoxicosis and is managed accordingly.

VOLATILE NITRITES

Volatile nitrites such as amyl nitrite have been used for the relief of angina pectoris for over a century. Alteration of mood and behavior are not unusual if sufficient amounts have been inhaled.

History

1) Amyl nitrite is sold in small thin glass capsules covered by webbing so that it can be crushed between the fingers and the fumes inhaled when a patient suffers anginal pain.

2) Volatile nitrites are sold in various "head shops," pornographic stores, novelty shops and through mail order houses under a number of names including Poppers, Heart-On, Toilet water, Gas, Bullet, Rush, and Aroma of Men.

3) Sometimes nitrous oxide is taken directly from the bottle through a single or double nasal inhaler.

4) Volatile nitrites have been used extensively to expand creativity, promote abandonment in dancing and art and to intensify both hetro- and homosexual experiences.

5) As with all drug intoxication states, the clinical picture represents an interaction of the amount of drug taken, the setting, the effect of concurrent physical illness, the personality structure of the user, the expectations of the user, and the pharmacology of the drug. (Sigell, et al. 1978).

Symptoms

1) Light-headedness
2) Nausea
3) Weakness
4) Fluctuating levels of consciousness
5) Disorientation
6) Dysattention
7) Pulsatile headaches and short-lived nitrite headaches
8) Syncope
9) Cutaneous flushing

Signs

1) Ataxia
2) Hypotension
3) Tachycardia
4) Transient changes on the electrocardiogram (e.g. inverted T waves and depressed ST segments)

Management

1) Symptoms generally pass with cessation of use of volatile nitrites.

WITHDRAWAL FROM PSYCHOTROPIC MEDICATION

Subjective behavioral and physiologic changes follow abrupt cessation of antidepressants, anticonvulsants, stimulants, antianxiety and antipsychotic medication. Acute organic mental syndromes, grand mal seizures, and prolonged coma have been reported following sudden withdrawal of large amounts of benzodiazepines such as diazepam (Valium) (DeBard, 1979). Delirium may develop as long as eight days after diazepam withdrawal consistent with the observation that symptoms are generally slower to develop following cessation of benzodiazepines than following discontinuation of alcohol or barbiturates. People with histories of chronic sedative or alcohol abuse are particularly prone to develop symptoms on cessation of benzodiazepines. Withdrawal from lesser amounts may lead to gastrointestinal upset, dysphoria, weight loss, increase in orthostatic pulse rate and physical discomfort.

Severe depression may follow cessation of stimulant drugs such as methylphenidate (Rosenfeld, 1979). Discontinuation of anticonvulsants have been reported in some instances to lead to psychotic symptoms in the context of a clear sensorium with markedly increased electroencephalographic abnormalities. Gastrointestinal dysfunction may result from abrupt cessation of antidepressants (Gualtieri and Staze, 1979).

Covert dyskinesias may appear upon discontinuation or reduction in dosage of antipsychotic medication which may mimic the symptoms of a psychotic exacerbation (Gardos, et al. 1978). These generally disappear in six to twelve weeks and are thought to reflect cholinergic overactivity and changes in dopamine-acetylcholine balance in the basal ganglia. Dyskinesia uncovered at the time of drug cessation may be an early sign of a developing tardive dyskinesia.

Management

Symptoms following abrupt cessation of benzodiazepines generally disappear if the drug is reinstated. Gradual rather than abrupt discontinuation is usually without untoward effect. The depression that follows discontinuation of stimulants may be so severe that antidepressant medication or electroshock is required. Suicide precautions are a required component of treatment if a patient's depression is so severe that they may take their own life. Reinstation of the anticonvulsants will bring about amelioration of psychotic symptoms erupting upon cessation of seizure medication. The gastrointestinal symptoms that appear following withdrawal of antidepressants are generally not of sufficient magnitude to merit recommencing the drug. If severe discomfort occurs, reinstitution of the medication and subsequent gradual withdrawal will handle the problem.

IV
BURN-OUT

When excessive demands are placed on individuals' energy, strength, or resources, they wear out or become exhausted. This situation is called burn-out (Freudenberger, 1975; Hall, et al. 1979; Pines and Maslach, 1978; Shuben, 1978). It is the occupational hazard of crisis psychiatric clinicians and other mental health professionals who must work with all pores open picking up and responding to nuances of patients' feelings. Unless a mental health professional learns early in his career how to counter this, therapists of potentially great talent are lost as they become inured to the great, sometimes magnificent and at other times painful, variety of the human experience.

Symptoms of Burn-out

1) Loss of charisma
2) Doubting ability to lead and to heal
3) Irritability
4) Dread of going to "work"
5) Exhaustion
6) Depression
7) Cynicism
8) Self-disgust
9) Disillusionment
10) Anger
11) Paranoia (e.g. fear someone will take your territory away if you are not careful)
12) Sense of isolation
13) Hyperexcitability (everything appears to be a crisis)
14) Headache
15) Indigestion

16) Dread of organization
17) Free floating anxiety
18) Undirected energy
19) Apathy
20) Emptiness
21) Confusion
22) Loss of innovativeness and creativity
23) Difficulty prioritizing activities
24) Negative job attitude
25) Negative self-image
26) Loss of concern and feeling for clients

Signs of Burn-out

1) Tearfulness
2) Ridicule of patients and other professionals
3) Defensiveness (to keep people away from seeing how burnt out one is)
4) Absenteeism (increased number of sick-leave days taken)
5) Sleeplessness
6) Diarrhea
7) Increase in patient drop out rate
8) Cancelling conferences capriciously
9) Declining appearance of self and work area
10) Inability to express oneself in writing and words
11) Not keeping up with paperwork or reading in one's field
12) Hystrionic responses to relatively minor stresses
13) More time spent talking with other employees than in patient care directed activity
14) Decreasing effectiveness at job
15) Inability to make decisions
16) Impairment of judgement
17) Fault finding in others and self
18) Detached concern
19) Intellectualization
20) Withdrawal
21) Compartmentalization

Causes of Burn-out

Pines and Maslach (1978) have identified in their research a number of factors which influence burn-out. These include:
1) Quality of staff-patient interactions: When staff-patient ratio

is sufficient to allow good staff-patient interaction, staff members report enjoying their work and feeling fulfilled in doing it.

2) Frequency of staff meetings: The greater the number of staff meetings, the more negative the attitudes toward patients.

3) Time out: Staff who could refocus their work efforts occasionally show a more favorable attitude toward patients.

4) Work schedule: Longer work hours are correlated with more staff stress and negative feelings toward work.

5) Time spent in direct contact with patients: The greater the contact with patients (save chronic schizophrenic patients) the less the burn-out.

6) Time spent with other staff members: Staff members who tend to spend more time with other staff members tend to rank themselves as tense and apathetic.

7) Time spent in administrative duties: Staff members who spend a great deal of time in administrative activities tend to like their work less and tend to like working with patients less.

8) Work sharing: Work is perceived as less stressful if it is shared. Sharing of work leads to increased freedom of expression and an increased feeling of personal power and of having a voice in institutional policy.

9) Formal education: Individuals with a high degree of formal education tend to desire more self-fulfillment than job satisfaction per se and in the absence of perceived individual growth tend to feel apathetic, powerless and weak.

10) Rank: Higher ranking mental health workers who tend to spend less time in direct patient care and more time in administration posses attitudes toward the mental health field which change negatively with time.

11) Years of practice: Individuals who have been in the mental health field longer tend to show a greater degree of burn-out.

12) Schizophrenic population: The greater the proportion of schizophrenics in a patient population, the greater the degree of burn-out.

Management

1) The most effective and self-gratifying way for a mental health professional to prevent burn-out is to cultivate the texture of both peoplescape and landscape. Too little attention is paid in training to how important it is for those who must daily face the vicissitudes of physical and mental health and illness to surround themselves with people who provide "soft landings" and a physical environment that

challenges their sensitivity to art, literature, nature and music. We, just like our patients, need to ventilate, to lance psychological abscesses so that they do not eat away at the essential core of our being. Each day must be fresh and each patient, like each new person we meet, be seen as and made to feel special. Art, music, nature and literature challenge us to be that which we all could be were it not for the layering of defenses against the realities of our molecular experiences. Art and nature have ways of getting at the core of our being in ways more intellectualized approaches do not. We relax, we laugh, and we cry as we savor texture and form and feel real substance.

2) Psychiatric clinicians should see a variety of patients. Clinicians become particularly burnt out when they see only one type of patient, especially if patients are chronic. Patient loads should be mixed to prevent burn-out and to help clinicians maintain a fresh approach to each patient.

3) Staff should be hired carefully. Individuals may come well credentialed but show, before commencing their new job, the insidious signs of burn-out such as apathy, overinvolvement with administrative minutia by history and a lack of innovativeness and creativity in their previous work.

4) Supervisors should get to know their staff as individuals and help each one develop a sense of specialness. It is good that staff members who have special interests such as alcoholism, spouse abuse and psychotherapy with adolescents be identified. These individuals should be encouraged to read, spend clinical time and attend conferences and other teaching exercises in their area of own interest. In addition, particularly talented clinicians should provide other staff members with case conferences and seminars for their area of interest and, if possible write on their subject for the popular press and scholarly journals.

5) Responsibilities should be rotated. Dealing with crisis patients is exhausting and must be a shared responsibility of all staff. The artificial separation between staff treating emergency patients and those working with inpatients and outpatients leads to burn-out and decreased creativity in both groups. Responsibility for all types of patients should be shared and rotated both to prevent burn-out as well as fatigue due to overwork. Staff members working with the more seriously ill patients tend to burn-out more rapidly.

6) People should not continue to work too long in areas which they have mastered. The lack of challenge leads to a stereotyping of both other staff and patients which is destructive to an organization and to themselves. Individuals need to be challenged to grow and

must sometimes move out of a high ranking position of leadership to allow someone newer with fresh enthusiasm and innovative ideas to take an organization through its next phase of growth.

7) Minimize administrative meetings. Staff burn-out is related to the number of administrative meetings attended. Administrative meetings should be short in duration and goal directed. They should not exceed one hour. Group psychotherapy is not a function of a staff meeting and long discussions over anger can lead to greater frustration and a greater sense of helplessness. One cannot get at core individual staff problems in a group and flirtation at the edge creates a sense of unfilled expectancy rather than therapeutic ventilation.

8) Patient-staff ratio should be low enough so that the staff may approach each patient with renewed optimism and individualized care. The greater the number of patients a staff member sees, the greater the sensory overload, and the more rapidly burn-out develops.

9) Work hours, especially in emergency psychiatry and crisis intervention, should be kept sufficiently low to prevent sleep deprivation and the attendant irritability, anger and lack of enthusiasm that comes from overwork.

10) Periodic staff retreats should be undertaken to review goals and increase the feeling of support and purpose among staff. Humanistic goals can become obfuscated when we do not step back to see the toll taken on even the most sensitive and idealistic clinician when repeatedly confronted with the realities of human pain and human limitation. It is imperative for successful crisis work that the clinician's eyes be set on finding strengths and bringing out human potential rather than focusing in on "psychopathology" and "illness."

11) Continuing education—Both staff and an institution must build in programs of continuing education to keep staff abreast of changes in the field and to review basic principles of evaluation and treatment.

12) Supervision—Staff must be adequately supervised. This allows both a monitoring of quality of care as well as an opportunity to ventilate anxiety over carrying suicidal and homicidal patients, psychotic patients, patients with diagnostic problems, and chronic patients, who frustrate clinician's desire to see evidence of great change over time. Supervision should be a time of support, education and quality control.

13) Early recognition of burn-out—The best approach to burn-out is primary prevention using such techniques as continuing education, supervision, rotation of duties, minimizing administrative

meetings, etc. When despite these approaches, the early symptoms of burn-out such as irritability and increased absenteeism occur, the staff members should be called aside by a supervisor and placed elsewhere in the institutional setting, either temporarily or permanently, to allow some renewal and reevaluation of where they are going and of their goals as mental health professionals.

V
DISASTER PLANNING

A disaster is defined by the Disaster Relief Act of 1974 as a hurricane, tornado, storm flood, high-water, wind-driven water, tidal wave, tsunami, earthquake, volcanic eruption, landslide, snowstorm, fire or other catastrophic occurrences in any part of the continental United States or its territories which causes damage of sufficient severity and magnitude to warrant disaster assistance. In summary, a disaster appears, by the definition, to be any situation which creates such widespread suffering and needs that victims cannot alleviate them without assistance beyond personal resources.

Planning for a disaster is an especially difficult task. Expertise in crisis intervention comes from training under those skilled in the field supplemented by practical experiences. The patient is always the best teacher. Comparably, expertise in management of disaster comes from both training under those who have been involved in disaster themselves and by field experience in a disaster. Unfortunately, (or perhaps better said fortunately) there are few who have such training in actual disasters because disasters are rare events. A disaster is simply not a multicar accident or a house burning with three families in it. It may involve whole communities, townships or even countries as in the hurricane in the Caribbean isle of Dominica where nearly ninety percent of the property was reported to have been destroyed. In instances where a disaster is more circumscribed, it may involve unfathomable human carnage such as in the Kentucky supper club fire outside of Cincinnati or the aircrash over San Diego in 1978. In the latter instance, the problem is not the lack of skills in physical or psychological medicine, but rather that the task has elements that counter all we are taught in the management of more specific individual crises.

In the management of a simple crisis such as sudden death of a loved one or a rape, we are called upon to be empathetic, sensitive and supportive. We ride the tide of feeling and listen with all our pores open to hear nuances of words and subtle distinctions of feeling. In a large disaster mental health clinicians are called upon to undertake tasks for which they have had no preparation and which they have never even imagined themselves doing. Following a large fire involving the death of over 100 people, they may be called upon to guide relatives and friends seeking someone who did not return home the night before who was reported to have been in the building that burned. The psychiatric clinician may have to view over 100 charred bodies with the relative before a ring on a charred hand or a scar or tattoo on a part of the chest not burned provides a clue to the identity of the victim. *Care givers* as well as friends and relatives of victims need support and time for ventilation in disaster work. Burnout may occur over months or years in crisis work. In disaster work, it can occur over hours.

Disasters provide, even for those accustomed to seeing multiated bodies and human violence, unprecedented tests to our fears of unexpected destruction and helplessness against the forces of nature or man (as in the explosion of a nuclear bomb, nuclear reactor or terrorist attack). The care giver is sometimes numbed as much as survivors. Mild (by comparison) disasters such as tornados, hurricanes and floods, which are accompanied by great property loss, but take less toll on human life, are easier to handle. Management skills in handling disasters such as floods, snowstorms and hurricanes requires leadership skills, the setting of priorities, and provision of social support, shelter, flood, clothing and medical assistance. The usual crisis techniques of ventilation and supportive psychotherapy coupled with the task of helping the victim leave the experience with a better eye to his values and better prioritization of life tasks is the usual approach.

In disasters with great loss of life and mutilation of bodies, sensitive-feeling psychotherapists may become a psychological casualty as will many sensitive firemen, policemen, clergy and other health professionals who empathize with the pain of the survivors and feel their own vulnerability and helplessness anew again and again as each new victim is found. The task of collecting fragmented body parts on a hot humid afternoon after an airplane crash over a city tests human limits. Those who handle it best are often those who do not think about the nuances and do not empathize with the horror of victim and survivor. This is just the opposite of who serves best in most other crisis intervention work.

There are a number of basic points that are helpful in planning the psychosocial component of a disaster plan for a community. These include:

1) *Enumeration of all the possible disasters that may occur in the area.* Snowstorms are usual in New England, but rare or unheard of in parts of California, while tidal waves and earthquakes are less unusual. Plane crashes and large fires could occur in both places. Explosion of nuclear reactors is limited to those areas where nuclear energy sources have been constructed. Each disaster has its own characteristics and requires specific planning for both the psychosocial and medical component of a disaster assistance program. Floods entail great property loss in a given community. Crisis intervention work focuses around unexpected loss, usually of property, rarely of life, and recruitment of physical, psychological, social and spiritual strengths to go on and begin anew from what little may remain. Disaster work for a large airplane crash may entail working with care givers rather than relatives of victims as victims may be from a number of cities both here and abroad and other than during the brief period entailed in claiming a body, the victim's relatives will need support at home in their own communities. Caregivers may, however, be overcome by the horror of human carnage and the feeling of the transience of life and man's helplessness. Psychiatric clinicians can play critical roles in structuring time schedules allowing adequate rest and nutrition and ventilation for caregivers. An important part of a disaster assistance program is the secondary prevention of psychiatric illness by early recognition of those who may become psychiatric casualties and their prompt removal from the scene of action.

2) *Individuals should be screened for work on disaster teams.* In the time of a major disaster, casualties due to an oversensitivity to the horror of the reality compound the work of disaster assistance teams. Well meaning individuals may volunteer but will not be able to be used in the task because they would decompensate. There are a number of films available that are used to train people in disaster assistance which are helpful in making the choice of who may best serve. In addition, some work in a large city, riding shift with a police officer, takes an individual into contact with serious injury and death in automobile accidents. This will in a small degree prepare the individual for the reality of death and bodily multilation seen in large airplane crashes and chemical explosions.

3) *An individual should be identified to coordinate the psychosocial aspect of a disaster assistance program.* It is important to have several people identified so that if one or more leadership people are not available at the time of an unexpected disaster, or lost as a vic-

tim, another may take leadership. On-call lists with all telephone numbers included (both listed and unlisted) must be in the hands of all leadership people. A clear administrative chain of command and alertness is essential for success of a disaster assistance program.

4) *Mock disaster assistance programs should be held to test out flaws in the organization and delivery of medical and psychosocial services.* A plan may look good on paper, but delays in arrival of staff or unavailability may be unanticipated. A mock disaster allows one to work out logistic problems. Unfortunately, the exercise usually does not sufficiently engender emotion to test the strength of team members to function in a disaster when flooded with unexpected emotion.

5) *Assistance to disaster victims and to casualties among the caregivers should be of a crisis oriented nature.* There are certain sample crisis principles which are essential for effective delivery of the psychosocial component of a disaster assistance plan:

a) Individual strengths rather than liability should be brought into focus.

b) Treatment should be given as near to the front lines as possible to reduce the potential for regression, dependency and guilt.

c) False assurances about loss of life or property or about extent of injuries should not be given.

d) Victims and families should be reunited as soon as possible.

e) Ventilation about the horror of the experience should be encouraged in a warm supportive atmosphere either with the psychiatric clinician alone or in groups with other victims.

f) Use drugs sparingly as they may delay working through of pent up emotion.

g) Help victims face realistically the extent of the disaster and its effect on their life.

h) Help individuals plan, given resources present, for what they must do over the ensuing days. This may include burying loved ones and finding shelter, food and medical assistance (e.g. diabetics needing insulin).

i) Information should be disseminated regarding the extent and severity of the disaster. This information should be updated as needed.

j) Victims who can still function should be encouraged to join in the task of reconstruction.

k) Shelter and food should be found for victims, if needed, with families or neighbors or with available social agencies in their own or neighboring community.

l) Patients should be provided with the expectation of recovery from the psychological crisis. Even though they may be flooded with anxiety, guilt, depression, anger, panic and shame for having survived, they should be helped to see it as but a moment in time. It, as other great sorrows and stresses, will pass even though at that moment the impact may be so predominant that they can see no tomorrow.

m) Community resources should be used rather than creating new ones. Crisis is a time for allowing individuals to find ways of coping within themselves that they may have had no idea existed before. So too, communities should be encouraged to find undiscovered resources as well as discovering new ways of using extant resources to manage crisis on a community level.

n) Records of individual contacts should be developed to coordinate and document services so that individuals may be referred for continued treatment if needed.

o) Physical facilities should be identified if hospitalization is needed as well as other shelters for the care of victims and their relatives.

p) Psychiatric clinicians and other caregivers should be appropriately identified by badges, armbands or other means.

q) Care should be provided for caregivers. We do not need to compound tragedy by tragedy. Food, shelter and sleep are needed as is careful evaluation and reevaluation to assure that the caregiver does not become part of the toll. The coordinator of the psychosocial component of the disaster assistance program should set clear time boundaries on all staff to prevent burnout and to maintain high quality assistance.

r) Always, a crisis is a time for value reassessment. Even in the worst of disasters it is possible to come out of the experience richer for the stress. Individuals who can find a "why" to live will be able to find a "how" to survive. We should help individuals at a time of disaster to find the "why" either in terms of human relationships or in terms of longer altruistic or spiritual goals.

VI
LEGAL AND ETHICAL ASPECTS OF EMERGENCY PSYCHIATRIC CARE

CONFIDENTIALITY

Privileged Communication

Definition

The patient has the right in many states to determine if information that he imparts to his physician during therapy can be disclosed by the physician at a judicial proceeding.

Origin

In order to be able to use this privilege there must be a state statute that provides for it. At the present time, over two-thirds of the states have statutes that recognize the confidentiality of personal information conveyed by a patient to his physician, and that this information cannot be divulged without the patient's consent.

Regarding federal courts, which do not for the most part operate under state statutes, the federal rules of evidence designed by the Supreme Court of the United States include a provision for privileged communication between patients and their psychotherapists. These rules apply only to federal courts.

Reason for Privilege

This is a societal decision which reflects a policy to encourage those in need of medical care to obtain help freely without the concern that information might be used in a civil or criminal court action.

Type of Information that is Privileged

The privilege covers information that is disclosed by a patient to a physician and that is connected with his illness. Because effective psychotherapy requires that the therapist become familiar with all aspects of the social and interpersonal history of the patient, nearly everything the patient discloses would be considered privileged.

For information to be privileged, there must be a therapist-patient relationship. As a result, information that a therapist learns outside of the treatment, for instance at a social gathering, about his patient would likely not be considered as privileged. In addition, if a physician is requested to examine a patient for the court or a third party the physician-patient relationship is not considered to have been established. However, as soon as the physician or therapist administers treatment, he essentially creates the relationship.

Therapist Obligated Under Privileged Communication

According to the statutes of most of the states, the rule on privileged communication applies only to licensed physicians. Others who do not have a medical degree such as lay analysts, psychiatric social workers and nurses may be compelled to testify on the witness stand, except where it can be shown that they are functioning as "agent" of physicians in caring for specific patients.

Not all of the states limit the rule for privileged communication to licensed physicians. Some states, like New York, include others who must comply with privileged communication such as psychologists, nurses, and psychiatric social workers. When the patient desires that the mental health worker provide information at a court proceeding, the therapist cannot refuse this request because the privilege is vested in the patient.

Exceptions

The rule for privileged communication in many states is not held applicable if there is a strong public policy that would be served if information were disclosed. For example, if a patient is afflicted with a venereal disease, such as syphilis, then for the protection of society it may be important that this fact be revealed. Similarly, where the patient is involved in a hearing for custody of children, it would be to the benefit of society to know that he has engaged in abusive behavior, or that he is a chronic alcoholic. Included under exceptions to this rule would be the disclosure of information about a patient's criminal conduct, such as that he engaged in procuring narcotics unlawfully, where it would be essential for the fair and proper administration of justice.

Confidential Communication

Definition

The patient has both an ethical and legal right to expect that information imparted by him to a therapist is held confidential and not conveyed to a third party—family members, friends, government agencies, etc.

Origin

Ethical codes going back as far as the Hippocratic Oath specifically prohibit physicians from divulging personal information about a patient. In addition to ethical prohibition, a physician or other therapist may be legally culpable under one of the following legal theories for disclosing personal information without prior consent:

1) *Libel*—This occurs when information is revealed which creates an unfavorable and unjust impression about a patient.

2) *Slander*—A slanderous statement is one in which a false charge or gross misrepresentation is made which in effect damages a patient's reputation.

3) *Invasion of privacy*—This refers to another legal theory whereby the information revealed by a patient is protected because of the right of an individual to require that his personal and private affairs be kept from public scrutiny, unless he gives his consent. Hence, a therapist may be held legally responsible for providing information about a patient even though he did not disclose false facts or create an unjust impression.

Reason for Privilege

Similar to the reason for the rule of privileged communication, the rule for confidentiality of communication reflects to some extent society's recognition of the importance of professional services, like psychiatric care, and the desire to avoid conflicts that might hinder the use of such services. Perhaps more importantly, the theories of law that are used to protect the confidentiality of communication emerged out of the common law tradition, unlike the rule for privileged communication which was created by a definite legislative act in the states where it is operative. The common law tradition has long recognized the right of an individual to be left alone, free from unwarranted publicity, and consequently to live without unjustified interference by the public in areas that should be outside the scope of public concern. The right to privacy, therefore, is the primary reason for the rule on confidentiality of communication.

Type of Information That is Confidential

As with the rule on privileged communication, nearly everything the patient discloses to his therapist would be considered confidential, whether it is connected to the therapy or not. The Hippocratic Oath prohibits the disclosure of any information "in connection with my professional practice or not in connection with it." For the most part, the legal rules against disclosure would consider information confidential if the patient has reason to believe it would not be revealed to a third party and if it was conveyed in the course of the physician or therapist-patient relationship.

Therapist Obligated Under Confidential Communication

Some states like California specifically prohibit in statutes a physician from disclosing confidential material about a patient to a third party. It is safe to assume, however, that any therapist who enters into a therapist-patient relationship would be potentially legally responsible under the theories of libel, slander or invasion of privacy, despite the presence of a statute or a code of ethics for the specific professions.

Exceptions

The rule for confidential communications can be circumvented if the disclosure of private information is necessary to protect the welfare of the individual patient or of the society at large. In any case, there are still restrictions on what information can be revealed and to whom. Only that amount of personal information may be revealed which is necessary to achieve the purpose for the disclosure. Furthermore, the information can be conveyed only to those persons or agencies that must be informed in order to achieve the purpose of disclosure either for the patient or the community. The following illustrate circumstances that would justify the conveying of private information about a patient:

1) *Conveying Information To A Spouse*—For the most part physicians, and probably other therapists, can inform a spouse of the medical condition of their husband or wife, as many courts have held that a spouse has the right to know if their partner is afflicted by a disease. There are circumstances that might militate against disclosure under this condition. For example, if the couple is involved in a separation or divorce proceeding, or if they are involved in a custody hearing, then it might be argued strongly that there in no justification in disclosing information to the other "spouse." Each situation has to be carefully evaluated in terms of the parties involved, the nature of the disclosure and the state of the marital relationship.

2) *Disclosure to legitimate agencies*—Courts have usually maintained that a physician or therapist does not violate confidentiality if he turns over the medical records of a patient to an agency, such as a school or employer, which has a strong reason for obtaining the information.

3) *Informing about contagious diseases*—A physician may inform those intimately involved with a patient that he has a contagious disease. This would include not only family members but employers, school officials and others who might be exposed to the patient while he is ill. If a patient has a venereal disease most states require that the physician inform the department of health of this condition. Similarly, in many states a physician must report those who are dependent on drugs to the health commissioner.

4) *Duty to warn potential victims*—The Tarasoff case, decided in 1976 by the California Supreme Court, places an affirmative obligation on psychotherapists to use reasonable care to protect the intended victim, including warning him as well as notifying the police. This ruling applies only to California, but a similar decision has been made in at least one additional state, and others are seriously considering this requirement.

Obtaining the Patient's Consent

Because of the particular stigma attached in this society to mental illness and the potentially injurious consequences that can result from indiscriminate disclosure of mental or emotional problems, the mental health professional is obligated to make every effort to obtain the patient's consent before disclosing confidential information.

If the patient is not mentally able to give consent and there is a compelling reason to reveal personal information about him, then the consent of the closest family member should be obtained if at all possible. It is best to be over-protective of the patient's rights to confidentiality of personal information where mental disease is involved, even if the therapist has a strong and legitimate reason to disclose specific facts about the patient. In addition, consent from family members should be sought as a last resort because of the possibility that they would not have the best interests of the patient in mind when giving consent.

MALPRACTICE

Medical Malpractice

Definition

This is a legal concept that refers to those happenings in medical practice that result in injury to the patient and that can be shown to be due to the therapist's negligence, carelessness, or incompetence. In order for there to be malpractice, three features in addition to injury to the patient must be present:

1) There must be a therapist-patient relationship.

2) There must be lack of skill and care on the part of the therapist.

3) There must be a proof of the standard of care by which the therapist is measured.

Standard of Care

Malpractice suits, in effect, serve as a legal device for regulating the medical profession. The standard of care by which individual acts are measured must be as objective as possible. In many jurisdictions, the locality rule is operative. This rule states that a therapist has been negligent or incompetent if he did not provide that level of care or skill that would be exercised by an ordinary psychiatrist in the community in which he practices. In 1968 a landmark case was decided in Massachusetts that essentially held that the level of care and skill that determines good medical practice is that of the average specialist in the field taking into account current medical advances and community resources. This case effectively over-ruled the "locality" rule in Massachusetts, and it is likely to set a precedent for similar decisions in other states. In addition, there are other systems being developed, most particularly the Professional Standards Review Organizations (PSRO's) which should create, in time, a concept of national standards of care for each medical specialty. The law on standard of care is in a state of flux, and although the "locality" rule still may be the predominant standard, certainly for the general practitioner, it will likely be applied in frequency where specialists are concerned.

Responsibility for Malpractice

When a physician or primary therapist commits an act which is considered by the court to be malpractice, he is generally responsible for his negligence. There are situations where he can be held responsible for the actions of his subordinates, or by the same token where the institution in which he works can be held liable for his actions.

1) Responsibility for delegated functions — When a psychiatrist has non-physician clinicians working under him he can be held liable for their negligent actions. The law applies a theory called "respondeat superior" or the "captain-of-the-ship" doctrine, which, in effect, means that an employer (the psychiatrist) is liable for the negligent and injurious acts of his employees. It is argued that the employer hires the employee and is in the position to select on the basis of competence. Furthermore, he is obligated to provide supervision and should therefore know what functions are within the capabilities of the employee.

2) Responsibility of institutions—Until the early 1940s hospitals were virtually exempt from legal liability for malpractice. However, since that time there has been a change in policy regarding the culpability of institutions and they are now vulnerable under at least two legal theories:

a) *Corporate negligence*—Traditionally, the concept of corporate negligence meant that hospitals, like corporations, should be held responsible for their administrative tasks, such as selecting and training competent personnel, making sure that adequate supervision is provided and above all maintaining the equipment and buildings appropriately. It had been felt until only very recently that corporations or hospitals could not be held responsible for the medical practice conducted under its domain. This distinction between administrative functions and medical practice broke down in a major case in 1965 in Illinois, when the Supreme Court of that state held a hospital liable for violating medical duties it had to patients because it allowed an unqualified physician to practice orthopedic surgery which resulted in injury to the patient. This case, in effect, held that the setting of standards of good patient care are the joint obligation of the practitioner and the institution. There have been several cases that have followed the same decision as the Darling case in 1965, and it is most likely that a trend has been started that will result in a nationwide re-evaluation of the role of the institution in the practice of medicine.

Hospitals are particularly susceptible to liability for patients injured while receiving emergency care, because they must often rely on physicians from the local community who are inadequately trained to handle a wide range of emergencies—from surgical to psychiatric.

b) *Vicarious liability*—Hospitals as employers can be held responsible for the negligent acts of its individual employees such as nurses and maintenance staff. Some states still consider nonprofit hospitals as exempt from this liability under a doctrine called, "Charitable immunity." But, in recent years the courts have discarded this special status so that now nearly all jurisdictions allow hospitals to be sued for the negligent acts of their employees. There is a shift away from the concept that the physician is the "captain-of-the-ship" and responsible for the careless acts of hospital employees, to that of viewing the hospital in this role.

Malpractice in Psychiatry

Inadequate Care

This term is used loosely to refer to situations when the type of care seemed appropriate but it was either inadequate or negligently executed or terminated before the course of treatment had been completed.

1) *The Suicidal Patient*—The suicidal patient is one of the most difficult emergency problems. If the therapist should reasonably have suspected that a patient was suicidal then he could be held liable for not instituting immediate emergency measures, such as placing the patient in the hospital where he can be carefully observed and, if necessary, be treated with effective psychoactive medication. In addition, instruments which might be used for effecting a suicide must be kept from the patient's reach. The law recognizes that suicides occur in spite of the most careful precautions.

However, the therapist is obligated to institute all available measures to prevent the death. Hospitals are also vulnerable to suits, particularly if it can be shown that inadequate efforts were made to restrain or control the patient, or that the hospital failed to adequately observe the suicidal patient.

2) *Abandonment of the Patient*—Abandonment can only occur if a therapeutic relationship has been established. A therapist is not obligated to take on a patient in therapy, but once he does so he must follow the patient either until the patient is placed in the care of another therapist, or until treatment is no longer necessary. If the therapist decides on his own to stop treating a patient who still requires treatment, he is essentially abandoning the patient. If, however, he provides adequate notice to the patient so that the patient can find another therapist, or he obtains the consent of the patient, he is no longer liable for abandonment. When therapists terminate treatment because they feel the patient no longer requires their attention, they do so at their own risk and could possibly be held responsible for abandonment. Abandonment does not in itself indicate that a therapist has committed malpractice. There must also be a showing that an injury has occurred that can be directly related to the abandonment.

3) *Psychiatric Procedures*—Three psychiatric procedures are particularly involved in malpractice suits:

a) *Wrongful commitment*—For the most part, courts have come out in favor of the psychiatrist where suits have been brought for wrongful commitment. To begin with, when a psychiatrist examines a patient for commitment he is not considered to be involved in a therapeutic relationship, and therefore owes no special duty of care to the patient. There have been some court decisions against psychiatrists particularly where the psychiatrist has inadequately examined the patient, or completely avoided examining the patient and instead relied on the opinion of the family members.

b) *Psychotherapy*—This is a very difficult area in which to establish malpractice. It is particularly hard to show that inadequate care has been given. For the most part, suits in this area have involved the use of unconventional techniques, such as using physical contact, and situations where the therapist became socially involved with the patient and the patient was injured as a result.

c) *Chemical and mechanical therapies*—Before the introduction of sedatives and paralyzing agents, electroshock and insulin shock therapies had significant risks of complications.

Most commonly patients suffered from fractures of the bones and spine and claimed that they were inadequately restrained during the treatment. Also, there have been several cases where patients alleged that they were not fully informed of the risks of shock therapy. Suits in the future will probably be concerned with whether preparatory medications were properly administered before the shock treatment. In addition to shock treatment, there have been suits involving drug reactions, particularly those from the phenothiazines. As more and more drugs become available for the care of psychiatric patients, adverse drug reactions (especially the tardive dyskinesias) will become more frequent and will inevitably end in many malpractice suits. It will be important that the therapist can show that he adequately diagnosed the condition and took the necessary steps to counteract it.

Inappropriate Care

This term refers to situations where techniques are used that have not been demonstrated to be appropriate or helpful in the treatment of a particular psychiatric condition. This concept must be distinguished from the use of an experimental procedure which, though it may not have been demonstrated clinically to be effective in the treatment of a condition, seems to be justified on the basis of preliminary laboratory and clinical findings as well as adherence to a reasonable and acceptable theoretical framework. Inappropriate care means that it does not fit into either category of those treatments that are recognized as proper or into those that have experimental merit.

1) *Illustrative Examples*—The following are two examples that illustrate inappropriate care in psychiatric practice:

a) *The use of mescaline to treat sociopaths*—There is no evidence that this drug has any place in psychiatric treatment of sociopathy. Furthermore, this drug, as with other hallucenogens, is potentially very dangerous to patients. In addition, at the present time there is no evidence in the psychiatric literature to support its use in an experimental trial. Hence, on the basis of existing information about sociopathy, the use of this drug would be strongly contraindicated and contrary to good clinical judgement.

b) *Physical abuse of the patient during psychotherapy*—Although there is a wide range of techniques that would be appropriate within the psychotherapeutic relationship, inflicting physical harm on the patient would not be considered by any approach to be acceptable therapy. There would also be no strong experimental reason for using this unusual technique that could justify the significant potentiality of harm to the patient.

2) *Professional and Legal Violations*—The therapist who engages in inappropriate treatment that results in harm to the patient may be faced with the following legal and professional sanctions:

a) *Legal Sanctions*—The therapist may be sued for a tort or wrongdoing in a civil procedure or he may be charged with a criminal offense.

1) *Tort or malpractice:* The patient may assert that the therapist performed an unauthorized procedure by not receiving informed consent, or that he conducted the therapy in a negligent manner. Similar to what would happen in the bulk of suits involving the adequacy of treatment, if the therapist loses he would be expected to pay for the damages caused by his malpractice.

2) *Criminal conduct:* The therapist could have criminal charges brought against him if the procedure were perceived as evidence of negligence that was so gross as to effectively amount to a reckless disregard of the rights and safety of another person. Should it be possible to prove that the therapist had the intent to harm the patient, then he could be charged with offenses such as criminal assault and even murder.

b) *Professional Sanctions*—By performing inappropriate procedures the therapist may have violated the standards of professional conduct defined by state statute and his license to practice may be denied, suspended or revoked. This decision would be made by the state licensing agency.

Obtaining The Patients' Consent

Definition

The concept of informed consent is difficult to define in a way that can be used as a guide for the physician or researcher who is interested in protecting the rights of his patients. Simply stated, informed consent means that the patient has been fully informed about a procedure which is to be performed on him, comprehends the risks and benefits of the procedure, and freely gives his consent. The problem with "informed consent" is in determining how much information should be presented to the patient, and the extent of the patient's capacity to fully comprehend the risks and benefits inherent in the medical procedure, as well as the alternatives that are available.

Circumstances that Require Consent

Informed Consent is required in both treatment and experimentation:

1) *Treatment*—The patient should be informed of the risks, benefits, and alternatives of specific psychiatric procedures. In the past, there have been suits against psychiatrists for not informing the patient about the risks of ECT or insulin shock. There have been recent cases in some states that require that the therapist inform the patient of risks associated with psychiatric treatment even if he does not request this information. The safest course of action is to fully inform patients of the risks, benefits, and alternatives of all treatment.

2) *Experimentation*—It is mandatory that patients be carefully informed of all the risks and benefits that may result from an experimental procedure. Unlike the treatment situation, the subject of an experiment often stands to benefit little if at all. This makes the need for "informed consent" even more important.

Limits of Informed Consent

Because of the difficulties of "informed consent," that is determining how much information to convey and the capability of the patient to understand fully the risks of procedures, other instruments are being proposed to supplement the protection afforded by informed consent. One such device is the "protection" or "consent" committee notion. These committees would serve and overview role and evaluate experiments before thay are conducted to determine if they should be allowed. The target population that would be benefited most by these committees would be particularly vulnerable groups like the mentally ill and retarded, prisoners and children.

VOLUNTARY HOSPITALIZATION

Admission to Hospital

Definition

An admission to a mental facility is voluntary if it is at the request of the patient himself, or a guardian in the case of a minor or mentally retarded patient. Even though the patient desires admission to a mental institution, this does not in itself guarantee that he will be admitted. The directors of facilities for the mentally ill have broad powers to admit or reject patients based on their perception as to whether an individual is an appropriate candidate for this treatment. Furthermore, limitations of resources often prevent hospitals from admitting patients who might otherwise benefit from treatment.

Types of Admission

A voluntary admission to a mental health facility can be either informal or formal:

1) *Informal*—An informal admission to a mental hospital is one in which the patient merely indicates his desire to be hospitalized without completing and submitting a formal written application.

2) *Formal*—A formal admission requires that the patient submit a written application. This application is usually witnessed and implies in effect that the patient is aware that he needs psychiatric care and that he will comply with the rules and regulations of the institution, which are restricted to some extent by state statutes.

Release From Hospital

Definition

The fact that a patient voluntarily admitted himself to a treatment facility does not mean that he can leave whenever he desires to terminate hospitalization. The right to leave a mental institution is, for the most part, conditioned by state statutes and depends on whether the patient was informally admitted or admitted through written application.

Types of Release

1) *Informal*—A patient who enters a hospital without submitting a written application has considerable freedom to end treatment when he desires to. Most statutes provide that a patient informally admitted can leave a hospital anytime during the business hours of that institution. In effect he can simply walk out of the hospital anytime between 8:30 or 9:00 in the morning to 5:00 or 5:30 at night. In some states that provide for informal admissions this includes weekends.

2) *Formal*—A patient who enters a hospital through a formal application is under legal obligation to follow specific procedures before he can terminate his hospitalization. Some states allow the patient to be discharged immediately upon his submitting a written request for release. Others require that he remain hospitalized for a period of time after he submits notice that he desires to be released. This period of detainment can be anywhere from 2 days, as in the District of Columbia, to as much as 2 weeks in some states. Many states, however, protect the patient from unnecessary hospitalization by limiting the period of time that he can be voluntarily hospitalized. For example, Pennsylvania sets a maximum period for confinement, after which the patient must be released unless he requests that hospitalization continue. For the most part, hospital authorities are also not legally obligated to inform a patient that according to the statutes of the state he can request release either immediately or after being hospitalized for a minimum period of time. Consequently, many patients do not even know that they have the right to request release from the hospital and that this request must be granted after a certain prescribed period of time.

Non-Protested Admissions

Definition

A non-protested admission similar to a voluntary "formal" hospitalization is brought about through a written application; however, this is not initiated by the patient, but by a relative, close friend or health authority. The admission is not involuntary in that it does not require certification by two or more medical persons nor does it result in a formal determination of mental illness. By the same token, it is not strictly a voluntary admission in that the patient has not requested it. What makes this admission "non-protested" is that the patient does not object to the admission as would be the case generally with an involuntary commitment.

Release

A patient can terminate treatment after a non-protested admission much the same way that he would terminate hospitalization following a voluntary 'formal' admission. He would simply state his desire in writing to terminate treatment and depending on the state statute would be released anywhere from 2 days to 14 days following the submission of this request.

INVOLUNTARY HOSPITALIZATION

Commitment to Hospital

Definition

A patient is generally committed to a mental institution if it is felt that he requires hospitalization because of the seriousness of his condition—specifically, he may be potentially dangerous to himself or to others—and he refuses to consent to treatment on a voluntary basis.

Types of Commitment

An involuntary commitment to a mental facility can be either for a determinate or an indeterminate period of time. For the most part indeterminate confinement has been a device used for committing sex offenders and dangerous offenders. Increasingly, however, indeterminate confinement is not viewed on favorably, predominately on policy grounds and the trend has been distinctly in the direction of minimizing the application of this form of commitment. Determinate commitment is clearly the predominate form for civil commitment of patients to mental facilities.

Determinate—A determinate commitment is usually for a designated period of time. Since the early 1970s and particularly following the *Lessard* decision in Wisconsin the trend has been distinctly in the direction of reducing the period of determinate commitment. The following types of hospitalization fit within this category:

1) *Emergency hospitalization*—Most of the states have provi-

sion in their statutes for the emergency detention of patients in order to control an immediate threat such as suicide or homicide. A formal application is required and usually made by a health officer or a law enforcement official. This form of hospitalization is to be used only until proper legal steps, such as a judicial hearing, are followed to determine if additional hospitalization is necessary. The length of time that a patient may be detained under emergency hospitalization is clearly limited by statute. Since the Lessard decision, many states allow a physician to commit a patient for 24 to 48 hours at the end of which time the decision for confining the patient must be reviewed to determine whether there is "probable cause" for detaining the patient further up to approximately 15 days at which time a judicial hearing is required to detain the patient further, and then usually only an additional 30 days. New York State allows a physician under emergency conditions to commit a patient for up to 15 days on the basis of "dangerousness to self and others" but requires that within 48 hours of the time of admission, the patient must be examined by another physician who is a member of the psychiatric staff of the hospital, and if that physician concurs in the judgment of the emergency room physician the patient may be detained up to 15 days. Beyond 15 days, the statute requires a new admission on an application supported by two new examining physicians' certificates, unless of course the patient enters on a voluntary basis in the interim.

2) *Temporary or observational hospitalization*—Many states have procedures for the hospitalization of patients where there is no clear emergency but where observation of the patient is warranted. This form of hospitalization is for a definite period of time and it avoids the formal procedures associated with judicial commitment that can be quite time consuming.

3) *Medical certification*—In most of the jurisdictions in this country hospitalization for a determinate period can be achieved by a certification that the patient is mentally ill and requires hospitalization. Depending on the requirements of the individual state statutes this certification for the most part is made by two physicians who have examined the patient. Some states require additionally that the decision of the physicians be reviewed and possibly approved by a judge, but this review is not the same as would occur in a judicial commitment. The judge's concern would be focused on the qualifications of the physicians who signed the medical certificate and the authenticity of the documents. After the patient has been committed through this mechanism, the state either grants him the right to be released after he submits a request for

release following a short period of detainment or the right to have the certification reviewed by a court from the standpoint of the merits of the decision of the physicians to commit the patient. In New York State the patient also has the right to contact the Mental Health Information Service which is a court agency independent of the treatment facility which would provide the patient with protective services and legal assistance as well as information regarding his hospitalization. Interestingly enough in New York State, the criteria for commitment of a patient through a two physician certification is broader than that through emergency commitment. In the former, the physician must attest to the fact that the person has a mental illness which requires care and treatment in a hospital as "essential to his welfare" and that the patient is so impaired in his judgment that "he is unable to understand the need for such care and treatment." As we already stated above, the criteria for emergency admission is the objective one of likelihood of "dangerousness to self and others."

4) *Judicial commitment*—This form of commitment is still the most common form of involuntary hospitalization as it is provided for in the statutes of nearly all of the states. In effect, this procedure involves the determination of whether a patient is mentally ill and should be hospitalized. This decision is made mostly by a judge and, less often, a jury on the basis of medical evidence. Since the Lessard decision, many states require that after 15 or more days of hospitalization a judicial hearing be conducted to justify further confinement. For the most part, a judicial determination of the need for hospitalization results in a commitment for a limited period of time, in some states 30 and other states 60 days. There have been strong moves recently to impose further safeguards for the patient against indiscriminate hospitalization, and include the requirements of continuing judicial review of the patient's progress. Judicial commitment begins with a petition or application which is usually signed and submitted by a close relative, friend, or physician who knows the patient. Along with the petition the court usually requires a medical certificate that states the patient has been examined by a physician and found to be mentally ill. Once the petition and medical certificate are submitted to the court, notice is usually given to the patient that the hearing will be held in the near future to determine if the patient should be committed for psychiatric treatment. This affords the patient an opportunity to obtain legal counsel should he desire to contest the commitment. The hearing is usually held before a judge who determines on the basis of the information presented if the patient should be committed for a further period of time.

5) *Administrative procedure*—This form of commitment is probably infrequently used. The procedure involves a board that consists primarily of the physician. The board holds the hearing to determine if commitment is necessary. In some states, an attorney or a judge is required to be a participant on the administrative board of the hospital.

Notice Of Rights

Many states provide the patient with a statement of notice of status and rights surrounding their admission to a hospital. Such statements exist for voluntary, emergency, and involuntary admissions in New York State. An example of such a form is seen with the "Notice of Status and Rights" for emergency admission in New York. The form reads "you have been admitted to this hospital for the mentally ill on an emergency basis for immediate observation care and treatment. Within 48 hours of the time of your admission you will be examined by another member of the psychiatric staff. If his finding confirms the initial finding of the admitting physician, you may then be retained for a period of up to 15 days from the date of your admission to this hospital. During this 15-day-period you may be released, asked to remain as an informal or voluntary patient, or be admitted as involuntary patient. You, your relatives, and your friends should feel free to ask members of the hospital staff about your condition, your status and your rights, and the rules and regulations of the hospital. If you, your relatives, or friends feel that you do not need immediate observation, care and treatment, you and they may request a court hearing. Copies of any written request for a court hearing will be forwarded by the hospital director to the appropriate court and the mental health information service". In addition to this information the form also includes a brief description of the Mental Health Information Service and its role in providing assistance to the hospitalized patient. The "Notice of Status and Rights" for involuntary admission, as well as voluntary admissions contains similar information that deals with the patients' and families' rights to contest the commitment.

Release From Hospital

Definition

If a patient is involuntarily committed to a mental institution, he is not allowed to leave the hospital whenever he desires. The decision to release a patient from a hospital resides for the most part with the treating psychiatrist or the administrator of the hospital. However, the statutes of most states considerably limit the extent to which the patient may be confined. This depends to some extent on the type of commitment. A hearing before a judge soon after commitment may be required as well as a right to be represented by counsel.

Types of Release

The laws that limit the amount of time a patient can be confined in a mental institution are generally specific for the type of commitment that brought the patient into the hospital. As we have already discussed, indeterminate commitments are presently in disrepute and consequently the majority of patients are admitted under a determinate form of commitment, with perhaps the exception of sexual or dangerous offenders.

1) *Determinate*—As we have already discussed, determinate commitments are for a designated period of time and include emergency hospitalization, temporary or observational hospitalization and involuntary commitment.

    a) *emergency hospitalization*—Most of the states that provide for emergency hospitalization limit the period of confinement to five or possibly up to fifteen days after which the patient must be released unless a judicial hearing for long term commitment is arranged. A few states following the *Lessard* decision require a preliminary hearing within 24 to 48 hours after the patient has been detained to determine if there is probable cause for detaining the patient for up to a further fifteen days before a judicial hearing. A few states limit commitment to as little as twenty-four hours, whereas some permit thirty or more days under emergency conditions.

    b) *temporary or observational hospitalization*—Commitment under this provision is usually for thirty or more days, after which a formal hearing is required to confine the patient for a longer period. Because of the non-emergency nature of this commitment, a hearing before a judge is necessary in some states for confinement even for the statutorily defined thirth or more days limit. Other states may require that a patient be committed through this procedure before a decision is made through a judicial procedure to commit him for a more substantial period of time. When the time limit has expired, the patient can agree to convert to a voluntary status in which case he would remain hospitalized. This applies both to temporary and emergency hospitalization.

c) *medical certification*—The states that allow involuntary admission on the basis of two physician certificates for the most part limit the number of days in which the patient can be detained. At any time during the confinement in New York State, for example, a patient, relative or friend may request a court hearing. Usually at the end of a specified period, the hospital must seek a judicial review to confine the patient for a longer period of time if they deem it necessary.

d) *judicial commitment*—The decision regarding the release of a patient committed through a hearing is often up to the court, which may oversee the hospitalization and require continuing review. However, many states even specify the length of time that the patient can be committed through a judicial proceeding.

e) *administrative procedure*—This infrequently used method of involuntary commitment is similar to judicial commitment in that the administrative board often retains the power to decide when the patient can be released, but most states stipulate some limit to how long the patient can be detained or confined without a further proceeding. In both forms of commitment—judicial or through an administrative board—the patient often has more difficulty in obtaining release than if he were committed through a medical certification. However, as we shall shortly see, mechanisms do exist whereby a patient can secure his release even under these conditions.

Mechanisms for Patient Release:

1) *Administrative Discharge*—The medical authorities involved with the care of the patient may decide to release him from hospitalization through discharge. This decision may be based on the conclusion that the patient recovered from his mental condition or that he will likely not improve additionally and is not potentially injurious to himself or others. Many state statutes provide criteria that are to be used by hospital authorities to determine if the patient should be discharged. These are generally focused on establishing that the patient will not be detrimental to his community.

2) *Writ of Habeas Corpus*—Since an administrative discharge is a decision of the medical staff of a hospital, the patient has little control over this mechanism. The most he can do is ask his therapist to consider discharging him. A writ of habeas corpus, on the other hand, provides the patient with a powerful tool against inappro-

priate commitment. This writ in effect allows a patient who feels he is being unjustly deprived of his liberty to have the issue examined by a court. In some jurisdictions, the writ is limited for mental patients to reviewing the appropriateness of the original confinement. Where this is the policy, the court will avoid the issue of whether continued hospitalization is warranted. The trend, however appears to be in the direction of expanding the scope of the writ of habeas corpus, so that many states may allow the court to examine the propriety of continuing hospitalization as well as the original decision to commit the patient. A writ of habeas corpus is available to anyone who feels he is being unjustly detained; it is not limited to use by mentally ill patients.

3) *Judicial Discharge*—Nearly all of the states have statutes which provide for judicial discharge of a committed patient. The patient, his family and even his friends can initiate this procedure if they feel that the patient is inappropriately hospitalized. This procedure, unlike the writ of habeas corpus, always examines the issue of whether the patient should be detained in the hospital. In addition, it requires that a medical certificate be submitted, either before or at the time of the hearing, that states that the patient has been examined and does not appear to need continued hospitalization. On the basis of the medical information provided, the court ultimately decides whether the patient should be discharged.

Criteria For Commitment

Definition

The criteria for commitment vary from state to state. Some of the statutes view commitment as serving primarily the benefit of society, whereas others focus on the needs of the patient. Following the colonial period, the states passed laws regarding commitment. The criteria were narrow and restricted to application for those persons who were potentially harmful to themselves or others. A gradual expansion of those criteria has occurred, so that many classes of persons are now considered potentially commitable by some of the statutes. This may change to some extent by virtue of the U.S. Supreme Court ruling in the Donaldson case, decided June 26, 1975. In this case the court held that patients cannot be involuntarily confined in mental institutions and without treatment if they are not dangerous to anyone and are able to survive in society. The court did not deal with whether those who are not dangerous and able to survive in society can be committed to receive treatment, or whether dangerous and mentally ill patients have a right to be treated when committed. The following however, are some of the important criteria currently used for commitment:

1) *Suicidal and Homicidal Behavior*—Conduct which is potentially harmful to others or to the patient himself has been the major reason for commitment of the mentally ill. There are many states that limit commitment to this criterion. On the other hand, some state statutes no longer use the explicit language "harmful to himself or others" in the conditions for commitment. Nonetheless, suicidal and homicidal patients would be considered commitable even in these states. Furthermore, as we have already seen in the section on malpractice, a therapist who reasonably suspects that a patient is suicidal (or homicidal) could be held liable for malpractice if he does not use emergency measures, including hospitalization. Since the *Lessard* decision, many states have adopted a principally objective criterion for determining commitments. This criterion is essentially the degree to which the patient is *dangerous to himself or others*. A recent Supreme Court case, the *Addington* case, held that there must be a demonstration of clear and convincing evidence (approximately 75% or better) that a patient is mentally ill and dangerous to himself or others. In the *Lessard* case, the element of dangerousness to self and others must be based on the presence of an imminent overt act such as assaultive behavior by the patient. In addition to this purely objective criterion, the *Lessard* case also introduced the right of the patient to 5th Amendment rights against self incrimination and the concept of "least restrictive alternative," that is to say, that all other avenues for the proper treatment of the patient must be explored before commitment is relied on.

2) *Drug and Alcohol Abuse*—Patients suffering from narcotics addiction are commitable in many states. This is achieved through a judicial hearing for the most part. In many of the states, the patient is confined to a mental institution until he is either cured or greatly improved. Where facilities exist for the treatment of the drug addict, he may be committed to these centers. The states differ on what they consider to be drug addiction for commitment purposes. Some states define the drug addict as one who is habituated and has a tolerance for a drug. Others define an addict as one who uses drugs to the point of becoming a danger to the health, safety and morals of the public. And still others define the addict as one who takes specific drugs, such as heroin or morphine, and is unable, as a consequence, to exert reasonable control over his actions.

Similar to the commitment of the drug addict, there are many states which have procedures for the commitment and treatment of seriously ill chronic alcoholics. Alcoholics can be committed through medical certification or judicial decision. In addition in many states they can apply for voluntary admission to a treatment facility. As with the narcotics addict, there is much variety in the states regarding the definition of commitable alcoholism. Many states require that the degree of alcoholism reach the level where the individual can no longer control his drinking and is also potentially dangerous to himself or others. Some states actually require that before he can be considered commitable the alcoholic should have been convicted, possibly more than once, for being a public intoxicant. The majority of states, however, have decriminalized acute alcoholic intoxication, but still allow for the acutely intoxicated patient to be detained for 24 to 36 hours during this phase when he can physically endanger himself until he sobers up. In most cases this period of detainment for acute intoxication is of a very limited period. In contrast the chronic alcoholic when committed may be subjected to long-term hospitalization, anywhere from 60 days to as long as 6 months and in some states up to 2 years.

3) *Other:*

a) *sexual psychopath*—Starting in the late 1930s, laws were passed in many states to provide for the involuntary hospitalization rather than imprisonment of persons who repeatedly engage in antisocial or criminal acts involving sexual conduct. Nearly thirty states have enacted such statutes under the assumption that sexual psychopaths are essentially mentally ill and do not seem to benefit from incarceration, whereas they would possibly achieve some benefit from psychiatric treatment. Various psychiatric conditions are known to be highly associated with psychopathic behavior—most prominently, psychoneurosis, alcoholism, mental retardation and psychosis. Not all of these conditions are responsive to psychiatric intervention, particularly psychopathic behavior and mental retardation, but psychosis, alcoholism and psychoneurosis to some extent are benefitted by psychiatric treatment. Equally important as the benefit that treatment has for the sexual psychopath, involuntary hospitalization is an effective means of protecting society from criminal offenders.

b) *persons in "need of treatment"*—The original criterion of "dangerousness to self or others" has been expanded considerably in almost twenty states to include validating involuntary commitment for those in "need of treatment" and the "gravely disabled. The statues of the states that include this provision are sometimes vague on the definition of what constitutes being "in need of treatment". As a result, a wide range of conditions, depending on the interpretation of this phase, can be potentially commitable.

c) *aged and infirm*—A few states actually include under the definition of mental illness for commitment purposes the aged and the infirm. Some statutes are less definite and provide for commitment if it is for the welfare of the individual or of society. The danger of such vague wording is that it legally allows the confinement of those who are not potentially injurious to themselves or others but are simply unable to conform to the norms of the community. The U.S. Supreme Court's decision in the Donaldson case should provide protection for the aged, infirmed and others against unwarranted confinement.

Filling Out Forms

For illustration purposes the following forms are based primarily on those used in the state of New York for voluntary admission (Form 472 OMH-4/79) and involuntary commitment (emergency admission: Form 474 OHM-2/79, and two physician certificates: Form 471 DMH-1/73). The rules for admission or commitment are very clearly spelled out for the patient and are similar to those of other states. The major difference in New York is that there is a Mental Health Information Service which provides legal assistance and information about admission and termination procedures as well as patient's rights, such as the right to legal counsel, independent psychiatric opinion and judicial review on the issue of confinement. This information service is a major advance in protecting patients against unwarranted or indiscriminate retention in mental hospitals.

Voluntary Admission Forms

According to most states, the prospective patient completes the written application for admission. If the patient is under a certain age—sixteen or eighteen years of age—the parent, guardian or next of kin can make the application. In New York, the applicant must have the ability to understand that he is applying for admission to a hospital for the mentally ill, that by submitting the written form he is making an application for admission, and that he is governed by certain provisions regarding release or possible conversion to involuntary status. It is the responsibility of the admitting physician to certify that the patient meets these requirements for admission.

The form for voluntary admission is generally in several parts. Part "A" would be filled out by the patient if he applies for voluntary admission. If the patient is a minor then a guardian or parent must make the application; and they would fill out Part "B". These parts usually read as shown in Figures 1 and 2.

I, _____, hereby apply for voluntary admission to
_____ hospital for the mentally ill.

My reasons for requesting care and treatment are as follows: (In New York this is answered in Part C)

_____

_____

I understand the nature of the voluntary status and the rules regarding release or possible conversion to involuntary status.

_____ Date: _____

Signature of Patient

FIGURE 1 — PART A

I, _____, acting for my _____ ,

                       (Relationship)

_____, _____, hereby apply for his admission to

   (Name)   *(Age)*

_____ hospital for the mentally ill.

My reasons for requesting care and treatment are as follows: (In New York this is answered in Part C)

_____

_____

_____

I have been notified and understand the nature of voluntary status and the rules pertaining to release or possible conversion to involuntary status.

_____ Date: _____

*Signature of parent, guardian or next of
kin of minor patient*

FIGURE 2 — PART B

The next part of the voluntary form (Part D with the New York form) usually asks for identifying data about the patient—name, address, place of birth, citizenship, relatives, previous medical and psychiatric hospitalizations and treatment, ethnic and religious background, occupation, marital status, etc. Following this section, there is a part to be completed by the staff physician who certifies that the applicant has the ability to understand the provisions of voluntary hospitalization and is suitable for voluntary status.

I have examined the above named patient, and find that he is in need of immediate care and treatment for mental illness. Hospital admission is necessary for:

_____ Treatment which could be expected reasonably to improve the patient's mental condition

_____ Diagnostic purposes

I certify that the patient is suitable for the type of admission requested in this application.

_____
Signature, Admitting Physician

FIGURE 3

According to the New York provision on voluntary admission, if a patient notifies the director of the hospital that he desires to be released, the director must release him immediately or may detain him for a maximum of seventy two hours by which time he must apply to a court for an order allowing the involuntary confinement of the patient. If the court concurs with the hospital director's request, the patient will be committed for a maximum of sixty days unless an application is made for further retention. Other states may allow the director of the hospital to medically certify a patient for involuntary admission without an immediate court determination on the issue of commitability. The New York voluntary provision also requires that the patient be given a special notice of his rights on admission and every 120 days thereafter.

Involuntary Commitment Form

The application for involuntary commitment of a patient is usually made by a family member, close friend, physician who knows the patient, or director of hospital or other facility in which the patient resides. The applicant for the most part may not be a physician who examines the patient for commitment. The examining physicians must usually be licensed to practice medicine in the state where the institution is located. In many states the physician need not be a psychiatrist, but he cannot be a relative of either the applicant or the patient. In New York the patient can be committed for 60 days under a two physician certificate or for 48 hours where immediate care is critical based on the dangerousness of the patient to himself or others and the patient is committed by a psychiatrist to an approved hospital.

Where two physicians are involved each physician must fill out and submit a separate certificate indicating that he examined the patient and found him to be commitable. In the case of the emergency 48 hour commitment, a psychiatrist may commit the patient but he must be released after 48 hours unless he willingly converts to voluntary status or unless another physician examines the patient and supports the original physician's position on the need for commitment, in which case the patient can be retained for a maximum of 15 days. To retain the patient beyond 15 days, a new admission on an application supported by two new examining physicians' certificates is required, unless he agrees to remain as a voluntary patient. Furthermore, if the patient requests a court hearing before the 60 days are up, it will usually be granted and he may be released. Again the criteria for emergency admission is the presence of mental illness and dangerousness to self or others, whereas the criteria for two physicians' certificates include the presence of a mental illness, the fact that care and treatment in a hospital is essential for his welfare, and the existence of seriously impaired judgment.

The form for involuntary commitment is in several parts, like the voluntary form. Part "A" is the application usually made by a relative, friend or physician in the case of a two physicians' certificates (See Figure 4) and by a director of community services where emergency commitment is desired (this one physician certificate in New York is not as widespread among the states as the two physicians' certificates). Part "B" is usually the statement outlining the reasons for hospitalization and often requiring the citing of behavior, etc., that suggests the presence of a mental illness. These parts of the form usually read as shown in Figure 5.

The next part of the involuntary form (Part C with the New York form) usually asks for identifying data about the patient similar to that already discussed on the voluntary form. Part D of the New York form is to be completed by the hospital indicating that the patient has been examined and is in need of treatment. (See Figure 6) In New York, if the hospital is a proprietary facility

I hereby request that _____ be admitted to
_____. This request is made because of the
circumstances stated in Part B, and on the attached physician certificates. I
attest that the information supplied on this application is true to the best of my
knowledge and belief.

_____   _____
Signature of Applicant   Date

_____   _____
Relationship to Patient   Address

FIGURE 4 — PART A

APPLICATION: Two Physicians Certificate Admission

Part B STATEMENT — reasons for requesting hospitalization citing behavior,
statements and changes in character that tend to show
the presence of mental illness.

_____

_____
_____

FIGURE 5

Part D — To Be Completed by Hospital

I have examined the above named patient and find that he is in need of
immediate care and treatment in an institution for the mentally ill because:

_____ Alternate care would be inadequate
OR
The following adequate alternatives are not available

_____ Psychiatric Day Care
_____ Nursing Home or Extended Care Facility
_____ Treatment in Psychiatric Unit, General Hospital
_____ Outpatient Treatment
_____ Other
Hospital admission is medically necessary because

_____ Diagnostic purposes
_____ Treatment could be expected reasonably to improve the patient's
mental condition

_____
Signature, Admitting Physician

FIGURE 6

neither of the examining physicians can be on the staff. In some states, there is a requirement that the patient being committed on a two physician certificate be examined by a physician at the institution where he is to be confined and if that physician disagrees with the appropriateness of the commitment, the patient must be discharged.

In addition to the major parts of the Application for Admission of Patient, the two physicians who examine the patient must also fill out a certification that he should be involuntarily committed. That form usually resembles the New York form which is similar to Figure 7, on the following page.

ETHICAL ISSUES IN EMERGENCY PSYCHIATRIC CARE

General Concepts

Definition of Ethics

Ethics as it relates to emergency psychiatry deals with conflicts in relates to medical care, particular attention is placed on the underlying values of the profession that determine its concept of moral responsibility, duty and obligation. Ultimately ethics focuses on how these values may affect others in society, especially the patient and consumer.

The Nature of Concerns

Thics as it relates to emergency psychiatry deals with conflicts in the desires and objectives of individuals and those of others who are involved in either the providing or consuming of health care services. A critical feature of this is how power for important decisions is used and distributed to fulfill the goals of improving the health of the individual patient and society. If the values of consumers and providers are commensurable, that is to say if no distinction exists between them, then there are essentially no moral or ethical issues. The difficulty occurs when conflicts exist or when the options that are available are different for different people so that underlying values become determinative in such decisions. In the case of emergency psychiatric care, such decisions might arise in triaging various patients to a treatment facility that is of high quality and effective for a particular condition versus one that is not. Patients may be treated differently at this stage based on such factors as whether they are wealthy or poor, acutely disturbed or chronically ill, etc.

CERTIFICATE OF EXAMINING PHYSICIAN
(MENTAL ILLNESS)   Patient Name

_____

Address

_____

_____

_____

CERTIFICATION

I, _____, do certify as follows:
   (name of physician)
   a.   I am physician licensed to practice medicine in _____ State.
   b.   On this date I have *personally* examined with care and diligence
        _____ , at _____
        (name of person examined)   *(place of examination)*

        _____
                          (address)

   c.   I find that this person:
        1. has a mental illness
        2. requires for his welfare care and treatment as a
           patient in a hospital
        3. is impaired in his judgment so that he is unable to
           understand the need for care and treatment
   d.   I have considered alternative forms of care but believe they are
        inadequate or are not available to provide for this person's needs
   e.   My opinion has been formed on the basis of my examination of the
        person and information I have obtained.
   f.   The facts stated are to the best of my knowledge true.

_____   _____

   (Signature)   *(date)*

_____   _____

   (printed name)   *(address)*

(statement of reasons for opinion on certification)

_____

_____

_____

_____

FIGURE 7

Reason For Concern

The mentally ill, along with children and prisoners, are a particularly vulnerable group for abuse. Even those who are not mentally ill are vulnerable to subtle and often not so subtle coercions during periods of emergency and crisis. The mentally ill, because of the nature of their diseased condition, often lack the competency or the ability to be able to protect themselves in the face of other people's objectives and desires. Hence, the ethical issues involving the mentally ill are in many ways more complicated and pervasive than those affecting patients who suffer from physical conditions.

Ethics and Emergency Psychiatry

The ethical issues involving emergency psychiatric care fall within the traditional clusters of concerns—conflicts involving the therapist-patient relationship, issues of distributive justice, and the obligations and responsibilities of psychiatry as a profession to society as a whole.

Therapist-Patient Relationship

There has been considerable attention in recent years devoted to the nature of the therapist-patient relationship. The emphasis has been placed primarily on equalizing the decision-making balance between the therapist and the patient to whatever extent possible given the limitations that the patient may have in understanding the full range of his options. The important concerns in the therapist-patient relationship relevant to emergency psychiatric treatment are the following:

1) *Informed Consent:* (this has been discussed in some detail in the beginning section of this chapter dealing with legal issues.) Informed consent as a concept is difficult when dealing with mentally ill patients because of the varying degrees of competency of such patients to understand the benefits, risks and alternatives to treatment. In the context of an emergency informed consent is even more problematic because the patient in acute distress is even less likely to understand or seriously consider the information presented to him. Furthermore even under less traumatic conditions as in the case of the voluntary patient being admitted to a hospital, studies have demonstrated that such patients often do not fully comprehend what they are agreeing to and accepting. In the emergency room the acutely distraught patient may agree to a specific course of diagnosis and

treatment without understanding the implications of this consent or the alternatives that might be available. The patient should be informed of the variety of treatment options that exist for his condition and to whatever extent possible the relative efficacy of each. When the patient is not able to understand this information, then the next of kin or guardian should be given the opportunity to review and decide on the therapist's treatment plan.

2) *Consumer Education and Responsiveness:* Psychiatric emergency treatment facilities should provide information for patients and consumers of health services of what treatments exist for the care of acute psychiatric problems and what facilities (inpatient and outpatient) in the area can be used for providing follow-up treatment. In addition, consumers should be informed of the relative benefits of neuropsychiatric evaluation and the types of treatment available—medications, electroshock, individual and group psychotherapy, etc. An emergency care facility should be responsive to the needs of the community. For example if the majority of the community is Spanish speaking, then interpreters should be available to serve that critical role. Furthermore, the hours for providing evaluation and treatment should be accommodated as much as possible with the working schedule of the members of the community. This last point is particularly important for crisis intervention where the schedules of family and friends can be determinative of the patient's ability to attend treatment sessions.

3) *Labeling:* Labeling is the process by which an individual patient is placed in a certain category or class of diseases which may affect his treatment while engaged with the mental health facility. There are significant dangers with labeling, particularly when it occurs in the emergency room context where the time constraints might result in a quick leap to the most convenient category. Some of these dangers are as follows:

a) Once labeled all changes or alterations in the patient's mental condition may be easily and inappropriately attributed to the process implied by the label.

b) Patients who are labeled with serious diseases may receive less respect or attention by therapists.

c) Mislabeling can lead to specious conclusions about the course of the untreated illness, what treatments would be appropriate, and how effective they are.

In the emergency room the primary emphasis should be on accurate assessment and treatment of the acute condition. A therapist should provide a listing of possible diagnostic classes, but not arrive at a definitive conclusion. There must be considerable flexibility and willingness to alter the diagnosis once the patient's condition stabilizes.

4) *The Right to Refuse Treatment:* This area with regards to psychotropic medications is only now developing in the law. There have been some cases recently that provide at least a limited prerogative to patients to refuse psychotropic medications. Generally, in the case of an emergency, medications can be given particulary if they are for the purpose of tranquilizing the patient during the acute stage and stabilizing his condition. The right to refuse treatment cases are dealing now with the right of patients to refuse psychotropic medication when involuntarily committed but not acutely disturbed. Patients or next of kin, when patients are incompetent, must give their informed consent before they can be treated by what are considered more intrusive therapies, i.e. ECT, behavioral modification, and psychosurgery.

Issues of Distributive Justice

Issues of distributive justice deal essentially with question of *who* gets *what* quality and type of psychiatric treatment—more specifically, how accessible is the treatment to the average person; what is the range of psychiatric treatments; what population groups are recipient of its benefits; and lastly, how much of the public funds are spent on psychiatric care, especially on the development of emergency psychiatric treatment programs. The following is a more complete discussion of some of the most important issues under distributed justice:

1) *Provision of Care*—This issue deals with the accessibility of psychiatric treatment to various segments of the population. Certain subgroups of patients, particularly the severely psychiatrically ill, may not be able to comply as readily with traditional treatment programs. An emergency psychiatric treatment center has an obligation to set up its programs so as to increase the accessibility of what it has to offer to all segments of the population. Preventive psychiatric measures are especially unknown to lower socio-economic groups. The primary care and emergency psychiatric programs must reach out to provide information on preventive measures to this population. In addition, the training and expertise of the clinicians dealing with patients with major psychiatric conditions as well as lower socio-economic groups should be equivalent to those who are providing services for other segments of the population. The tendency may be to spend less time with the seriously psychiatrically ill, such as the chronic deteriorating schizophrenic, rather than invest the

time and energy to work out the most effective and appropriate treatment program for such patients.

2) *The Mental Health Professionals*—The training of mental health professionals is of primary importance for a high quality emergency treatment program. Such individuals, including the physician, should be keenly aware of the neurophychiatric evaluation of the patient, social and economic issues that may affect the capacity of the family to respond sensitively to his immediate needs and the broader social support system available to assist this patient during the acute emergency stage. It may be necessary to hospitalize a patient, not so much because his condition is so serious, but because the social supports do not exist to assist this patient to obtain proper treatment on an out-patient basis. The training of the mental health team is critical; they should be oriented to provide consumers with the highest quality of care at all stages of their treatment. The emergency room is one of the most important parts of a psychiatric treatment program, as it is often the first point of contact and therefore determines in large measure the way in which the patient is treated within the system.

3) *The Mental Health Care Budget*—The way money is spent for psychiatric treatment has to be assessed not only in terms of what parts of the psychiatric program receive financial support, but also what schools or philosophies of psychiatry are being promoted. The emergency treatment program, a primary care program of a hospital, is one of the most important features of a hospital and should be of a high priority for receiving financial and other resources. The kind of information that a psychiatrist must master for emergency triaging is predominantly based on a neuropsychiatric evaluation and requires that the emphasis be placed on that aspect of a resident's training. Being astute in the nuances of psychoanalytic theory is of minimal help in the triaging of seriously psychiatrically ill patients in the emergency room system. The allocation of funds must not only be seen in terms of developing emergency systems, but also in providing for the training of mental health professionals knowlegeable and sensitive to the full range of needs of their patients. A significant part of the increase in the allocation of resources for various aspects of psychiatric care is the need to evaluate the efficacy of such programs. Programs like suicide prevention, for example, have yielded somewhat questionable results. In emergency psychiatric treatment it is essential that appropriate follow-up be conducted to evaluate the services that may be necessary for the community, as well as the effectiveness of the services that do exist.

The Issues of Psychiatry and Society

These issues deal with the broader ethical or justice issues of psychiatry as a profession establishing its responsibilities and accountability to society. The following ethical considerations are particularly important in the defining of psychiatry as a profession.

1) *Psychiatry and Control*—Psychiatry can be highly abusive as a mechanism for controlling human behavior. Especially in the Soviet Union psychiatry has been used for the purposes of controlling dissident political beliefs by defining the advocate as mentally ill and thereby justifying confinement. In our system of psychiatry, control can exist by the way in which psychiatry ends up adopting the prevailing values of society in its development of a taxonomy of mental illness. Social-economic determinants may in large part be responsible for much of psychiatry's characterization of behaviors as deviant. In the emergency room it is necessary to be constantly aware of the social and cultural dimensions of the patient, approaching each patient with flexibility so that diagnoses will be based on objective criteria, rather than on conflicts of values.

2) *Psychiatry and Regression*—Psychiatry can also be abusive by "normalizing" unique or divergent features of the individual's personality. To quell anxiety per se may be detrimental to the personal development of a patient. Furthermore, it can result in the loss of creativity and ethical sensitivity. It is important in the evaluation of a patient in the emergency room to be aware of those elements of the personality which though deviant from the majority may reflect special characteristics that should be protected. In deciding the appropriate disposition of a patient the therapist should reflect on some of the negative effects that might be achieved through long-term psychotherapy, drug treatment, psychoanalysis or even behavioral modification, as these treatments may adversely affect creative elements of the patient.

3) *Integrity and Psychiatric Theory*—The way in which psychiatry conceptualizes the etiology and development of mental illness can have a major impact on the way in which acceptable social behavior is defined and structured. Psychiatric norms greatly influence how individuals evaluate their personal development and success in their respective social roles. At one time much attention was placed on the role of the family in the development of schizophrenia. Often statements like "double binding," "skewed," "pseudo-mutuality" were applied to families of schizophrenic children. Now with increasing awareness of the genetic implications in

the transmission of schizophrenia, the former concepts of disturbance in the family have become much less important. Nonetheless,
they were influential on the ways in which families, especially
mothers and fathers, viewed themselves, and resulted in much pain
and consternation for the parents of seriously ill mental patients.

Integrity of psychiatric theory reaches down to the very practical
level of the obligations of the profession to periodically assess the
efficacy, the effectiveness and cost of its treatment modalities. In the
emergency context, the types of treatment offered for specific conditions must be evaluated over a period of time to determine if they are
effective, if in fact the conditions have been properly diagnosed and
have merited such treatment, and if the cost of the treatment has
been prohibitive for a just distribution of health resources.

4) *Education*—The emergency room psychiatrist has the responsibility of educating others on the mental health professional
team, as well as consumers, of the varieties of presenting neuropsychiatric illnesses, the role of psychosocial factors in the genesis of
psychological and organic illness, and the characteristics of help-
seeking behavior. Many consumers of health care are not aware that
when they develop disorders of mood, thought and behavior these
may relate to the medication that they are taking for some other
organic dysfunction.

Mental health professionals are trained often to think in terms of
the historical basis for crisis and conflicts without focusing on the
organic changes that may be occurring because of other kinds of
medication, or because there is a positive family history of depression, mania, suicide, or alcoholism that may predispose people
to this kind of reaction. In addition, many nonpsychiatric clinicians
have not been taught the appropriate doses that are needed to treat
certain psychiatric illnesses, particularly depression, or how long the
medication should be given before the patient can be considered a
non-responder.

Many patients coming into the emergency room are already under treatment for their condition, but the medication may not have
worked effectively at the time that they are seen in the emergency
room. It is important that psychiatrists, whose area of expertise is
the diagnosis and treatment of these disorders, see their role as that
of training other professionals, and the consumer, with reliable information about what is known about the condition. Emergency room
clinicians need to be at the forefront of knowledge about the psychosocial and neuro-psychiatric basis of mental illness and particularly
the points of differentiation between those conditions which are
medical and neurologic and those which are predominantly psychiatric.

BIBLIOGRAPHY

Abel, G.G.; Barlow, D.H.; Blanchard, E.B.; Guild, D.: The components of rapists' sexual arousal. *Arch Gen Psychiat*, 34:895-903, 1977.

Aden v. Younger, 57 Cal. App. 3d 662, 129 Cal. Rptr. 535 (1976).

Addington v. Texas—U.S.—47 L.W. 4473 (April 30, 1979).

ALI Model Penal Cose (1955) Section 4.01 (1) (Tent. Draft No. 4).

Allen, R.M.; Young, S.J.: Phencyclidine–induced psychosis. *Am J Psychiat*, 135:1081-1084, 1978.

American Bar Association, Commission of the Mentally Disabled: Mental Disability. *Law Reporter*, 2:337-354, September-December, 1977.

Ananth, J.; Solyom, L.; Bryntwick, S.; Krishnappa, U.: Chlorimipramine therapy for obsessive-compulsive neurosis. *Am J Psychiat*, 136:700-701, 1979.

Andersen, W.H.; Kuehnle, J.C.: Strategies for the treatment of acute psychosis. *JAMA*, 229:1884, 1974.

Aquilera, D.C.; Messick, J.M.; Farrell, M.S.: *Crisis Intervention: Theory and Methodology*. St. Louis, C.V. Mosby, 1970.

Arnold, L.E.; Christopher, J.; Huestis, R.; Smettzer, D.J.: Methylphenidate vs. dextroamphetamine vs. caffeine in minimal brain dysfunction: Controlled comparison for placebo workout design with Bayes' Analysis. *Arch Gen Psychiat* 35:463-473, 1978.

Arnold, W.H.: *The techniques of withdrawal of opiates and barbiturate-sedatives*. Mimeo, Lexington, Kentucky, 1961.

Aronowitz, R.: Civil commitment of narcotics addicts. *Columbia L Rev*, 67:405, 1967.

Avery, D.; Winokur, G.: Suicide, attempted suicide, and relapse rates in depression. Occurrence after ECT and antidepressant therapy. *Arch Gen Psychiat*, 35:749-753, 1978.

Azar, J.; Turndorf, H.: Paroxysmal left bundle branch block during nitrous oxide anesthesia in a patient on lithium carbonate. A case report. *Anesth Anal*, 56:868-870, 1977.

Bacher, N.M.; Lewis, H.A.: Addition of reserpine to antipsychotic medication in refractory chronic schizophrenic outpatients. *Am J Psychiat*, 135:488-489, 1978.

Bach-Y-Rita, G.; Habitual violence and self-mutilation. *Am J Psychiat*, 131:1018, 1974.

Bach-Y-Rita, G.; Veno, A.: Habitual violence: a profile of 62 men. *Am J Psychiat*, 131:1015, 1974.

Barke, J.D.; White, H.S.; Havens, L.L.: Which short-term therapy? Matching patient and method. *Arch Gen Psychiat*, 35:177-186, 1979.

Barkley, R.A.; Cunningham, C.E.: The effects of methylphenidate on the mother-child interactions of hyperactive children. *Arch Gen Psychiat*, 36:201-208, 1979.

Barnhart, C.C.; Bowden, C.L.: Toxic psychosis with cimetidine. *Am J Psychiat*, 136:725-726, 1979.

Bartolucci, G.; Drayer, C.S.: An overview of crisis intervention in the emergency rooms of general hospitals. *Am J Psychiat*, 130:753, 1973.

Bazelon, D.L.: Psychiatrists and the adversary process. *Sci Am*, 230:18, 1974.

Beck, A.T.: *Depression: Clinical, Experimental and Theoretical Aspects.* New York, Harper and Row, 1967.

Beck, A.T.; Beck, R.; Kovacs, M.: Classification of suicidal behaviors; I. Quantifying intent and medical lethality. *Am J Psychiat*, 132:285-287, 1975.

Becker, R.: The historical background. *Psychiatr Ann*, 3:8, 1973.

Beecher, H.K.: *Research and the Individual Human Studies.* Boston, Little, Brown & Co., 1970.

Bellak, L.; Small, L.: *Emergency Psychotherapy and Brief Psychotherapy.* New York, Grune and Stratton, 1965.

Belmaker, R.H.; Lehrer, R.; Epstein, R.P.; Lettik, H.; Kugelmoss, S.: A possible cardiovascular effect of lithium. *Am J Psychiat*, 136:577-579, 1979.

Biederman, J.; Lerner, Y.; Belmaker, R.H.: Combination of lithium carbonate and haloperidol in schizo-affective disorders: a controlled study. *Arch Gen Psychiat*, 36:327-333, 1979.

Bien, R.D.: Cogwheel rigidity early in lithium therapy. *Am J Psychiat*, 133:1093-1094, 1976.

Biggs, J.T.; Spiker, D.G.; Petit, J.M.; Ziegler, V.E.: Tricyclic antidepressant overdose: Incidence of symptoms. *JAMA*, 238:135-138, 1977.

Birch, N.J.: "A note of animal and human studies of possible kidney damage caused by lithium" in Johnson, F.N.; Johnson, S.: *Lithium in Medical Practice.* Baltimore, University Park Press, 1978.

Blachly, P.; Disher, D.; Roduner, G.: Suicide by Physicians. *Bulletin of Suicidology.* Washington, D.C., U.S. Government Printing Office, December, 1968.

Blackwell, B.; Marley, E.; Price, J.; et al.: Hypertensive interactions between MAOI's and foodstuffs. *Brit J Psychiat*, 113:349-365, 1967.

Blackwell, B.; Stepopoulos, A.; Endess, P.; Kunma, R.; Adolphe, A.: Anticholinergic activity of two tricyclic antidepressants. *Am J Psychiat*, 135:722-724, 1978.

Block, S.H.: The grocery store high. *Am J Psychiat*, 135:126-127, 1978.

Bowers, M.B.: Psychoses precipitated by psychotomimetic drugs. A follow-up study. *Arch Gen Psychiat*, 34:832-835, 1977.

Bows, J.F.; Anostasi, M.; Casoni, R.; Russo, R.D.; DiMascio, L.; Fusco, L.; Rubenstein, J.; Snyder, M.: Psychotherapy in the goldfish bowl: The role of the indigenous therapist. *Arch Gen Psychiat*, 36:187-190, 1979.

Braden, W.: Response to lithium in a case of L-dopa-induced psychosis. *Am J Psychiat*, 134:808-809, 1977.

Brakel, S.J.; Rock, R.S.: *The Mentally Disabled and the Law* (rev. ed.). Chicago, University of Chicago Press, 1971.

Branchey, M.H.; Charles, J.; Simpson, E.M.: Extrapyramidal side effects in lithium maintenance therapy. *Am J Psychiat*, 133:4444-4451, 1976.

Breed, W.: Suicide, migration and race: a study of cases in New Orleans. *J Soc Issues*, 22:30-43, 1966.

Brenner, F.: Bromism: Alive and well. *Am J Psychiat*, 135:857-858, 1978.

Brenner, I.; Rheubon, W.J.: The catatonic dilemma. *Am J Psychiat*, 135:1242-1243, 1978.

Briggs Law (The), Mass. Gen. Laws c 123, Sec. 100A, (Ter Ed) (1932).

Brill, H.; Malzberg, B.: *Statistical report based on the arrest record of 5354 male ex-patients released from New York State Mental Hospitals during the period 1946-48*. Mimeo, New York, New York, 1950.

Brill, N.Q.; Storrow, H.A.: Social class and psychiatric treatment. *Arch Gen Psychiat*, 3:340, 1960.

Brinkley, J.R.; Beitman, B.D.; Friedel, R.O.: Low-dose neuroleptic regimens in the treatment of borderline patients. *Arch Gen Psychiat*, 36:319-326, 1979.

Brown, G.M.; Stancer, H.C.; Moldofsky, H.; Harman, J.; Murphy, J.T.; Gupta, R.H.: Withdrawal from long-term high-dose desipramine therapy. *Arch Gen Psychiat*, 35:1261-1264, 1978.

Burgess, A.W.; Holmstrom, L.: Rape trauma syndrome. *Am J Psychiat*, 131:981, 1974.

Burgess, A.W.; Holmstrom, L.: *Rape, Victims of Crisis*. Bowie, Md., Robert J. Brady, 1974.

Butler, R.N.: Psychiatry and the elderly: An overview. *Am J Psychiat*, 132:893-900, September, 1975.

Cadoret, R.J.: Psychopathology in adopted-away offspring of biologic parents with antisocial behavior. *Arch Gen Psychiat*, 35:176-184, 1978.

Caffeinism. *Pharmacy Newsletter of the Connecticut Mental Health Center*, Department of Pharmacy Services, 1:22, 1974.

Caine, E.D.; Hunt, R.D.; Weingartner, H.; Ebert, M.H.: Huntington's dementia: clinical and neuropsychological features. *Arch Gen Psychiat*, 35:377-384, 1978.

Caldwell, J.M.: "Military Psychiatry" in *Comprehensive Textbook of Psychiatry*. A.M. Freedman, H.I. Kaplan, H.S. Kaplan, eds. Baltimore, Williams and Wilkins, 1967.

Cal. Welf. & Inst'ns Code Section 5325(f) (W. Supp. 1973)—Statute that gives the patient the right to refuse electroshock treatment. Calif. Welf. & Inst'ns Code (West 1966) (Supp. 1968) Section 5276.

Cantwell, D.P.; Sturzenberger, S.; Burroughs, J.; Salkin, B.; Green, J.K.: Anorexia nervosa: an affective disorder? *Arch Gen Psychiat*, 34:1087-1093, 1977.

Caplan, G.: *An Approach to Community Health*. New York, Grune and Stratton, 1961.

Caplan, G.: *Concepts of Mental Health and Consultation*. Washington, U.S. Dept. of Health, Education and Welfare, Children's Bureau, 1959.

Caplan, G.: *Manual for Psychiatrists Participating in the Peace Corps Program*. Washington, Medical Program Division, Peace Corps, 1962.

Caplan, G.: *Principles of Preventive Psychiatry*. New York, Basic Books, 1964.

Carlson, G.A.; Davenport, Y.B.; Jamison, K.: A comparison of outcome in adolescent and late-onset bipolar manic-depressive disease. *Am J Psychiat*, 134:919-922, 1977.

Carpenter, W.T.; Bartko, J.J.; Strauss, J.S.; Hawk, A.B.: Signs and symptoms as predictors of outcome: a report from the international pilot study of schizophrenia. *Am J Psychiat*, 135:940-945, 1978.

Carter v. United States, 252 F.2d 608 (D.C. Cir. 1957).

Casey, D.E.; Rabins, P.: Tardive dyskinesia or a life-threatening illness. *Am J Psychiat*, 135:486-488, 1978.

Casper, R.C.; Davis. J.M.: On the course of anorexia nervosa. *Am J Psychiat*, 134:974-978, 1977.

Cavenar, J.O.; Sullivan, J.L.; Maltbie, A.A.: A clinical note on hysterical psychosis. *Am J Psychiat*, 136:830-832, 1979.

Chayet, N.L.: Legal neglect of the mentally ill. *Am J Psychiat*, 125:785, 1968.

Chouinard, G.; Annable, L.; Ross-Chouinard, A.; Nestoros, J.N.: Factors related to tardive dyskinesia. *Am J Psychiat*, 136:79-83, 1979.

Christy v. Saliterman, 288 Minn 144, 179 NW 2d 288 (1970).

Civil Commitment of the Mentally Ill. De Paul L Rev, 23:1276-97 (Spring, 1974).

Clark v. State, 12 Ohio Rep 483 (1843).

Cocozza, J.J.; Steadman, H.J.: Some refinements in the measurement and prediction of dangerous behavior. *Amer J Psychiat*, 131:1012, 1974.

Cohen, L.H.; Freeman, H.: How dangerous to the community are state hospital patients? *Connecticute State Medical Journal*, 9:E97, 1945.

Committee on Trauma—*American College of Surgeons: Emergency Care.* Philadelphia, W.B. Saunders, 1966.

Comprehensive Textbook of Psychiatry. A.M. Freedman and H.I. Kaplan, eds. Baltimore, Williams and Wilkins, 1967.

Comroe, B.I.: Follow-up study of 100 diagnosed as neurosis. *J Nerv Ment Dis*, 83:679-684, 1936.

Conn Gen Stat Sec 17-206d (1974).

Conn Gen Stat Sec 17-183 (1975).

Craig, J.; Abu-Saleh, M.; Smith, B.; Evans, I.: Diabetes mellitus in patients on lithium. *Lancet*, ii:1028, 1977.

Craig, T.J.; Van Natta, P.A.: Influence of demographic characteristics on two measures of depressive symptoms: the relation of prevalence and persistence of symptoms with sex, age, education and marital status. *Arch Gen Psychiat*, 35:149-154, 1979.

Crane, G.E.: The prevention of tardive dyskinesia. *Am J Psychiat*, 134:756-758, 1977.

Croughan, J.L.; Woodruff, R.A.; Reich, T.: The management of patients with undiagnosed psychiatric illness. *Arch Gen Psychiat*, 36:341-346, 1979.

Crowe, M.J.; Lloyd, G.G.; Bloch, S.; Rosser, R.M.: Hypothyroidism in patients treated with lithium: a review and two case reports. *Psychol Med*, 3:337-342, 1973.

Cutler, N.R.; Anderson, D.J.: Proven asymptomatic esoinophilia with imipramine. *Am J Psychiat*, 134:1296-1297, 1977.

Daggett, L.R.; Rolde, E.J.: Decriminalization of public drunkenness: the response of suburban police. *Arch Gen Psychiat*, 34:937-941, 1977.

Darbonne, A.: Crisis: a review of theory, practice and research. *Int J Psychiat*, 6:371, 1968.

Darling v. Charleston Memorial Hospital, 33 III 2nd 326, 211 N.E. 2d 253 (1965); cert. denied 383 U.S. 946 (1966).

Davidson, H.A.: *Forensic Psychiatry* (2nd ed). New York, The Ronald Press, 1965.

Davidson, J.; McLeod, M.; Law-Yone, B.; Limoila, M.: A comparison of electro-convulsive therapy and combined phenelzine-amitriptyline in refractory depression. *Arch Gen Psychiat*, 35:630-642, 1978.

Davidson, M.; Hutt, C.: A study of 500 Oxford Student Psychiatric Patients. *Brit J Soc Clin Psychol*, 3:175-185, 1964.

Davies, D.W.: Physical illness in psychiatric outpatients. *Brit J Psychiat*, 111:27-33, 1965.

Davis, K.L.; Berger, P.A.; Hollister, L.E.: Deanol in tardive dyskinesia. *Am J Psychiat*, 134:807, 1977.

Dawidoff, D.J.: The malpractice of psychiatrists. Springfield, Illinois, Charles C Thomas, 1973.

Dawidoff, D.J.: The malpractice of psychiatrists. Duke L Journ 1966:696.

DeBard, M.L.: Diazepam withdrawal syndrome: a case with psychosis, seizure, and coma. *Am J Psychiat*, 136:104-105, 1979.

Dekret, J.J.; Maany, I.; Ramsey, T.A.; Mendels, J.: A case of oral dyskinesia associated with imipramine treatment. *Am J Psychiat*, 134:1297-1298, 1977.

Delworth, V.; Rudow, E.H.; Taub, J.: *Crisis Center/Hotline*. Springfield, Illinois, Charles C Thomas, 1972.

Demers-Desrosiers, L.A.; Nestoros, J.N.; Vaillancourt, P.: Acute psychosis precipitated by withdrawal of anticonvulsant medication. *Am J Psychiat*, 135:981-982, 1978.

Demers, R.; Lukesh, R.; Prichard, J.: Convulsion during lithium therapy. *Lancet*, ii:315-316, 1970.

Dershowitz, A.N.: Dangerousness as a criterion for confinement. *Bulletin of the American Academy of Psychiatry and the Law*, 2:172-179 (September, 1974).

Detre, T.P.; Jarecki, H.G.: *Modern Psychiatric Treatment*. Philadelphia, J.P. Lippincott Co., 1971.

Deutsch, H.: Some forms of emotional disturbance and their relationship to schizophrenia. *Psychoanal Q*, 11:301, 1942.

Diagnostic and Statistical Manual of Mental Disorders, Third Edition (DSM-III), Washington, D.C., American Psychiatric Association, 1980.

Dimsdale, J.E.: Emotional causes of sudden death. *Am J Psychiat*, 134:1361-1366, 1977.

Disclosure of confidential information. *JAMA*, 216:385, April 12, 1971.

District of Columbia Alcoholic Rehabilitation Act (1968): P.L. 90-452, 82 Stat 618.

Donlon, P.T.; Hopkin, J.; Tupin, J.P.: Overview: efficacy and safety of the rapid neuroleptization method with injectable haloperidol. *Am J Psychiat*, 136:273-278, 1979.

Donlon, P.T.; Tupin, J.P.: Successful suicides with thioridazine and mesoridazine: a result of probable cardiotoxicity. *Arch Gen Psychiat*, 34:955-957, 1977.

Dorpat, T.; Anderson, W.F.; Ripley, H.S.: "The relationship of physical illness to suicide" in *Suicidal Behaviors*. H.L.P. Resnick, ed. Boston, Little, Brown & Co., 1968.

Driver v. Hinnant, 356 F. 2d 761 (4th Cir. 1966).

Drug Interactions—a review. *Pharmacy Newsletter of the Connecticut Mental Health Center*, Department of Pharmacy Services, 1:21, 1974.

Dubey, J.: Confidentiality as a requirement of the therapist: Technical necessities for absolute privilege in psychotherapy. *Am J Psychiat*, 131:1093-1096, 1974.

Dublin, L.: Suicide: a public health problem in E.S. Schneidman, ed.: *Essays in Self-Destruction*. New York, Science House, 1967.

Dunn, C.G.; Gross, D.: Treatment of depression in the medically ill geriatric patient: a case report. *Am J Psychiat*, 134:448-450, 1977.

Durham v. United States, 214 F. 2d 862 (D.C. Cir. 1954).

Durkheim, E.: *Le Suicide: Etude de Sociologic*. Paris, Alcan, 1897.

Dysken, M.W.; Chan, C.H.: Diazepam withdrawal psychosis: a case report. *Am J Psychiat*, 134:573, 1977.

Easter v. District of Columbia, 361 F. 2d 50 (D.C. Cir. 1966).

Emergency Psychiatric Care: *The Management of Mental Health Crises*, H.L.P. Resnik and H.L. Ruben, eds. Bowie, MD., Charles Press, 1975.

Endicott, J.; Cohen, J.; Nee, J.; Fleiss, J.L.; Herz, M.I.: Brief vs. standard hospitalization. For Whom? *Arch Gen Psychiat*, 36:706-712, 1979.

Ennis, B.J.: Emerging legal rights for the mentally handicapped. *The Bulletin of the American Academy of Psychiatry and the Law*, 2:185 (1974).

Ennis, B.J.; Litwack, T.R.: Psychiatry and the presumption of expertise: Flipping coins in the courtroom. *California L Rev* 62:693-754, May, 1974.

Erikson, E.: *Childhood and Society*. New York, W.W. Norton Co., 1950.

Ethics of Health Care. L.R. Tancredi, Ed. Washington D.C. National Academy of Sciences, 1973.

Faquet, R.A.; Rowland, K.F.: "Spice cabinet" intoxication. *Am J Psychiat*, 135:860-861, 1978.

Farberow, N.L.; Shneidman, E.S.: *The Cry for Help*. New York, McGraw-Hill, 1965.

Favazza, A.R.; Martin, P.: Chemotherapy of delirium tremens: a survey of physician's preferences. *Am J Psychiat*, 131:1031, 1974.

Feighner, J.P.; et al.: Diagnostic criteria for use in psychiatric research. *Am J Psychiat*, 26:57, 1972.

Feirstein, A; Weisman, G.; Kamas, C.: "A Crisis Intervention Model for Inpatient Hospitalization" in *Current Psychiatric Therapies*, Vol. 11 J.H. Masserman, ed. New York, Grune and Stratton, 1971.

Feldman, S.; Goldstein, H.H.: Community mental health centers in the United States: An overview. *Int J of Nursing Studies*, 8:247-257, 1971.

Females Lead Suicide Attempts. *NAMH Reporter*, Winter, 1972/3.

Fenichel, U.: *The Psychoanalytic Theory of Neurosis*. New York, W.W. Norton Co., 1945.

Flaherty, J.A.; Lahmeyer, H.W.: Laryngeal-pharyngeal dystonia as a possible cause of asphyxia with haloperidol treatment. *Am J Psychiat*, 135:1414-1415, 1978.

Forrest, N.J.; Cohen, J.D.; Torretti, J.; et al.: On the mechanism of lithium induced diabetes insipidus in man and the rat. *J Clin Invest*, 53:1115, 1974.

Forster, F.M.: *Synopsis of Neurology*. St. Louis, C.V. Mosby Co., 1962.

Fowler, R.C.; Kronfol, Z.A.; Perry, P.J.: Water intoxication, psychosis, and inappropriate secretion of antidiuretic hormone. *Arch Gen Psychiat*, 34:1097-1099, 1977.

Frankel, M.: Narcotic addiction, criminal responsibility and civil commitment. *Utah L Rev*, 1966:581.

Frankl, V.E.: *The Doctor and the Soul*. New York, Knopf, 1955.

Frankl, V.E.: *Man's Search for Meaning*. New York, Washington Square Press, 1963.

Franks, R.D.; Richter, A.J.: Schizophrenia-like psychosis associated with anti-convulsant toxicity. *Am J Psychiat*, 136:973-974, 1979.

Fras, I.; Karlavage, J.: The use of methylphenidate and imipramine in Gilles de la Tourette's disease in children. *Am J Psychiat*, 134:195-197, 1977.

Dr. Frederick Notes Suicide Increase During Spring. *ADAMHA News*, April 30, 1976.

Frederick, C.J.: *Current Trends in Suicidal Behavior in the United States*. Paper presented in abridged form at Thirteenth National Scientific Meeting of the Association for the Advancement of Psychotherapy, Toronto, Canada, May 1, 1977.

Frederick, C.J.: *Ecological Aspects of Self Destruction: Some Legal, Legislative and Behavioral Implications in Health and Human Values*. A. Jefcoat, ed. New York, John Wiley and Sons, 1972.

Frederick, C.J.: The present suicide taboo in the United States. *Mental Hygiene*, 55:178-183, 1971.

Frederick, C.J.: The role of the nurse in crisis intervention and suicide prevention. *J Psychiat Nursing*, 11:27-31, 1973.

Frederick, C.J.: The school guidance counselor as a preventive agent to self-destructive behavior. *New York State Personnel and Guidance Journal*, 5:1-5, 1970.

Frederick, C.J.; Farberow, N.L.: Group psychotherapy with suicidal persons: a comparison with standard group methods. *Int J Soc Psychiat*, 16:103-111, 1970.

Frederick, C.J.; Lague, L.: *Dealing with the Crisis of Suicide*. New York, Public Affairs Pamphlet No. 406A, 1972. Copyright Public Affairs Committee, Inc., Eight printing revised November, 1978.

Frederick, C.J.; Resnik, H.L.P.: How suicidal behaviors are learned. *Am J Psychotherapy*, 25:37-55, 1971.

Frederick, C.J.; Resnik, H.L.P.: Interventions with suicidal patients. *J Contemporary Psychotherapy*, 2:103-109, 1970.

Freedman, R.; Schwab, P.J.: Paranoid symptoms in patients on a general hospital psychiatric unit: implications for diagnosis and treatment. *Arch Gen Psychiat*, 35:387-390, 1978.

Freud, S.: Mourning and melancholia, in *Collected Papers IV*. London, Hogarth Press, 1925.

Freud, S.: *Beyond the Pleasure Principle*. London, Hogarth, 1950.

Freudenberger, H.J.: The staff burn-out syndrome in alternative institutions. *Psychotherapy: Theory, Research and Practice*, 12:73-82, 1975.

Friedman, I.; Von Mering, O.; Hinko, E.N.; Intermittent patienthood. *Arch Gen Psychiat*, 33:386, 1976.

Gaitz, C.M.; Varner, R.V.; Overall, J.E.: Pharmacotherapy for organic brain syndrome in late life. Evaluation of an Ergot derivative vs. placebo. *Arch Gen Psychiat*, 34:839-845, 1977.

Garbutt, J.; Malepoar, B.; Brunswick, O.; Jonmalagadda, M.R.; Jolliff, L.; Podolak, R.; Wilson, F.; Prange, A.: Effects of triiodothyromine on drug levels and cardiac function in depressed patients treated with imipramine. *Am J Psychiat*, 136:980-982, 1979.

Gardos, G.; Cole, J.O.: Weight reduction in schizophrenics by molindone. *Am J Psychiat*, 134:302-304, 1977.

Gardos, G.; Cole, J.O.; Tarsy, D.: Withdrawal syndromes associated with antipsychotic drugs. *Am J Psychiat*, 135:1321-1324, 1978.

Gelenberg, A.J.; Mandel, M.R.: Catatonic reactions to high-potency neuroleptic drugs. *Arch Gen Psychiat*, 34:947-950, 1977.

Gerle, B.: Clinical observations on the side effects of haloperidol. *Acta Psychiatr Scand*, 40:65, 1964.

Glass, A.J.: Psychotherapy in the combat zone. *Am J Psychiat*, 110:725, 1954.

Glassman, A.H.; Perel, J.M.; Shostak, M.; Kantor, S.J.; Fleiss, J.L.: Clinical implications of imipramine plasma levels for depressive illness. *Arch Gen Psychiat*, 34:197-204, 1977.

Glassman, A.H.; Giardina, E.V.; Perel, J.M.; et al.: Clinical characteristics of imipramine-induced orthostatic hypotension. *Lancet*, i:468-472, 1979.

Glick, I.; Hargreaves, W.A.; Drues, J.; Showstack, J.A.; Katzow, J.J.: Short vs. long hospitalization: a prospective controlled study. VII. Two-year follow-up results for nonschizophrenics. *Arch Gen Psychiat*, 34:314-317, 1977.

Goffman, E.: *Asylums*. New York, Anchor, 1961.

Gold, M.: *Psychiatric Emergencies*. Unpublished mimeo. Summit, New Jersey, Fair Oaks Hospital, 1979.

Golden, K.M.: Voodoo in Africa and the United States. *Am J Psychiat*, 134:1425-1427, 1977.

Goldstein, J.; Windle, C.: *Ideas for Improving Telephone Emergency Services*. Unpublished mimeo available from C. Windle, Room 11-C-03, NIMH, 5600 Fishers Lane, Rockville, Maryland, 20857.

Goldstein, M.J.; Rodnick, E.H.; Evan, J.R.; May, P.R.A.; Steinberg, M.R.: Drug and family therapy in the aftercare of acute schizophrenics. *Arch Gen Psychiat*, 35:1169-1177, 1978.

Good, M.I.: Primary affective disorders, aggression, and criminality. A review and clinical study. *Arch Gen Psychiat*, 35:954-960, 1978.

Good, M.I.; Shoder, R.I.: Behavioral toxicity and equivocal suicide associated with chloroquine and its derivatives. *Arch J Psychiat*, 134:798-801, 1977.

Goodman, L.S.; Gilman, A.: *The Pharmacological Basis of Therapeutics*, Fourth Edition. New York, MacMillan, 1970.

Gordon, J.S.: The runaway center as community mental health center. *Am J Psychiat*, 135:932-935, 1978.

Greaves, G.; Ghant, L.: Comparison of accomplished suicides with persons contacting a crisis intervention clinic. *Psychol Rep*, 3:390, 1972.

Greden, J.F.: Anxiety or caffeinism: a diagnostic dilemma. *Am J Psychiat*, 131:1089, 1974.

Greenblatt, M.: Efficacy of ECT in affective and schizophrenic illness. *Am J Psychiat*, 134:1001-1005, 1977.

Greilsheimer, H.; Groves, J.E.: Male genital self-mutilation. *Arch Gen Psychiat*, 36:441-446, 1979.

Grinker, R.R.; Werble, B.; Drye, R.: *The Borderline Syndrome: A Behavioral Study of Ego Functions*. New York, Basic Books, 1968.

Gross, M.: Pseudoepilepsy: a study in adolescent hysteria. *Am J Psychiat*, 136:210-213, 1979.

Groves, J.E.; Mandel, M.R.: The long-acting phenothiazines. *Arch Gen Psychiat*, 32:893-900, 1975.

Gualtieri, C.T.; Staze, J.: Withdrawal symptoms after abrupt cessation of amitriptyline in an eight-year-old boy. *Am J Psychiat*, 136:457-459, 1979.

Gunderson, J.G.; Singer, M.T.: Defining borderline patients: an overview. *Am J Psychiat*, 132:1, 1975.

Guttmacher, M.; Weihofen, H.: *Psychiatry and the Law*. New York, W.W. Norton, 1952.

Guze, S.B.: The validity and significance of the clinical diagnosis of hysteria. Briquet's Syndrome. *Am J Psychiat*, 132:138, 1975.

Hadl, J.: *Short Term Therapy: A Personal Exposition and a Historical Perspective* (Unpublished mimeo). Bethesda, Maryland, 1979.

Hales v. Petit, 75 Eng. Rep. 387 (KB) (1562).

Hall, R.C.W.; Gardner, E.R.; Perl, M.; Stickney, S.K.; Pfefferbaum, B.: *Psychiatric Opinion*, pp. 12-17, 1979.

Hall, R.C.W.; Popkin, M.K.; Devaul, R.A.; Faillace, L.A.; Stickney, S.K.: Physical illness presenting as psychiatric disease. *Arch Gen Psychiat*, 35:1315-1320, 1978.

Hall, R.C.W.; Popkin, M.K.; McHenry, L.E.: Angel's trumpet psychosis: a central nervous system anticholinergic syndrome. *Am J Psychiat,* 134:312-314, 1977.

Halliday, J.L.: Principles of aetiology. *Brit J Med Psychol,* 19:367, 1943.

Hammer v. Rosen, 7 NY 2d 376, 165 NE 2d 756, 198 NYS 2d 65 (1960).

Hargreaves, W.A.; Glick, I.D.; Drues, J.; Showstack, J.A.; Feigénbaum, E.: Short vs. long hospitalization: a prospective controlled study. VI. Two-year follow-up results for schizophrenics. *Arch Gen Psychiat,* 34:305-311, 1977.

Harkoff, L.D.: *Emergency Psychiatric Treatment. A Handbood of Secondary Prevention.* Springfield, Charles C Thomas, 1969.

Harrow, M.; Grinker, R.R.; Holzman, P.S.; Kayton, L.: Anhedonia and schizophrenia. *Am J Psychiat,* 134:794-797, 1977.

Hausman, A.; Rioch, D.M.: Military psychiatry. *Arch Gen Psychiat,* 16:727, 1967.

Heiser, J.F.; Wilbert, D.E.: Reversal of delirium induced by tricyclic antidepressant drugs with physostigmine. *Am J Psychiat,* 131:1275, 1974.

Heller, S.S.; Kornfeld, D.S.; Frank, K.A.; Hoar, P.F.: Postcardiotomy delirium and cardiac output. *Am J Psychiat,* 136:337-339, 1979.

Henderson, J.: *Emergency Medical Guide.* New York, McGraw-Hill, 1963.

Hendin, H.: *Suicide and Scandinavia.* New York, Grune and Stratton, 1964.

Hendin, H.: *"Suicide" in Comprehensive Textbook of Psychiatry.* A.M. Freedman; H.I. Kaplan, eds. Baltimore, Williams and Wilkins, 1967.

Henry, A.F.; Short, J.F.: *Suicide and Homicide: Some Economic, Sociological and Psychological Aspects of Aggression.* New York, Free Press, 1954.

Henslin, J.M.: Problems and prospects in studying significant others of suicides. *Bull Suicidology,* No. 8, Fall, pp. 81-84, 1971.

Herrero, F.A.: Lithium carbonate toxicity. *JAMA,* 226:1109-1110, 1973.

Herridge, C.F.: Physical disorders in psychiatric illness: A study of 209 consecutive admissions. *Lancet,* 2:949-951, 1960.

Herz, M.I.; Endicott, J.; Gibbon, M.; Brief hospitalization. Two-year follow-up. *Arch Gen Psychiat,* 36:701-705, 1979.

Hestbech, J.; Mansen, H.E.; Amdisen, A.; Olsen, S.: Chronic renal lesions following long-term treatment with lithium. *Kidney International,* 12:205-213, 1977.

Hill, D.: Discussion on surgery of temporal lobe epilepsy. Indications and contra-indications to temporal lobectomy. *Proc Roy Soc Med,* 51:610, 1958.

Himmelhoch, J.M.; Detre, T.; Kupfer, D.J.; et al.: Treatment of previously intractable depressions with tranylcypromine and lithium. *J Nerv Ment Dis,* 155:216-220, 1972.

Hoch, P.; Polatin, P.: Pseudoneurotic forms of schizophrenia. *Psychiat Q*, 23:248, 1949.

Hoffman, W.H.; Chodoroff, G.; Piggott, L.R.: Haloperidol and thyroid storm. *Am J Psychiat*, 135:485-486, 1979.

Hollingshead, A.B.; Redlich, F.C.: *Social Class and Mental Illness*. New York, Wiley, 1958.

Hollister, LE.: Psychiatric Disorders in G.S. Avery (ed). *Drug Treatment*. Seaforth, Australia, ADN Press, 1976.

Horney, K.: *Self-Analysis*. New York, W.W. Norton, 1942.

Horwitz, D.; Lovenberg, W.; Engelman, K.; et al.: Monoamine oxidase inhibitors, typramine, and cheese. *JAMA*, 188:1108-1110, 1964.

Hunt, R.G.: Social class and mental illness: some implications for clinical theory and practice. *Am J Psychiat*, 116:1065, 1960.

Hussain, M.Z.; Khan, A.G.; Chandry, Z.A.: Aplastic anemia associated with lithium therapy. *Can Med Asso J*, 108:724-728, 1973.

Husserl, E.: *Ideas*. New York, Macmillan, 1931.

Hutt, P.B.; Merrill, R.A.: *Criminal responsibility and the right to treatment for intoxication and alcoholism*. Georgetown L J 57:835, 1969.

Iversen, B.M.; Willassen, Y.; Bakke, O.: Charcoal haemoperfusion in nortriptyline poisoning. *Lancet*, i:388-389, 1978.

Jacobson, G.F.: Crisis theory and treatment strategy. Some sociocultural and psychodynamic considerations. *J Nerv Ment Dis*, 141:209, 1965.

Jacobson, G.; Strickler, M.; Morley, E.: Generic and individual approaches to crisis intervention. *AJPH*, 58:339, 1968.

Jaffe, C.M.: First-degree atrioventricular block during lithium carbonate treatment. *Am J Psychiat*, 135:88-89, 1977.

Janis, I.L.: *Psychological Stress: Psychoanalytical and Behavioral Studies of Surgical Patients*. New York, Wiley, 1958.

Jefferson, J.W.: Central nervous system toxicity of cimetidine: a case of depression. *Am J Psychiat*, 136:346, 1979.

Jefferson, J.W.; Greist, J.H.: *Primer of Lithium Therapy*. Baltimore, The Williams and Wilkins Co., 1977.

Jellinek, E.M.: *European Seminar on Alcoholism*, October, 1951.

Jeste, D.V.; Potkin, S.G.; Sinha, S.; Feder, S.; Wyatt, R.J.: Tardive Dyskinesia—reversible and persistent. *Arch Gen Psychiat*, 36:585-590, 1979.

Jobson, K.; Linnoila, M.; Gillam, J.; Sullivan, J.L.: Successful treatment of severe anxiety attacks with tricyclic antidepressants: a potential mechanism of action. *Am J Psychiat*, 135:863-864, 1978.

Johnson, D.A.W.: The evaluation of routine physical examination in psychiatric cases. *Practitioner*, 200:686-691, 1968.

Johnson, G.F.S.; Leeman, M.M.: Analysis of familial factors in bipolar affective illness. *Arch Gen Psychiat*, 34:1074-1083, 1977.

Jus, A.; Pinean, R.; Lachance, R.; et al.: Epidemiology of tardive dyskinesia. *Dis Nerv Syst*, 37:210-214, 1976.

Kane, J.; Quitkin, F.; Rifkin, A.; Klein, D.F.: Comparison of the incidence and severity of extrapyramidal side effects with fluphenazine enanthate and fluphenazine decanoate. *Am J Psychiat*, 135:1539-1542, 1978.

Kane, J.; Rifkin, A.; Quitkin, F.; Klein, D.: Extrapyramidal side effects with lithium treatment. *Am J Psychiat*, 135:851-853, 1978.

Kantor, S.J.; Bigger, J.; Glassman, A.H.; et al.: Imipramine-induced heart block. *JAMA*, 231:1364-1366, 1975.

Kaplan, D.M.; Mason, E.A.: Maternal reactions to premature birth viewed as an acute emotional disorder. *Am J Orthopsychiat*, 30:539, 1960.

Kardiner, A.: *The Traumatic Neurosis of War*. Washington, National Research Council, 1941.

Kelley, J.G.; Snowden, L.R.; Munnoz, R.F.: Social and Community Interventions in M.R. Rosenzweig and L.W. Porter (eds.): *Annual Rev Psychol*, 28:323-361, 1977.

Kelly, W.A.: Suicide and psychiatric education. *Am J Psychiat*, 130:463-468, 1973.

Kendler, K.S.: Amitriptyline-induced obesity in anorexia nervosa: a case report. *Am J Psychiat*, 135:1107-1108, 1978.

Kernberg, O.: Borderline personality organization. *J Am Psychoanal Assoc*, 15:641, 1967.

Ketai, R.: Psychotropic drugs in the management of psychiatric emergencies. *Postgraduate Medicine*, 58:87-93, 1975.

Kirk, L.; Baastrup, P.C.; Schou, M.: Propranolol treatment of lithium-induced tremor. *Lancet*, ii:1086-1087, 1973.

Kirstein, L.; Prusoff, B.; Weissman, M.; Dressier, D.M.: Utilization review of treatment for suicide attempters. *Am J Psychiat*, 132:22-27, 1975.

Kittrie, N.: *The Right to be Different*. John Hopkins Press, Baltimore, 1971.

Klawans, H.L.: The pharmacology of tardive dyskinesia. *Am J Psychiat*, 130:82-85, 1973.

Kleber, H.D.: *Withdrawal from barbiturates and sedatives*. Mimeo, New Haven, CT, 1974.

Kleber, H.D.: *Withdrawal from opiates*. Mimeo, New Haven, CT, 1974.

Kleber v. Stevens, 39 Misc 2d 712, 241 NYS 2d 497 (Sup. Ct.) Aff'd 20 App. Div. 2d 896, 239 NYS 2d 668 (1964).

Knight, R.: Borderline states. *Bull Menninger Clin*, 17:1, 1953.

Kobazaski, R.M.: Drug therapy of tardive dyskinesia. *New Engl J Med*, 296:257-260, 1977.

Kobazaski, R.M.: Orofacial dyskinesia: Clinical features, mechanisms, and drug therapy. *West J Med*, 125:277-288, 1976.

Koranyi, E.K.: Morbidity and rate of undiagnosed physical illnesses in a psychiatric clinic population. *Arch Gen Psychiat*, 36:414-419, 1979.

Kozol, R.; Boucher, R.; Garoflao, R.: "The diagnosis and treatment of dangerousness." *Crime and Delinquency*, 19:371-392, 1972.

Kramer, B.A.: Sleep disturbance associated with fluphenazine HCI: a case report. *Am J Psyciat*, 136:977-978, 1979.

Krauthammer, C.; Klerman, G.L.: Secondary mania. Manic syndromes associated with antecedent physical illness or drugs. *Arch Gen Psych*, 35:1333-1339, 1978.

Lamb, H.R.: The new asylums in the community. *Arch Gen Psychiat*, 36:129-134, 1979.

Lapierre, Y.D.: A controlled study of penfluridol in the treatment of chronic schizophrenia. *Am J Psychiat*, 135:956-959, 1978.

Leighton, A.: *My Name is Legion, Vol. 1. The Stirling County Study of Psychiatric Disorder and Sociocultural Environment*. New York, Basic Books, 1963.

Leighton, D.C.; et al.: *The Character of Danger, Vol. III. The Stirling Study of Psychiatric Disorder and Sociocultural Environment*. New York, Basic Books, 1963.

Lessard v. Schmidt, 349 Supp. 1078 (E.D. Wisc. 1972); vacated and remanded, 94 S. Ct. 713 (1974).

Lester, D.: *Effects of Suicide Prevention Centers on Suicide Rates in the United States*. Health Services Reports, 89:37-39, 1974.

Lester, D.: The myth of suicide prevention. *Comparative Psychiat*, 13:555-560, 1972.

Lester, D.; Brockopp, G.W.: *Crisis Intervention and Counseling by Telephone*. Springfield, Illinois, Charles C Thomas, 1973.

Levar, I.; Greenfield, H.; Baruch, E.: Psychiatric combat reactions during the Yom Kippur War. *Am J Psychiat*, 136:637-641, 1979.

Levenstein, S.; Klein, D.F.; Pollack, M.: Follow-up study of formerly voluntary psychiatric patients: The first two years. *Am J Psychiat*, 122:1102, 1966.

Lieb, J.; Lipsitch, I.I.; Slaby, A.E.: *The Crisis Team: A Handbook for The Mental Health Professional*. New York, Harper and Row, 1973.

Lieb, J.: Degraded protein-containing food and monoamine oxidase inhibitors. *Am J Psychiat*, 134:1444-1445, 1977.

Lieb, J.; Slaby, A.E.: *Integrated Psychiatric Treatment*. New York, Harper and Row, 1975.

Lieberman, M.A.; Solow, N.; Bond, G.R.; Reibstein, J.: The psychotherapeutic impact of women's consciousness-raising group. *Arch Gen Psychiat*, 36:161-168, 1979.

Liebowitz, M.R.; Wuetzel, E.J.; Bowser, A.E.; Klein, D.F.: Phenelzine and delusions of parasitosis: a case report. *Am J Psychiat*, 135:1565-1566, 1978.

Lief, H.I.; et al.: Low dropout rate in psychiatric clinic. *Arch Gen Psychiat*, 5:200, 1961.

Lifschutz (In re), 2 Cal. 3d 330 (1970).

Lindemann, E.: Symptomatology and management of acute grief. *Am J Psychiat*, 101:141, 1944.

Lindemann, E.: The Wellesley Project for the Study of Certain Problems in Community Mental Health, in *Interrelationships between Social Environment and Psychiatric Disorders*. New York, Milbank Memorial Fund, 1953.

Linder v. United States, 268 U.S. 5 (1925).

Locke, S.: *Neurology*. Boston, Little, Brown and Co., 1966.

Liss, L.; Frandes, A.: Court-mandated treatment: Dilemmas for hospital psychiaatry. *Am J Psychiat*, 132:924-927, 1975.

Litwack, T.R.: The role of counsel in civil commitment proceedings: Emerging problems. *California L Rev*, 62:816-839, May, 1974.

Loranger, A.W.; Levine, P.M.: Age at onset of bipolar affective illness. *Arch Gen Psychiat*, 35:1345-1348, 1978.

Lyman, J.L.: Student suicide at Oxford University. *Student Medicine*, 10:218, 1961.

MacMahon, B.; Johnson, S.; Pugh, T.F.: Relation of suicide rates to social conditions. *Public Health Rep*, 78:285, 1963.

Maguire, G.P.; Granville-Grossman, K.L.: Physical illness in psychiatric patients. *Brit J Psychiat*, 115:1365-1369, 1968.

Maldonado, R.R.; DeFrancisco, C.P.; Tamajo, L.: Lithium dermatitis. *JAMA*, 224:1534, 1973.

Malmquist, C.P.: Can the committed patient refuse chemotherapy. *Arch Gen Psychiat*, 36:351-354, 1979.

Man, P.L.; Chen, C.H.P.: Rapid tranquilization of acutely psychotic patients with haloperidol and chlorpromazine. *Psychosomatics*, 14:59, 1973.

Manual of Medical Therapeutics (20th Edition). C.M.G. Rosenfeld, ed. Boston, Little, Brown and Co., 1971.

Markusk, R.E.; Schwab, J.J.; Farris, P.; Present, P.A.; Holzer, E.E.: Mortality and community mental health. *Arch Gen Psychiat*, 34:1393-1401, 1977.

Marsden, C.D.; Tarsy, D.; Baldessarini, R.J.: Spontaneous and drug-induced movement disorders in psychiatric patients. In Benson, D.F.; Blumer, D.; eds.: *Psychiatric Aspects of Neurological Disease*, New York, Grune and Stratton, 1975.

Marshall, H.: Incidence of physical disorders among psychiatric inpatients. *Brit Med J*, 2:468-470, 1949.

Martin, R.L.; Cloninger, R.; Guze, S.B.: Female criminality and the prediction of recidivism: a prospective six-year follow-up. *Arch Gen Psychiat*, 35:207-214, 1978.

Marx, A.J.; Test, M.S.; Stein, L.I.: Extra-hospital management of severe mental illness. *Arch Gen Psychiat*, 29:505, 1973.

Mass. Gen. Laws Ch. 123 ss 7, 8, 12 (1971).

McCoid, A.H.: A reappraisal of liability for unauthorized medical treatment. *Minnesota L Rev*. 41:381, 1957.

McCurdy, L.: Lorazepam, a new benzodizepine derivative, in the treatment of anxiety: a double-blind clinical evaluation. *Am J Psychiat*, 136:187-190, 1979.

McDonald v. United States, 114 U.S. App. D.C. 120, 312 F. 2d 847 (en banc) (1962).

McGarry, A.L.; H.A. Kaplan: Overview: Current trends in mental health law. *Am J Psychiat*, 130:621-630 (1973).

McGee, R.K.: *Crisis Intervention in the Community*. Baltimore, University Park Press, 1974.

McLean, P.; Casey, D.E.: Tardive dyskinesia in an adolescent. *Am J Psychiat*, 135:969-971, 1978.

McNeil v. Director, Patuxen Institution, 407 U.S. 245 (1972).

Mechanic, D.: The concept of illness behavior. *J Chron Dis*, 15:189, 1962.

Mendel, W.M.; Rapport, S.: Determinants of the decision for psychiatric hospitalization. *Arch Gen Psychiat*, 20:321, 1969.

Menninger, K.: *Man Against Himself*. New York, Harcourt Brace, 1938.

Menninger, W.C.: *Psychiatry in a Troubled World*. New York, Macmillan, 1948.

Merritt, H.H.: *A Textbook of Neurology*. Fourth Edition. Philadelphia, Lea and Febiger, 1967.

Miller, F.T.; Mazade, N.A.: *Crisis Intervention Services in Comprehensive Community Mental Health Centers in the United States*. Unpublished mimeo, 1978, available through Dr. Mazade at The Staff College, National Institute of Mental Health, 5635 Fishers Lane, Rockville, Maryland, 20857.

Minkoff, K.; Bergman, E.; Beck, A.T.; Beck, R.: Hopelessness, depression, and attempted suicide. *Am J Psychiat*, 130:455-459, 1973.

Minnesota ex rel Pearson v. Probate Court, 309 U.S. 270 (1940).

Mintz, R.S.: A pilot study of the prevalence of persons in the City of Los Angeles who have attempted suicide. Presented at the 120th Annual Meeting of the American Psychiatric Association, Los Angeles, May 4, 1964.

M'Naghten Case: House of Lords, 1843, 8 *Eng Rep*, 718 (HL), 1843.

Monahan, J.: Prediction research and the emergency commitment of dangerous mentally ill persons: a reconsideration. *Am J Psychiat*, 135:198-201, 1978.

Moore, D.C.: Amitriptyline therapy in anorexia nervosa. *Am J Psychiat*, 134:1301-1304, 1977.

Morris, G.H.: Institutionalizing the rights of mental patients: Committing the legislature. *California L Rev*, 62:816-839, 1974.

Morse, H.N.: The tort liability of the psychiatrist. *Baylor L Rev*, 19:208, 1971.

Moskovitz, C.; Moses, H.; Klawans, H.L.: Levadopa-induced psychosis: a kindling phenomenon. *Am J Psychiat*, 135:669-675, 1978.

Motto, J.A.: Evaluation of a suicide prevention center by sampling the population risk. *Life-threatening Behavior*, 1:18-22, 1971.

Muller, O.E.; Goodman, N.; Bellet, S.: The hypotensive effect of imipramine hydrochloride in patients with cardiovascular disease. *Clin Pharmacol Ther*, 2:300-307, 1961.

Murphy, G.E.; Armstrong, J.W.; Hermele, S.L.; Fischer, J.R.; Clendenin, W.W.: Suicide and alcoholism: interpersonal loss confined as a predictor. *Arch Gen Psychiat*, 36:65-69, 1979.

Myers, J.K.; Bean, L.L.: *A Decade Later: A Follow-up of Social Class and Mental Illness*. New York, John Wiley and Sons, 1968.

Myers, M.J.: Informed consent in medical malpractice. *California L Rev*, 55:396, 1967.

National Research Council Committee in Clinical Evaluation of Narcotic Antagonists: Clinical evaluation of naltrexone treatment of opiate-dependent individuals. *Arch Gen Psychiat*, 135:335-340, 1978.

Neil, J.F.; Himmelhoch, J.M.; Licata, S.M.: Emergency of myasthenia gravis during treatment with lithium carbonate. *Arch Gen Psychiat*, 33:1090-1092, 1976.

Nelson, J.C.; Bowers, M.B.: Delusional unipolar depression. Description and drug response. *Arch Gen Psychiat*, 35:1321-1328, 1978.

Nelson, J.C.; Bowers, M.B.; Sweeney, D.R.: Exacerbation of psychosis by tricyclic antidepressants in delusional depression. *Am J Psychiat*, 136:574-576, 1979.

Neuringer, C.; Lettieri, D.J.: Cognition attitude and affect in suicidal individuals. *Life-Threatening Behavior*, 1:106-124, 1971.

New Hampshire v. Jones, 50 NH 369, (1869).

New Hampshire v. Pike, 49 NH 399 (1869).

New York Civil Rights Law, Act 45, Section 4501, 4507, 4508 (1972).

New York Mental Hygiene Law, McKinney, 1951, Supp. 1970.

New York Mental Hygiene Law Sections 15, 29, 31 (McKinney Supp. 1973).

New York State Department of Mental Hygiene: *Application for Admission of Patient*. Form 471 DMH, 1/73.

New York State Department of Mental Hygiene: *Notice of Status and Rights—Emergency Admission*. Form OMH 474 (11-78).

New York State Department of Mental Hygiene: *Notice of Status and Rights—Involuntary Admission*. Form 461 DMH (5-73).

New York State Department of Mental Hygiene: *Notice of Rights—Voluntary or Minor Voluntary Admission.* Form OMH 460 (4-78).

New York State Department of Mental Hygiene: *Record of Emergency Admission.* Form OMH 474 (2-79).

New York State Department of Mental Hygiene: *Voluntary Request for Hospitalization.* Form 472 DMH, 1/73.

Newton, R.W.: Physostigmine salicylate in the treatment of tricyclic antidepressant overdosage. *JAMA,* 231:941-944, 1975.

Nies, A.; Robinson, D.S.; Friedman, M.J.; Green, R.; Cooper, T.B.; Ravaris, C.L.; Ives, J.O.: Relationship between age and tricyclic antidepressant plasma levels. *Am J Psychiat,* 134:790-793, 1977.

Note: Developments in the Law—"Civil commitment of the mentally ill." *Harvard L Rev,* 87:1190, April, 1974.

Note: Overt dangerous behavior as a constitutional requirement for involuntary civil commitment of the mentally ill. *University of Chicago L Rev,* 44:562, 1977.

Noyes, R.; Clancy, J.; Crowe, R.; Hoenk, P.R.; Slymen, D.J.: The familial prevalence of anxiety neurosis. *Arch Gen Psychiat,* 35:1057-1059, 1978.

O'Brien, J.P.: Increase in suicide attempts by drug ingestion: the Boston experience, 1964-1974. *Arch Gen Psychiat,* 34:1165-1169, 1977.

O'Connor v. Donaldson, 422 U.S. 563, 95 S. Ct. 2486 (1975).

Ogden, M.; Spector, M.I.; Hill, C.A.: Suicides and homicides among Indians. *Pub Health Rep,* 85:75-80, 1970.

Okin v. Rogers, U.S. Ct. of Appeals 1st cir. (No. 77-1201). See also "Okin v. Rogers," *Mental Disability Law Reporter,* 2:43-50, 1977.

Okrasinski, H.: Lithium acne. *Dermatologica,* 154:251-253, 1977.

Olin, G.B.; Olin, H.S.: Informed consent in voluntary mental hospital admissions. *Am J Psychiat,* 132:938-941, September, 1975.

Paffenbarger, R.S.; King, S.H.; Wing, A.C.: Chronic disease in former college students: IX characteristics in youth that predispose to suicide and accidental death in later life. *AJPH,* 59:900-908, 1969.

Palmer, A.B. and Wohl, J.: Voluntary admission forms: does the patient know what he is signing? *Hospital and Community Psychiatry,* 23:38-40, 1972.

Parad, H.J., ed.: *Crisis Intervention: Selected Readings.* New York, Family Service Association of America, 1965.

Parad, H.J.; Caplan, G.; A Framework for studying Families in Crisis, in *Crisis Intervention: Selected Readings.* New York, Family Service Association of America, 1965.

Parham v. J.L.—U.S.—47 LW. 4739 (June 20, 1979).

Pariser, S.F.; Pinta, E.R.; Jones, B.A.: Mitral valve prolapse syndrome and anxiety neurosis/panic disorder. *Am J Psychiat,* 135:246-247, 1978.

Parrish, H.: Cause of death among college students: a study of 209 deaths at Yale University, 1920-1955. *Public Health Rep*, 71:1081-1085, 1956.

Parrish, H.M.: Epidemiology of suicide among college students. *Yale J Biol Med*, 29:585, 1957.

Pasamanik, B.; Scarpitti, F.; Dinitry, S.: *Schizophrenics in the Community*. New York, Appleton-Century-Crofts, 1967.

Paulose, K.P.; Shaw, A.A.: Rapidly recurring seizures of psychogenic origin. *Am J Psychiat*, 134:1145-1146, 1977.

Peck, M.; Schrut, A.: Suicidal behavior among college students. *HSMHA Health Reports*, 86:149-156, 1971.

Pederson, A.M.; Aruad, G.A.; Kindler, A.R.: Epidemiological differences between white and nonwhite suicide attempters. *Mental Health Digest*, 5:27-29, 1973.

People v. Gorsehn, 51 Cal. 2d 716, 336 P. 2d 492 (1959)

People v. Wells, 33 Cal. 2d 330, 202 P. 2d 53 (1949).

Perris, C.: Morbidity suppressive effect of lithium carbonate in cycloid psychosis. *Arch Gen Psychiat*, 35:328-331, 1978.

Persild, H.; Madsen, S.N.: Hansen, J.E.M.: Irreversible myxedema after lithium carbonate. *Brit Med J*, 1:1105-1109, 1978.

Peszke, M.D.: Is dangerousness an issue for physicians in emergency commitment? *Am J Psychiat*, 132:825-828, 1975.

Peterson, M.W.: Imipramine treatment for hypersomnia. *Am J Psychiat*, 136:984-985, 1979.

Pevnick, J.S.; Jasinski, D.R.; Haertzen, C.A.: Abrupt withdrawal from therapeutically administered diazepam. Report of a case. *Arch Gen Psychiat*, 35:995-998, 1978.

Physician's Desk Reference, 28th Edition. Oradell, N.J., Medical Economics Co., 1974.

Pines, A.; Maslach, C.: Characteristics of staff burnout in mental health settings. *Hospital & Community Psychiatry*, 29:233-237, 1978.

Pitts, F.N.; Schuller, A.B.; Rich, C.L.; Pitts, A.F.: Suicide among U.S. Women Physicians, 1967-1972. *Am J Psychiat*, 136:694-696, 1974.

Plante, M.L.: An analysis of 'informed consent.' *Fordham L Rev*, 36:639, 1968.

Platman, S.R.: A comparison of lithium carbonate and chlorpromazine in mania. *Am J Psychiat*, 127:351-353, 1970.

Plaut, E.A.: A perspective on confidentiality. *Am J Psychiat*, 131:1021-1024, 1974.

Plotkin, R.: Limiting the therapeutic orgy: Mental patient's right to refuse treatment. *Northwestern University L Rev*, 72:461, 1977.

Pollit, J.; Young, J.: Anxiety state or masked depression? A study based on the action of monoamine oxidase inhibitors. *Brit J Psychiat*, 119:143-149, 1971.

Porter, R.A.: Crisis intervention and social work models. *Community Mental Health Journal*, 2B:13, 1966.

Prien, R.F.; Point, P.; Caffey, E.M.; et al.: Comparison of lithium carbonate and chlorpromazine in the treatment of mania. *Arch Gen Psychiat*, 26:146-153, 1972.

Principles of Internal Medicine, Fourth Edition. T.R. Harrison, et al., ed. New York, McGraw-Hill, 1962.

Privileged communication, *JAMA*, 297:257, 1966.

Projects: Civil commitment of the mentally ill. *UCLA L Rev*, 14:822, 1967.

Prusoff, B.A.; Williams, D.H.; Weissman, M.M.; Astrachan, B.M.: Treatment of secondary depression in schizophrenia: a double-blind, placebo-controlled trial of amitriptyline added to perphenozine. *Arch Gen Psychiat*, 36:569-575, 1979.

Psychiatric News. Survey shows many community mental health centers lack emergency services. *Psychiatric News*, February 2, 1977.

Psychiatric News, New CMHC survey shows better emergency service. August 19, 1977.

Quitkin, F.; Rifkin, A.; Gochfeld, L.; Klein, D.F.: Tardive dyskinesia: are first signs reversible? *Am J Psychiat*, 134:84-87, 1977.

Quitkin, F.; Rifkin, A.; Kane, J.; Ramos-Lorenzi, J.F.; Klein, D.F.: Long-acting oral vs. injectable antipsychotic drugs in schizophrenics. A one-year double-blind comparison in multiple-episode schizophrenics. *Arch Gen Psychiat*, 35:889-892, 1978.

Rachlin, S.; Fam, A.; Milton, J.: Civil liberties versus involuntary hospitalization. *Am J Psychiat*, 132:189-192, 1975.

Rainey, J.M.: Disulfiram toxicity and carbon disulfide poisoning. *Am J Psychiat*, 134:371-378, 1977.

Rampling, D.: Aggression: A paradoxical response to tricyclic antidepressants. *Am J Psychiat*, 135:117-118, 1978.

Rapaport, L.: The State of Crisis: Some Theoretical Consideration, in *Crisis Intervention: Selected Readings*. H.J. Parad, ed. New York, Family Service Association of America, 1965.

Rapaport, R.: Normal crisis, family structure, and mental health. *Family Process*, 2:68, 1963.

Raphael, B.: Preventive intervention with the recently bereaved. *Arch Gen Psychiat*, 34:1450-1454, 1977.

Rappolt, R.T.; Gay, G.R.; Farris, R.D.: Emergency management of acute phencyclidine intoxication. *JACEP*, 8:68-76, 1979.

Ravaris, C.L.; Nies, A.; Robinson, D.S.; et al.: A multiple-dose, controlled study of phenelzine in depression-anxiety states. *Arch Gen Psychiat*, 33:347-350, 1976.

Raymond, M.; Slaby, A.; Lieb, J.: *The Healing Alliance*. New York, W.W. Norton and Co. 1975.

Reasons Sought for Adolescent Suicide Increase. *The Washington Post*, Friday, June 4, 1976.

Reich, W.: Soviet psychiatry on trial. *Commentary*, 40-48, January, 1978.

Reichard, C.C.; Elder, S.T.: The effects of caffeine on reaction time in hyperkinetic and normal children. *Am J Psychiat*, 134:144-148, 1977.

Remick, R.A.; Wada, J.A.: Complex partial and pseudoseizure disorders. *Am J Psychiat*, 136:320-323, 1979.

Rennie v. Klein, 476 F. Supp. 1294 (D.N.J. 1979).

Rennie v. Klein, 462 F. Supp. 1131 (1978).

Resnik, H.L.P.: Erotized repetitive hangings: a form of self-destructive behavior. *Am J Psychotherapy*, 26, 4-21, 1972.

Resnik, H.L.P.: *Suicidal Behavior: Diagnosis and Management*. Boston, Little, Brown and Co., 1968.

Resnik, H.L.P.; Dizmang, L.H.: Observations on suicidal behavior among American Indians. *Am J Psychiat*, 127:882-887, 1971.

Resnik, H.L.P.; Wittlin, B.J.: Abortion and suicidal behaviors: observations on the concept of "endangering the mental health of the mother." *Mental Hygiene*, 55:10-20, 1971.

Reusch, J.: Social Factors in Therapy, in *Psychiatric Treatment*. Vol. 31. S.B. Wortis, M. Herman, and C.C. Hare, eds. Association for Nervous and Mental Diseases. Baltimore, Williams and Wilkins, 1953.

Rieger, W.; Brady, J.P.; Weisberg, E.: Hematologic changes in anorexia nervosa. *Am J Psychiat*, 135:984-985, 1978.

Rifkin, A.; Quitkin, F.; Kane, J.; Struve, F.; Klein, D.F.: Are prophylactic antiparkinson drugs necessary? A continued study of procyclidine withdrawal. *Arch Gen Psychiat*, 35:483-489, 1978.

Rifkin, A.; Quitkin, F.; Rabiner, C.J.; Klein, D.F.: Fluphenazine decanoate, fluphenazine hydrochloride given orally, and placebo in remitted schizophrenics. I. Relapse rates after one year. *Arch Gen Psychiat*, 34:43-47, 1977.

Rights of the mentally ill during incarceration: The developing law. (Note), *U Fla L Rev*, 25:494, 1973.

Robins, E.; Gentry, K.A.; Munoz, R.A.; Marten, S.: A contrast of the three more common illnesses with the ten less common in a study and 18-month follow-up of 314 psychiatric emergency room patients. I. Characteristics of the sample and methods of study. *Arch Gen Psychiat*, 34:259-265, 1977.

Robins, E.; Gentry, K.A.; Munoz, R.A.; Marten, S.: A contrast of the three more common illnesses with the ten less common in a study and 18-month follow-up of 314 psychiatric emergency room patients. II. Characteristics of patients with the three more common illnesses. *Arch*

Gen Psychiat, 34:269-281, 1977.

Robins, E.; Gentry, K.A.; Munoz, R.A.; Marten, S.: A contrast of the three more common illnesses with the ten less common in a study and 18-month follow-up of 314 psychiatric emergency room patients. III. Findings at follow-up. *Arch Gen Psychiat*, 34:185-291, 1977.

Robinson v. California 370 U.S. 660 (1962).

Robinson, D.S.; Nies, A.; Ravaris, C.L. et al.: The monoamine oxidase inhibitor, phenelzine, in the treatment of depressive-anxious states. *Arch Gen Psychiat*, 29:407-413, 1973.

Rogers v. Okin, 478 F. Supp. 1343 (1979).

Rosen, A.: Case report: symptomatic mania and phencyclidine abuse. *Am J Psychiat*, 136:118-119, 1979.

Rosen, D.H.: Suicide Survivors—a follow-up study of persons who survived jumping from the Golden Gate and San Francisco-Oakland Bay Bridges. *West J Med*, 122:289-294, 1975.

Rosenfeld, A.A.: Depression and psychotic regression following prolonged methylphenidate use and withdrawal: case report. *Am J Psychiat*, 136:226-228, 1979.

Ross, H.A.: Commitment of the mentally ill: problems of law and policy. *Michigan L Rev*, 57:945, 1959.

Roth, L.H.; Meisel, A.; Litz, C.W.: Tests of competency to consent to treatment. *Am J Psychiat*, 134:279, 1977.

Rouse v. Cameron, 373 F. 2d 451 (1962).

Roy v. Hartogs, 173 (52) NYLJ (3-18-75) 17, Col. 7F (1975).

Sainsburg, P.: *Suicide in London*. London, Chapman and Hall, 1955.

Sangiovanni, F.; et al.: Rapid control of psychotic excitement states with intramuscular haloperidol. *Am J Psychiat*, 130:1155, 1973.

Satterfield, J.H.; Cantwell, D.; Schell, A.; Blaschke, T.: Growth of hyperactive children treated with methylphenidate. *Arch Gen Psychiat*, 36:212-217, 1979.

Schatzberg, A.F;; Cole, J.O.: Benzodiazepines in depressive disorders. *Arch Gen Psychiat*, 35:1359-1365, 1978.

Schless, A.P.; Mendels, J.: The value of interviewing family and friends in assessing life stresses. *Arch Gen Psychiat*, 35:565-567, 1978.

Schmideberg, M.: The borderline patient, in *American Handbook of Psychiatry*. S. Arieto, ed. New York, Basic Books, 1959.

Schmidt, H.S.; Clark, R.W.; Hyman, P.R.: Protriptyline: an effective agent in the treatment of the narcolepsy-cataplexy syndrome and hypersomnia. *Am J Psychiat*, 134:183-185, 1977.

Schou, M.; Juel-Nielsen, N.; Stromgren, E.; et al.: The treatment of manic psychoses by the administration of lithium salts. *J Neurol Neurosurg Psychiat*, 126:1306-1310, 1970.

Schuckit, M.A.: *Drug and Alcohol Abuse: A Clinical Guide to Diagnosis and Treatment*. New York, Plenum Medical Book Co., 1979.

Schuckit, M.A.; Morrissey, E.R.: Drug abuse among alcoholic women. *Am J Psychiat*, 136:607-611, 1979.

Schwartz, A.: Civil liability for causing suicide: a synthesis of law and psychiatry. *Vanderbilt L Rev*, 24:217, 1971.

Seiden, R.: *Suicide among Youth*. Washington, D.C.; U.S. Government Printing Office, 1969.

Shader, R.I.; et al.: *Psychotic Drug Side Effects*. Baltimore, Williams and Wilkins, 1970.

Shah, S.A.: Dangerousness and civil commitment of the mentally ill: Some public policy considerations. *Am J Psychiat*, 132:501-505, 1975.

Shear, M.K.; Sacks, M.H.: Digitalis delirium: report of two cases. *Am J Psychiat*, 135:109-110, 1978.

Sheehy, L.M.; Maxmen, J.S.: Phenelzine-induced psychosis. *Am J Psychiat*, 135:1422-1423, 1978.

Shephert, J.T.; Whiting, B.: Beta-adrenergic blockade in the treatment of MAOI self-poisoning. *Lancet*, ii:1021, 1974.

Shneidman, E.S.; Faberow, N.L.: The Los Angeles Suicide Prevention Center: A demonstration of public health feasibilities. *Am J Public Health*, 55:21-26, 1965.

Shneidman, E.; Farberow, N.; Litman, R.: *The Psychology of Suicide*. New York, Science House, 1970.

Shneidman, E.S.; Mandelkom, P.: How to Prevent Suicide. New York Public Affairs Pamphlet No. 407, 1967.

Shopsin, B.; Gershon, S.: Cogwheel rigidity related to lithium maintenance. *Am J Psychiat*, 132:536-538, 1975.

Shopsin, B.; Klein, H.; Aaronson, M.; Collora, M.: Clozapine, chlorpromazine, and placebo in newly hospitalized, acutely schizophrenic patients: a controlled, double-blind comparison. *Arch Gen Psychiat*, 36:657-664, 1979.

Showalter, C.V.; Thorton, W.E.: Clinical pharmacology of phencyclidine toxicity. *Am J Psychiat*, 134:1134-1238, 1977.

Shubin, S.: Burnout: the professional hazard you face in nursing. *Nursing*, 8:23-27, 1978.

Siegel, R.K.: Cocaine hallucinations. *Am J Psychiat*, 135:309-314, 1978.

Sigell, L.T.; Kapp, F.T.; Fusaro, E.A.; Nelson, E.D.; Falck, R.S.: Popping and snorting volatile nitrites: a current fact for getting high. *Am J Psychiat*, 135:1216-1218, 1978.

Siris, S.G.; von Kammen, D.P.; Docherty, J.P.: Use of antidepressant drugs in schizophrenia. *Arch Gen Psychiat*, 35:1368-1377, 1978.

Skodol, A.E.; Karasu, T.B.: Emergency psychiatry and the assaultive patient. *Am J Psychiat*, 135:202-205, 1978.

Slaby, A.E.; Lieb, J.; Tancredi, L.R.: *Handbook of Psychiatric Emergencies: A Guide for Emergencies in Psychiatry*. Flushing, New York,

Medical Examination Publishing Co., 1975.

Slaby, A.E.; Perry, P.L.: Use and abuse of psychiatric emergency services. Paper presented at the meetings of the American Psychiatric Association, Chicago, May, 1979.

Slaby, A.E.; Tancredi, L.R.: *Collusion for Conformity*. New York, Jason Aronson, Inc., 1975.

Slaby, A.E.; Wyatt, R.J.: *Dementia in the Presenium*. Springfield, Charles C Thomas, 1974.

Slater, E.: The diagnosis of "hysteria." *Brit Med J*, I, 1395, 1965.

Slater, E.; Roth, M.: *Mayer-Gross Slater and Roth: Clinical Psychiatry*, Third Edition, London, Bailiere, Tindall and Cassell, 1969.

Slovenko, R. (ed): *Sexual Behavior and the Law*. Charles C Thomas, Springfield, Illinois, 1965.

Slovenko, Ralph: *Psychiatry and Law*. Little, Brown & Co., Boston, 1973.

Slovenko, R: Psychotherapist-patient testimonial privilege: A picture of misguided hope. *Catholic U L Rev*, 23:649-73, 1974.

Smart, R.G.; Gray, G.: Multiple predictors of dropout from alcoholism treatment. *Arch Gen Psychiat*, 35:363-367, 1978.

Snole, L.; et al.: *Mental Health in the Metropolis*. New York, McGraw-Hill, 1962.

Solomon, J.G.; Solomon, S.: Psychotic depression and bronchogenic carcinoma. *Am J Psychiat*, 135:859-860, 1978.

Solomon, K.: Phenothiazine-induced bulbar palsy-like syndrome and sudden death. *Am J Psychiat*, 134:308-311, 1977.

Souder v. Brennan, 367 F. Supp. 808 (D DC 1973).

Southwick, R.: Hospital's responsibility. Cleveland-Marshall L Rev, 17:156 (1968).

Specter, G.A.; Claiborn, W.L.: *Crisis Intervention*. New York, Behavioral Publications, 1973.

Spensley, J; Barter, J.T.; Werme, P.H.; Langsley, D.G.: Involuntary hospitalization: What for and how long? *Am J Psychiat*, 131:219-223, 1974.

Spiker, D.G.; Weiss, A.N.; Chang, S.S.; et al.: Tricyclic antidepressant overdose: Clinical presentation and plasma levels. *Clin Pharmacol Ther*, 18:539-546, 1975.

Spitzer, S.P.; Denzen, N.K.: *The Mental Patient: Studies in the Sociology of Deviance*. New York, McGraw-Hill, 1968.

Squire, L.R.: ECT and memory loss. *Am J Psychiat*, 134:997-1001, 1977.

Stanton, A.; Schwartz, M.: *The Mental Hospital*. New York, Basic Books, 1954.

State v. Thompson, Wright's Ohio Rep. 617 (1834).

Stewart, M.M.: MAOI's and food—fact and fiction. *Adverse Drug Reaction Bull*, 58:200-203, 1976.

Stinson, D.J.; Smith, W.G.; Amidjayo, I.; Kaplan, J.M.: Systems of care and treatment outcomes for alcoholic patients. *Arch Gen Psychiat*, 36:535-539, 1979.

Stockley, I.H.: Monoamine oxidase inhibitors: Interactions with sympathomimetic amines. *The Pharmaceutical J* (June 30):590-593, 1973.

Stone, A.: (Comment, on Peszke's: Is dangerousness an issue for physicians in emergency commitment?) *Am J Psychiat*, 132:829-831, 1975.

Stone, A.: The right to treatment and the medical establishment. *The Bulletin of the American Academy of Psychiatry and the Law*, 2:172, 1974.

Stone, Alan A.: *Mental Health and Law: A System in Transition*. National Institute of Mental Health, DHEW Publication No. (ADM) 75-176, Washington, D.C. 1975.

Stoner v. Miller, 377 F. Supp. 177 (EDNY 1974).

Stotsky, B.A.: Relative efficacy of parenteral haloperidol and thiothixene for the emergency treatment of acutely excited and agitated patients. *Diseases of the Nervous System*. 38:967-973, 1977.

Suicide: How to Keep Patients from Killing Themselves. Interviews with C.J. Frederick and H. Hendin. *Med World News*, pp. 86-95, July, 1976.

Suicide Rate for Young Rises Sharply. *The Washington Post*, April 28, 1975.

Summers, W.K.; Reich, T.C.: Delirium after cataract surgery: review and two cases. *Am J Psychiat*, 136:386-391, 1979.

Suspected rape. *ACOG Technical Bulletin*. No. 14, July, 1970.

Susser, M.: *Community Psychiatry: Epidemiologic and Social Themes*. New York, Random House, 1968.

Suzuki v. Quisenberry, 411 F. Supp. 1113 (D. Hawaii, 1976).

Swett, D.; Cole, J.O.; Hartz, S.C.; Shapiro, S.; Slone, D.: Hypotension due to chlorpromazine. Relation to cigarette smoking, blood pressure and dosage. *Arch Gen Psychiat*, 34:661-663, 1977.

Swett, C.; Cole, J.O.; Shapiro, S.; Slone, D.: Extrapyramidal side effects in chlorpromazine recipients: emergence according to benztropine prophylaxis. *Arch Gen Psychiat*, 34:942-943, 1977.

Sylph, J.A.; Kedward, H.B.: Alternatives to the mental hospital: Use of residential facilities for long-term psychiatric care. *Arch Gen Psychiat*, 34:909-912, 1977.

Szasz, T.S.: The communication of distress between child and parent. *Brit J Med Psychiat*, 32:161, 1959.

Tamminga, C.A.; Crayton, J.W.; Chase, T.W.: Improvement in tardive dyskinesia after muscimol therapy. *Arch Gen Psychiat*, 36:595-598, 1979.

Tamminga, C.A.; Smith, R.C.; Pandey, G.; Frohman, L.A.; Davis, J.M.: A neuroendocrine study of supersensitivity in tardive dyskinesia. *Arch Gen Psychiat*, 34:1199-1203, 1977.

Tancredi, L.R.; Lieb, J.; Slaby, A.E.: *Legal Issues in Psychiatric Care*. New York, Harper and Row, 1975.

Tancredi, L.R.; Woods, J.: "The social control of medical practice" in: *Economic Aspects of Health Care*. J. McKinlay, ed. New York, Prodist, 1973.

Tancredi, L.R.; Lieb, J.; Slaby, A.E.: *Legal Issues in Psychiatric Care*. New York, Harper & Row Publishers, 1975.

Tancredi, L.R.; Slaby, A.E.: "Ethical Issues in Mental Health Care" in Hiller, M.D.: *Medical Ethics and the Law: Implications for Public Policy*. Boston, Ballinger Press. (In press).

Tancredi, L.R.; Slaby, A.E.: *Ethical Policy in Mental Health Care: The Goals of Psychiatric Intervention*. New York, Prodist, 1977.

Tarasoff v. Regents of the University of California, 529 P. 2d. 553 (1974).

Tarasoff v. Regents of the University of California, 551 P. 2d. 334 (1976).

Tardiff, K.J.: A survey of psychiatrists in Boston and their work with violent patients. *Am J Psychiat*, 131:1008, 1974.

Taylor, M.A.; Abrams, R.: Catatonia: Prevalence and importance in the manic phase of manic-depressive illness. *Arch Gen Psychiat*, 34:1223-1225, 1977.

Tefft, B.M.; Pederson, A.M.; Babigian, H.M.: Patterns of death among suicide attempters; a psychiatric population, and a general population. *Arch Gen Psychiat*, 34:1155-1161, 1977.

Teicher, J.D.; Jacobs, J.: Adolescents who attempt suicide: preliminary findings. *Am J Psychiat*, 122:1248-1257, 1966.

Teicher, J.D.; Jacobs, J.: The physician and the adolescent suicide attempter. *J School Health*, 36:406-415, 1966.

Temby, W.D.: *Suicide in Emotional Problems of the Student*. G.B. Blaine and C.C. McArthur, eds. New York, Appleton-Century-Crofts, 1961.

Thomas, C.S.; Weisman, G.K.: Emergency planning: The practical and theoretical backdrop to an emergency treatment unit. *Int J Soc Psychiat*, 16:283, 1970.

Thomson, K.; Shou, M.: "The treatment of lithium poisoning" in *Lithium Research and Therapy*. F.N. Johnson, ed. New York, Academic Press, 1975.

Tonsic v. Wagner, 329 A.2d 497 (1974).

A Treatment Manual for Acute Drug Abuse Emergencies, P.G. Bourne, ed. Rockville, Md., National Clearinghouse for Drug Abuse Information, National Institute in Drug Abuse, NCDAI Publication, November 16, 1974.

Tsuang, M.T.: Suicide in schizophrenics, manics, depressives, and surgical controls: a comparison with general population suicide mortality. *Arch Gen Psychiat*, 35:153-155, 1978.

Tsuang, M.T.; Woolson, R.F.: Excess mortality in schizophrenia and affective disorders. Do suicides and accidental deaths solely account for this excess? *Arch Gen Psychiat*, 35:1181-1185, 1978.

Tyrer, P.; Candy, J.; Kelly, D.: Phenelzine in phobic anxiety: A controlled trial. *Psychol Med*, 3:120-124, 1973.

United States v. Brawner, 471 F. 2d 969 (1972).

United States v. George, 239 F. Supp. 752 (1964).

U.S.P.H.S.: Department of Health Education and Welfare, NIMH: Mental Health Statistics—Current Reports, Series MHB-H-7, January, 1963.

Van Patten, T.; May, P.R.A.: "Akinectic depression" in schizophrenia. *Arch Gen Psychiat*, 35:1101-1107, 1978.

Van Scheyen, J.D.; Van Kammen, D.P.: Clomipramine-induced mania in unipolar depression. *Arch Gen Psychiat*, 36:560-565, 1979.

Wald, D.; Lerner, J.: Lithium in the treatment of periodic catatonia: a case report. *Am J Psychiat*, 135:751-752, 1978.

Walker, W.R.; Parsons, L.B.; Skelton, W.D.: Brief hospitalization on a crisis service: a study of patient and treatment variables. *Am J Psychiat*, 130:896, 1973.

Wegner, J.T.; Struve, F.A.; Kantor, J.S.; Kane, J.M.: Relationship between the B-mitten EEG pattern and tardive dyskinesia: a pilot control study. *Arch Gen Psychiat*, 36:599-603, 1979.

Wehr, T.A.; Goodwin, F.K.: Rapid cycling in manic-depressives induced by tricyclic antidepressants. *Arch Gen Psychiat*, 36:555-559, 1979.

Weiner, M.F.: Haloperidol, hyperthyroidism, and sudden death. *Am J Psychiat*, 136:717-718, 1979.

Weisman, G.; Feirstein, A.; Thomas, C.: Three-day hospitalization—a model for intervention. *Arch Gen Psychiat*, 21:620, 1969.

Weiss, G.; Hectman, L.; Perlman, T.; Hopkins, J.; Wener, A.: Hyperactives as young adults: a controlled prospective ten-year follow-up of 75 children. *Arch Gen Psychiat*, 36:675-681, 1979.

Weissman, M.M.: The epidemiology of suicide attempts, 1960 to 1971. *Arch Gen Psychiat*, 30:737-746, 1974.

Weissman, M.; Fox, K.; Klerman, G.L.: Hostility and depression associated with suicide attempts. *Am J Psychiat*, 130:450-455, 1973.

Weissman, M.M.; Prusoff, B.A.; Dimascio, A.; New, C.; Goklaney, M.; Klerman, G.: The efficacy of drugs and psychotherapy in the treatment of acute depressive episodes. *Am J Psychiat*, 136:555-558, 1979.

Welner, A.; Morten, S.; Nochnick, E.; Davis, M.A.; Fishman, R.; Clayton, P.J.: Psychiatric disorders among professional women. *Arch Gen Psychiat*, 35:169-173, 1979.

White, J.H.; O'Shanick, G.: Juvenile manic-depressive illness. *Am J Psychiat*, 134:1035-1036, 1977.

Wiesert, K.N.; Hendrie, H.C.: Secondary mania? A case report. *Am J Psychiat*, 134:929-930, 1977.

Wilder, J.F.; Levin, G.; Zwerling, I.: A two-year follow-up evaluation of acute psychotic patients treated in a day hospital. *Am J Psychiat*, 122:1095, 1966.

Wilder, J.F.; Plutchnik, R.; Cente, H.R.: Compliance with psychiatric emergency room referrals. *Arch Gen Psychiat*, 34:930-933, 1977.

Winberg, B.G.; Goldstein, S.; Gepes, L.E.; Perel, J.M.: Imipramine and electrocardiographic abnormalities in hyperactive children. *Am J Psychiat*, 132:542-545, 1975.

Wing, J.K.: "Institutionalism in Mental Hospitals" in *Mental Illness and Social Process*. T. Scheff, ed. New York, Harper and Row, 1967.

Winokur, G.: Unipolar depression: Is it divisible into autonomous subtypes? *Arch Gen Psychiat*, 36:47-52, 1979.

Winters v. Miller, 466 F.2d 65 (1971).

Wittenborn, J.R.; Buhler, R.: Somatic discomforts among depressed women. *Arch Gen Psychiat*, 36:465-471, 1979.

Wis. Stat. Ann. Secs. 51.001 and 51.75 art. II(f) (Supp. 1973).

Woo, E.; Greenblatt, D.J.: Massive benzodiazepine requirements during acute alcohol withdrawal. *Am J Psychiat*, 136:821-823, 1979.

Woodrow, K.M.: Gilles de la Tourette's Disease—a review. *Am J Psychiat*, 131:1000, 1974.

Wyatt v. Stickney, 344 F. Supp. 373, 344 F. Supp. 387 (1972).

Yalles, S.F.: "Suicide: A Public Health Problem" in *Suicidal Behaviors*. H.L.P. Resnik ed. Boston, Little, Brown, 1968.

Yedder (In re), Northampton Co., Orphans Court, Penna (1972) No. 1973-433 (June 6, 1973: Unreported opinion, Judge Alfred T. Williams, Jr.)

Yesavage, J.A.; Tinklenberg, J.R.; Hollister, L.E.; Berger, P.A.: Vasodilators in senile dementias: a review of the literature. *Arch Gen Psychiat*, 36:220-223, 1979.

Young Suicides. Harper's Bazaar, June, 1976.

Zitrin, C.M.; Klein, D.F.; Woerner, M.G.: Behavior therapy, supportive psychotherapy, imipramine, and phobias. *Arch Gen Psychiat*, 35:307-316, 1978.

Zonana, H.; Henisz, J.E.; Levine, M.: Psychiatric emergency services a decade later. *Psychiat in Med*, 4:273, 1973.

Zusman, J.; Shaffer, S.: Emergency psychiatry hospitalization via court order: A critique. *Am J Psychiat*, 130:1323-1326, 1973.

Index

335